dupl

Ethology and Psychopharmacology

Cover illustrations by kind permission of E. J. Brill
Publishing Co., Leiden, The Netherlands

Ethology and Psychopharmacology

Edited by
S.J. COOPER
Professor of Psychology, University of Durham, UK

C.A. HENDRIE
Lecturer in Psychology, University of Leeds, UK

JOHN WILEY & SONS

Chichester • New York • Brisbane • Toronto • Singapore

Copyright © 1994 by John Wiley & Sons Ltd,
Baffins Lane, Chichester,
West Sussex PO19 1UD, England
Telephone: National Chichester (0243) 779777
International +44 243 779777

Other Wiley Editorial Offices

John Wiley & Sons, Inc., 605 Third Avenue,
New York, NY 10158-0012, USA

Jacaranda Wiley Ltd, 33 Park Road, Milton,
Queensland 4064, Australia

John Wiley & Sons (Canada) Ltd, 22 Worcester Road,
Rexdale, Ontario M9W 1L1, Canada

John Wiley & Sons (SEA) Pte Ltd, 37 Jalan Pemimpin #05-04,
Block B, Union Industrial Building, Singapore 2057

Library of Congress Cataloging-in-Publication Data

Ethology and psychopharmacology/edited by S.J. Cooper and C.A. Hendrie.
    p.   cm.
  Includes bibliographical references and index.
  ISBN 0 471 95213 3
  1. Psychopharmacology—Research—Methodology—Congresses.
2. Mental illness—Animal models—Congresses.   3. Animal behavior—Congresses.   I. Cooper,
S.J.   II. Hendrie, C.A.
  [DNLM: 1. Psychopharmacology—congresses. 2. Psychotropic Drugs—congresses. 3. Social
Behavior—congresses.   QV 77 E842 1994]
RM315.E87   1994
615'.78—dc20
DNLM/DLC
for Library of Congress   94-15718
                                                                                                                        CIP

British Library Cataloguing in Publication Data

A catalogue record for this book is available from the British Library

ISBN 0 471 95213 3

Typeset in 10/12pt Plantin by Keytec Typesetting Ltd, Bridport, Dorset.
Printed and bound in Great Britain by Biddles Ltd, Guildford, Surrey

Contents

Contributors

C.H.M. Beck
Department of Psychology, Bioscience Building, University of Alberta, Edmonton, Alberta T6G 2E9, Canada

D.C. Blanchard
Department of Anatomy, J.A. Burns School of Medicine, University of Hawaii at Manoa, Pacific Biomedical Research Center, Honolulu, Hawaii 96822, USA

R.J. Blanchard
Department of Psychology, University of Hawaii at Manoa, 2430 Campus Road, Honolulu, Hawaii 96822, USA

P.F. Brain
School of Biological Sciences, University College of Swansea, Singleton Park, Swansea SA2 8PP, Wales, UK

L.J. Carter
Department of Psychology, Bioscience Building, University of Alberta, Alberta T6G 2E9, Canada

P.G. Clifton
Laboratory of Experimental Psychology, School of Biological Sciences, University of Sussex, Brighton BN1 9QG, UK

M. Cobain
Department of Neuropharmacology, Wyeth Research (UK) Ltd, Huntercombe Lane South, Taplow, Maidenhead, Berks SL6 OPH, UK

J.C. Cole
Ethopharmacology Laboratory, Department of Psychology, University of Leeds, Leeds LS2 9JT, UK

S.J. Cooper
Department of Psychology, University of Durham, Science Laboratories, South Road, Durham DH1 3LE, UK

M.G. Cutler
Department of Biological Sciences, Glasgow Caldenonian University, Glasgow G4 OBA, UK

D. Della Seta
Dipartimento di Biologia e Fisiologia Generali, Università di Parma, 43100
Parma, Italy

P. Donát (deceased)
Department of Pharmacology, 3rd Medical Faculty, Charles University, Ruská
87, 100 00 Prague 10, Czech Republic

D. Eilam
Department of Zoology, Tel-Aviv University, Ramat-Aviv 69 978, Israel

P.F. Ferrari
Dipartimento di Biologia e Fisiologia Generali, Università di Parma, 43100
Parma, Italy

I. Golani
Department of Zoology, Tel-Aviv University, Ramat-Aviv 69 978, Israel

S. Grewal
Department of Neuropharmacology, Wyeth Research (UK) Ltd,
Huntercombe Lane South, Taplow, Maidenhead, Berks SL6 OPH, UK

S. Hansen
Department of Psychology, University of Göteborg, PO Box 14158, S-400 20,
Sweden

C.A. Hendrie
Department of Psychology, University of Leeds, Leeds LS2 9JT, UK

E.D. Kemble
Division of Social Sciences, University of Minnesota–Morris, Morris,
Minnesota 56267, USA

M. Kršiak
Department of Pharmacology, 3rd Medical Faculty, Charles University, Ruská
87, 100 00 Prague 10, Czech Republic

H. Kurishingal
School of Biological Sciences, University College of Swansea, Singleton Park,
Swansea SA2 8PP, Wales, UK

P.J. Mitchell
Department of Neuropharmacology, Wyeth Research (UK) Ltd,
Huntercombe Lane South, Taplow, Maidenhead, Berks SL6 0PH, UK

J. Mos
CNS Pharmacology, Solvay-Duphar b.v., PO Box 900, 1380 DA Weesp,
Holland

B. Olivier
CNS Pharmacology, Solvay-Duphar b.v., PO Box 900, 1380 DA Weesp, Holland, and Psychopharmacology Department, Faculty of Pharmacy, University of Utrecht, Utrecht, Holland

P. Palanza
Dipartimento di Biologia e Fisiologia Generali, Università di Parma, 43100 Parma, Italy

S. Parmigiani
Dipartimento di Biologia e Fisiologia Generali, Università di Parma, 43100 Parma, Italy

C.J. Restall
School of Biological Sciences, University College of Swansea, Singleton Park, Swansea SA2 8PP, Wales, UK

R.J. Rodgers
Ethopharmacology Laboratory, Department of Psychology, University of Leeds, Leeds LS2 9JT, UK

J. Shepherd
Department of Neuropharmacology, Wyeth Research (UK) Ltd, Huntercombe Lane South, Taplow, Maidenhead, Berks SL6 0PH, UK

A.P. Silverman
17 Links Road, Wilmslow, Cheshire SK9 6HQ, UK

A. Šulcová
Department of Pharmacology, Medical Faculty of Masaryk University, Brno, Czech Republic

J. Tolboom
Department of Statistics, Solvay-Duphar b.v., PO Box 900, 1380 DA Weesp, Holland

A. Troisi
Cattedra di Psichiatria, Università di Roma Tor Vergata, via Guattini 14, 00161 Rome, Italy

R. van Oorschot
CNS Pharmacology, Solvay-Duphar b.v., PO Box 900, 1380 DA Weesp, Holland

S.M. Weiss
Department of Psychology, University of Leeds, Leeds LS2 9JT, UK

K. Whiting
School of Biological Sciences, University College of Swansea, Singleton Park, Swansea SA2 8PP, Wales, UK

Preface

In April 1993, a two-day conference was held in the University of Birmingham (UK) to commemorate the outstanding pioneering work of a Birmingham group of scientists: M.R.A. Chance, E.C. Grant, J.H. Mackintosh, A.P. Silverman and their students. Thirty years ago, this group brought together, in an imaginative and enduring fashion, the disciplines of ethology and psychopharmacology. Its members provided a theoretical basis for the integration, a challenging programme of research, and a lexicon for describing and categorizing the social behaviour of common laboratory animals. Their work has been an inspiration to several subsequent generations of research workers, and it was the aim of the conference, and of this volume, to pay each member of the group the warmest of tributes for their outstanding contribution.

This volume was planned as a less ephemeral commemoration of the Birmingham group's work. Speakers at the conference were invited to contribute a chapter and the majority accepted. The experimental reports of this volume begin with three chapters, by Rodgers and Cole, Cutler and Shepherd *et al.*, respectively, dealing with the application of ethological principles to an understanding of the effects of anxiolytic drugs. These are followed by chapters dealing with the animal models of depression (Mitchell) and panic (Hendrie and Weiss). A group of chapters focus on offence and defence in rats (Blanchard and Blanchard, Mos and colleagues) and mice (Palanza and colleagues, Kemble, and Donát and colleagues).

A more varied assembly of chapters then follows. First, Brain and his colleagues consider ethopharmacology in relation to behavioural teratology. Eilam and Golani analyse amphetamine's effects in an original way, while Beck and colleagues emphasize the utility of the concept of behavioural variability in psychopharmacological investigations. Hansen writes about maternal behaviour, while Clifton considers ingestive behaviour. Troisi discusses the relevance of ethology for animal models of psychiatric disorders. Finally, looking to the future, Kršiak considers the contribution that ethological studies may make to human happiness and welfare.

Together, this international group of contributors provide authoritative and interesting accounts of contemporary studies in the interdisciplinary arena of ethology and psychopharmacology. Their achievements represent part of the fulfilment of the promise of the Birmingham programme of research begun 30 years ago. We consider ourselves fortunate in securing the agreement of Paul Silverman to provide a personal memoir of early days at the Uffculme Clinic, which provides interesting historical insight into the early origins of ethology and psychopharmacology. His contribution forms the first chapter of this volume.

This work should prove to be of great interest to research workers, graduate and senior undergraduate students who are engaged in work on ethology and psychopharmacology, or those who wish to assess current work in this important field.

We should like to thank all the contributors to this volume, for responding to editorial comment so promptly, and to thank the Wellcome Trust, Solvay-Duphar b.v., Sandoz Research Ltd and Wyeth Research (UK) Ltd for their kind support of the Birmingham conference. We should also like to thank our publisher for the efficient publication arrangements.

Finally, with deep sadness, we should like to record the recent death by accident of an esteemed and dear colleague, Petr Donát. We thought it fitting to include in this volume a short tribute and obituary prepared by his close colleague, Milos Kršiak. As editors, we offer this volume as a memorial to Petr's life and work.

July 1994   S.J. Cooper
                                                                            Birmingham
                                                                          C.A. Hendrie
                                                                                 Leeds

Petr Donát (1955–1994)

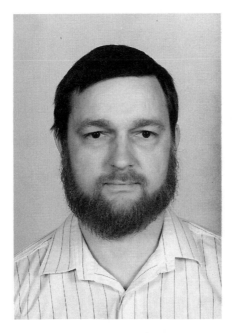

We have been most shocked by the news that our close friend Petr Donát died in a car accident in June 1994. He was only 39. Petr was a dedicated ethologist and ethopharmacologist.

For thirteen years he had been working at the Institute of Pharmacology at the Czechoslovak Academy of Sciences and the Charles University in Prague. His main professional interests were the ethological study of agonistic behaviour (his chapter in this volume is on this topic) and the use of computer and video technology in the measurement and quantitative analysis of behaviour. He had been in a close touch with many prominent world ethopharmacologists; for some time, he had also worked at the Department of Psychology at the Tufts University in Boston and at the University of Leeds. Petr was the chairman of the Czechoslovak Ethological Society and a principal organizer of the first international Ethopharmacological Conference which took place at Lísek in Bohemia in 1991.

Petr was exceptional in his many-sided gifts and capabilities, whatever he did he did with ease and well. He was physically strong, robust and fearless and at the same time he was very kind, friendly and good. Petr's death is a great loss to ethopharmacology and to all who could know him more closely.

1 A Memoir of Uffculme

A.P. SILVERMAN
Wilmslow, Cheshire, UK

When I arrived in Birmingham in October 1958, Michael Chance was a senior lecturer in pharmacology, known mostly for his wartime work on the toxicity of amphetamine. I do not think that anyone imagined a group with a collective name then, but the Uffculme story began with his observations.

Amphetamine had been widely used by RAF pilots to keep awake, but some of them took doses considered a bit risky. In fact, estimates of the lethal dose in mice differed enormously, and Michael Chance systematically sorted these until he found the main source of variance, namely whether the mice had been housed singly or in groups. A solitary mouse could survive a dose that killed mice confined in groups, though only after hours of stereotyped running round and round. Michael's interest in behaviour stemmed from this discovery. What did grouped mice actually do that potentiated the drug effect? Moreover, why did the lethal dose have such a wide variance in mice caged alone or in large groups, whereas mice in small groups died not only at a lower dose but also a much more uniform one?

When I arrived, John Mackintosh (supported by the Universities Federation for Animal Welfare) had started an MSc thesis showing that the latter phenomenon may well be general. Measuring the sleeping time from a standard anaesthetic dose of a barbiturate, he showed that if mice had been housed for a week in small groups (two to six or so, per cage), the variance in sleeping time was quite narrow. If the mice were still strangers to each other, or caged either singly or in large groups (eight or more), then the variance was very wide: some mice woke up in a few minutes, others not for hours. Mice presumably establish social relationships with familiar individuals which somehow promote physiological stability.

Ethology was hardly known in Britain until Tinbergen's *Study of Instinct* (1951) but Michael Chance, discovering the book after anthropological observations of rhesus monkeys at London Zoo, found it a revelation. The core of ethology lies in relating behaviour to ecology and evolution, and even if some of Tinbergen's detailed studies were laboratory based, they were referred back to behaviour in the wild. Chance realized that laboratory rodents, not domesticated from the wild until around 1900, must have a spontaneous behaviour of their own. To laboratory scientists at the time, this insight

Ethology and Psychopharmacology. Edited by S.J. Cooper and C.A. Hendrie
© 1994 John Wiley & Sons Ltd

seemed surprisingly original, even eccentric, though it can be deafeningly obvious. Try lingering quietly in the animal house for a few minutes in the evening, after everybody else has turned the lights out and gone home. Ethological study of laboratory rodents' 'natural' behaviour could be expected to throw light on all sorts of psychological and pharmacological experimental results, not least the group toxicity of amphetamine. In this context, 'natural' means that whether the behaviour is 'instinctive' or 'learned' (as we used to say), it was not deliberately and specifically conditioned, nor constrained by extreme confinement. Chance was persuasive enough (quite an achievement, even in the go-ahead 1950s) to get a new laboratory built at Uffculme Clinic.

Actually it was not quite a new laboratory. Uffculme was a small mansion built in the 1890s by a junior scion of the Cadbury family, and the story goes that in 1915 Grandma called young Cadbury home, and gave Uffculme to the city as a clinic for shell-shocked war heroes. Apparently there had been some friction with the young Chamberlain next door, and the wall between the mansions was built of concrete castings from 25-pounder shell cases. By the late 1950s, Uffculme was a pioneering and very successful mental hospital for out-patient and short-stay treatment. The clinic was able to spare some out-buildings for research, the coach-house for biochemistry and psychology (some operant conditioning that I regret I found practically incomprehensible), while the stables were expensively converted for the zoologists.

The Ethology Lab was a single-story building, and Michael had a comfortable little office at one end, and a part-time secretary, Mrs Therese 'T' Hadley, whose down-to-earth Brummie common sense kept us all going. The rest of us lived in a lab at the other end. In the middle was the animal room with racks of wire cages large enough for a litter of four to six adult rats, sitting on sawdust-covered trays. A horse-box-sized cubbyhole was full of bins of rat food (cubes of 'diet 41B') or sawdust. There were two strains of rats: some albinos but mostly a rather attractive wild-type brown strain. For a short time we had a third, brown-hooded strain, after a budgie-fancying assistant explored Mendelian genetics.

Caring for the rats was hard work: water bottles had to be filled every day (preferably including Sundays) and the sawdust changed once a week; more often if a polythene bottle leaked or (too close to the cage) got gnawed through. We reserved glass bottles for rats that acquired a taste for polythene. Two or three times while I was there, a mite infestation had to be treated, dipping every blessed rat by the tail into a bucket of warm solution of γ-BHC, drying them in a dishcloth and warming them for a time under a lamp.

There were three or four experimental rooms—window-less cubby-holes just big enough for shelves with a couple of dozen cages and a trolley to observe them on. But each room had 'reversed lighting', where white lights came on only at night. Red lights, which rats are relatively insensitive to, stayed on all day. So, as Michael never tired of informing visitors and grant-giving institutions, we observed the rats when we could expect these essentially nocturnal animals to be awake. There was also an especially rat-proof room where, for a few months, a pair of rats was left to run free. Observation of Carrot and Cabbage was a necessarily limited but enlightening supplement to that on caged animals, and we counted about 80 descendants when the experiment ended.

By 1958, Ewan Grant had been with Michael for about two years, and had helped him design the lab and the move to Uffculme, leaving John Mackintosh with the mice in the Medical School. The Medical School, built in 1920, was infested with wild and escapee mice, running unstoppably along the hot-water pipes and disrupting experiments. One or two albino females, housed singly for breeding in wire-mesh cages, managed to produce wild-type-coloured litters; our prurient minds boggled at the necessary murine gymnastics. Eventually it was possible to get a purpose-built lab for the study of mouse behaviour and keep the experiments under human control.

Ewan Grant's basic method, like the rest of us rodent-watchers after him, was the same as that of Lorenz, Tinbergen and all other ethologists: just watch. For long periods, again and again. At first, behaviour seems shapeless, elastic, and indeed for long periods nothing much seems to happen. Eventually regularities begin to emerge from the fog. You begin slowly to notice that you are seeing something that you have seen before. You begin to recognize a specific action or posture. You give it a name, and then you can begin to record the circumstances in which it appears, the elements (acts or postures) which precede and follow it; and if another animal is present, the cross-sequence, the elements in animal B before and after the element of interest in animal A.

This volume celebrates the classic Grant and Mackintosh (1963) paper describing all the elements they could identify (surely virtually all that exist, but see Silverman 1978b) after hundreds of hours observing laboratory rats and mice. It also compared the elements shown by these two species and, after rather less study, by golden hamsters and guinea-pigs. In a companion paper Grant (1963) meticulously analysed the commonest sequences of these elements in individual rats, and the commonest cross-sequence from one rat to another.

Ewan Grant had to calculate his results laboriously on a slow, noisy electro-mechanical calculator, using four-figure tables for square roots. Birmingham University did possess a computer then, but you had to queue up, and it was incredibly slow by modern standards. When, a year or two later, John Mackintosh wanted to analyse the comparable sequences in mice rigorously, he estimated that the computer would only have finished the number-crunching in time for his PhD deadline if his data-processing had started early in the Pleistocene.

The first element that Grant identified was the supine posture *submit*. If he had named it strictly according to objective, physical form, he would have called it *flat-on-back*. But then, he argued, he or readers of his paper might miss how it corresponds to the human 'OK, I give in.' The correspondence is real, since *submit* is active (i.e. not the result of a push) and ends a sequence of social activity; elements that lead to *submit* also lead to *retreat* and avoidance of social partners. Conversely, the cross-sequence shows that *dominate* is a response to *submit* ('I won!') and elements leading to it can (rarely) lead to *bite*.

As the names suggest, Grant's first thought (later modified) was that rats living in small groups adopt a dominant–subordinate hierarchy, which might help to explain the social stability of small groups. The first experiment which Michael asked me to do when I arrived at Uffculme was to look for any correlation between this hierarchy and the order in which rats emerge from a familiar cage onto an unfamiliar runway. Unfortunately there was none. I could not find a consistent order of emergence, and linear D/S relationships appeared to be an over-simplification in groups of four rats. This applied to the albino strain which Grant had used in the Medical School, and still more to the brown Uffculme rats which were less likely to adopt exclusively S or D type habits.

Whatever social structure consists of, it seems more subtle and flexible than a military-type linear hierarchy. To understand it, we need to know more of rodents in the wild (I included a review of this in my *Animal Behaviour in the Laboratory* (1978), as well as discussing all the main laboratory techniques). We also need modern ethological ideas, considering what individual animals do from the 'selfish gene' viewpoint. The interests of one individual (or, strictly, of his/her genes) may overlap those of another but are not identical. Male and female, parent and offspring, share an objective but the returns on their differing investments may also differ.

Incidentally it is remarkable how ethologists (utterly non-political though they are) have focused their attention and some concepts in parallel with the dominant political economists of the past decade or two. Perhaps we should look back a little, although we must not forget the 'selfish' reasons for social 'altruism' (worker bees usually do not mate but care for their mother queen's larvae; they share 75% of their sisters' genes, 50% of their own offsprings'). We might look more at how individuals benefit from their social context. Tinbergen's four questions are as relevant as ever: (1) the function (= survival value) of doing something (and not doing something else) in relation to the species' ecological niche; (2) the physiological mechanism (= motivation); (3) its developmental history in the individual; (4) its evolution in the species.

Back to Uffculme. The clinic was a satellite of All Saints Hospital on the other side of Birmingham, who also largely funded the ethology lab. They included a research assistant (me) and a technician, much to my profit. Michael Chance had offered me £500 a year, definitely more attractive than normal Research Council grants. 'I don't know where he plucked that figure from,' grumbled All Saints' finance officer to me, 'we'll have to pay you as a basic-grade biochemist.' £625. We had to send requisitions to All Saints for rat food, red light-bulbs, or hair-dye (to mark rats for identification), and the understandably bemused hospital stores clerks would phone us for clarification: 'Is that the rat house?' 'Yes,' we could hardly resist replying. 'Chief Rat speaking.'

If we were primarily interested in rat social behaviour, or more exactly, in behaviour shown by one rat in the presence of another, the main problem was to know when to watch. In the daytime or under bright, white light as explained above, rats are mostly asleep. For 10 minutes or so after nightfall, social activity in a group of rats is exuberant and intense. Then they settle down to exploring the cage, to washing and grooming themselves, and to breakfast. Social interactions occur intermittently but irregularly, and data take a long time to accumulate. The solution we adopted, for the most part, was to house rats singly for up to a week, to starve them of rodent companionship, so to speak, and then introduce one into the home cage of another for, say, 10 minutes. Ewan Grant made a point, however, of comparing previously isolated rats with grouped rats housed, Carrot-and-Cabbage-like, in open runs.

Two observers each watched one rat, and spoke the names of the elements onto a tape recorder. These would later be laboriously transcribed against an event-marker where observers had pressed buttons as they spoke, for timing and cross-sequence analysis. The original event-marker was that marvel of Edwardian engineering, a kymograph with a sooty smoked drum and varnish, but we managed to replace it by pen-and-paper tape, and one or the other made a permanent record of the raw data. A reel-to-reel tape recorder was the only practical way to record the observations; typing a two-letter code for each of the 40–50 recognized elements would have disturbed the rats, and would have been impossibly slow even for skilled touch-typists, given that we can observe an average of more than one element per second, and a peak of three or four. At least when I began to study drug effects on social behaviour, I could dispense with the sequence analysis. If a drug lowers the probability that element A leads to element B and raised that of C, then the proportions of B and C in unit time change accordingly.

I argued that, if the ethological analysis of behaviour is valid (a point not to be taken for granted in the peak era of operant-conditioning dogma), then a drug used in psychiatry to reduce anxiety, say, should reduce all elements related to *retreat*, *submit* and *crouch*. If it merely weakens muscle tone, then it would probably reduce all the varied elements where rats stand up on their hind legs. And if ethology is not valid, then I would not be able to make a coherent story out of drug effects on the element of rat social behaviour.

The work on drugs started when students of Professor Harold Steward in St Mary's Hospital, an old friend of Michael Chance, developed a series of opiate derivatives. One of them apparently made rats cataleptic: what did it do to behaviour? This was my opportunity. I found that, if rats were isolated a few days and introduced in random order on successive days to the same partner, the drug made them 'hold' postures for anything up to a minute or two after the stimulus—the partner—had walked away. But almost all the held postures indicated the 'flight' tendency (*submit*, *defensive upright*, *crouch*, etc.). Moreover nearly all 'flight' elements were increased, those involving approach to the partner (investigation as well as aggression, etc.) were reduced, while exploration of the cage and maintenance (eating, grooming, etc.) remained in proportion to the reduced 'total activity' observed. At a smaller dose (1 mg/kg instead of 4), no 'held postures' were seen and total activity was actually higher than in saline controls, but the changes in ratio of 'approach' to 'flight' elements remained.

The clear inference is that this pethidine derivative has a fairly direct influence on the physiological system (whatever it is) increasing what, in people, would be called anxiety. More surprisingly, I showed that chlorpromazine does much the same. The drug was well known to slow down all actions, and widely believed also to reduce responses to any sensory stimuli. After comparing chlorpromazine with other drugs, I could only account for the results if, in addition to these mechanisms, chlorpromazine also increased 'flight'. The surprise came because (when benzodiazepines were only beginning to come into use) neuroleptics like chlorpromazine were still marketed as 'major tranquillizers' to reduce anxiety. I now wonder (as I think Ewan Grant always did) if perhaps the drug does not so much make the animal fear another rat, as avoid all social contact ('Don't bother me, I want to be alone'). Yet the actual data consistently showed increases in *defensive upright*, *submit*, etc., as well as *evade*, *retreat*, *crouch*.

These experiments show the value of a behavioural method where several measures can be taken at the same time. It is difficult (and also laborious), for example, to condition animals to do two things at once. Normally only a single measure is practicable, which a drug can only increase or reduce. If you can reliably observe units of behaviour shown by all normally bred animals without deliberate conditioning, you find that different behavioural tendencies vary independently, in absolute terms as well as relative to the total observed activity. The hypothesis you propose to explain this may be wrong and certainly needs testing, but you are already several stages further along the research road than with a single measure—especially if a drug like chlorpromazine (known to block receptors for at least four different neurotransmitters) has multiple behavioural effects.

Admittedly the statistical method I had to use at Uffculme is suspect, but when I moved to the toxicology lab at ICI (now Zeneca) I was (quite easily) persuaded to use valid multivariate statistics, and these support the same conclusions. It is also true that isolating rats and introducing them to strangers can be counter-productive if repeated, since it seems to condition rats to behave in a stereotyped way, less sensitive to low doses. Serendipitously, I found a better method at ICI, housing rats in pairs, separating them for a few hours a day, and returning them home early in the red-light period. They seem to show their 'normal' bout of social activity at a time under experimental control. Certainly low-dose drug effects were repeatable—and reversible (i.e.

not conditioned)—in long-term experiments. Similarly John Mackintosh housed mice in pairs, separating them only long enough to cross-introduce a mouse from one cage to the stay-at-home partner of the other.

Anyway in 1964–65 I was awarded a PhD, became engaged, and began a new job. Two of the three achievements owe more than I then realized to the benign environment created by Michael Chance (not to mention his fund-raising techniques 20 years ahead of their time). But at least I realized how much benefit I had from all our debates (I even managed, twice, to bring together animal behaviour researchers from no less than four separate departments at Birmingham University: ourselves, and students of Philip Bradley, Peter Broadhurst and John Cohen).

Above all I needed the patient, good-humoured assistance of Christine Summerhill. She came about the same time as Eddie Chalk, when Malcolm Mogford left us to train as a teacher and Clive Young went back to his Herefordshire farm.

In my last year Michael Chance, with his new student David Humphries, started asking about rats' sensory perception. If rats get information mainly from their nose and vibrissae, is it their eyes which detect their partner's upright postures? Michael had the brilliant idea to find out by reversibly blinding them—with opaque contact lenses. Poor Eddie Chalk had to telephone every optician in the West Midlands to try and get them made. 'Contact lenses? Yes, we make them. For ... did you say, rats?? Where are you speaking from? Uffculme Mental Hospital ...?'

REFERENCES

Chance, M.R.A. (1946) *J. Pharmacol. Exp. Ther.* **87**, 214–219.
Grant, E.C. (1963) *Behaviour* **21**, 260–281.
Grant, E.C. and Mackintosh, J.H. (1963) *Behaviour* **21**, 246–259.
Silverman, P. (1978a) *Animal Behaviour in the Laboratory: Behavioural Tests and their Interpretation*. Chapman & Hall, London.
Silverman, A.P. (1978b) *Anim. Behav.* **26**, 1279–1281.
Tinbergen, N. (1951) *The Study of Instinct*. Clarendon Press, Oxford.

2 The Elevated Plus-maze: Pharmacology, Methodology and Ethology

R.J. RODGERS AND J.C. COLE

Department of Psychology, University of Leeds, UK

ANIMAL MODELS OF ANXIETY

Conceptual issues

Animal models are used in anxiety research for two principal reasons: as bioassays to screen for novel therapeutic agents, and as simulations to facilitate an understanding of underlying mechanisms (Green and Hodges, 1991; Lister, 1990; Treit, 1985). In view of traditional pharmacotherapy for anxiety, it is perhaps unsurprising that these models comprise physiological and/or behavioural responses which are to sensitive to benzodiazepine anxiolytics. Indeed, it has been argued that existing animal models of anxiety should more accurately be termed models of benzodiazepine psychopharmacology (Green and Hodges, 1991). However, sole reliance upon pharmacological validation of test procedures has been severely criticized by a number of authors, including Lister (1990), who commented that 'pharmacological validation alone does not make a test a model of anxiety'. This crucial point applies to all models, but is especially valid in respect to those which are employed in research on underlying mechanisms (Green and Hodges, 1991). After all, an effect produced by an anxiolytic in a particular procedure may have little, if anything, to do with the drug's antianxiety action. Furthermore, pharmacological validation *per se* provides distinct problems in the search for novel antianxiety compounds. Thus, where a particular model has been validated against the benzodiazepine 'gold standard', there is no *a priori* reason to assume that it will be sensitive to compounds which reduce anxiety by entirely novel mechanisms. Nowhere has this shortcoming been more apparent than in the failure of classical animal tests to detect the therapeutic potential of the novel and clinically effective anxiolytic, buspirone.

In principle, an animal model of anxiety should have not only predictive validity but also face validity and construct validity (Green and Hodges, 1991). Predictive validity refers to the sensitivity of the model to known anxiolytics,

Ethology and Psychopharmacology. Edited by S.J. Cooper and C.A. Hendrie
© 1994 John Wiley & Sons Ltd

but not to other types of psychoactive agent. Face validity implies that the model produces fear-like reactions in animals that are analogous to anxiety-related behaviours in humans. Construct validity is more difficult in that it implies homology, or direct correspondence, between the animal model and the condition being modelled. Unfortunately, while many models have a fair degree of face validity, they fall short on the criteria of predictive and construct validity. No single model selects anxiolytics without some false positives or false negatives, while attempts to assess construct validity are compromised by our incomplete understanding of human anxiety (Lister, 1990; Treit, 1985). As such, most workers in the area advocate a broad-based approach to anxiolytic psychopharmacology (Green and Hodges, 1991).

Of direct relevance to these issues is the diversity of human anxiety states. For example, DSM-III-R lists a range of anxiety disorders including generalized anxiety disorder, panic disorder, phobias, obsessive-compulsive disorder and post-traumatic stress disorder. These conditions can be differentiated on a number of dimensions, including symptomatology and therapeutic response, and it is particularly pertinent to note that benzodiazepines are mainly effective in patients with generalized anxiety disorder (Nutt, 1991). Against this background, there remains an implicit assumption in much of the animal literature that all models of anxiety are equivalent (Handley, 1991) and, hence, should yield similar results. That the latter is the exception rather than the rule suggests either that some of our models are invalid or that different models may be tapping different aspects of anxiety (File, 1992; Green, 1991; Handley, 1991; Treit, 1985). From this analysis, it is clear that the superficially simple criterion of predictive validity in animal modelling is actually rather complex. Using the benzodiazepine 'gold standard', high predictive validity might simply mean that a given procedure detects 'me-same' (i.e. benzodiazepine-like) compounds, thereby offering little hope of discovering truly novel agents. In this context, the question 'predictive of what?' clearly acquires profound significance. For this reason, several authors have cogently argued that animal models of anxiety should be examined very much more closely from a *behavioural* perspective (Green and Hodges, 1991; Handley, 1991; Lister, 1990; Treit, 1985). On this crucial issue, Barrett (1991) states that 'suitable and reliable models require extensive validation and a balance must be struck between the proliferation of newer models and the refinement of existing ones'.

The diversity of animal models of anxiety

At first glance, current animal models of anxiety present a bewildering array of procedures. However, they may be grouped into two general categories; namely, conditioned responses and unconditioned responses (File, 1992; Green and Hodges, 1991; Lister, 1990; Treit, 1985). Table 1 lists some examples of

Table 1 Examples of current animal models of anxiety. Available procedures may be differentiated on the basis of conditioned versus unconditioned responses

Conditioned responses	Unconditioned responses
Geller–Seifter conflict	Rodent social interaction
Vogel punished drinking	Separation-induced vocalization
Four-plate test	Primate social behaviour
Conditioned emotional response	Antipredator defence in rats
Defensive burying	Mouse light/dark exploration
Potentiated acoustic startle	ELEVATED PLUS-MAZE

these tests but is not intended to be an exhaustive catalogue. Conditioning models, such as the Geller–Seifter conflict procedure, require considerable training of subjects, food or water deprivation and/or the use of electric shock as an aversive stimulus. Other conditioning procedures, such as conditioned defensive burying, take advantage of the fact that animals show faster stimulus–response associations when faced with ecologically relevant (versus more arbitrary) environmental challenges (Lister, 1990; Treit, 1985; Treit, 1991). Tests based on spontaneous behaviour, such as the separation-induced ultrasonic vocalization test, have a high degree of ecological validity in that they rely upon unconditional reactions to stimulus situations which, although non-painful, nevertheless pose a threat to survival and are seen under feral conditions. A recent, and important, extension to such procedures is the elegant work of Blanchard and colleagues (1991) on antipredator defence in rats.

Handley (1991) has recently elaborated on the above traditional classification, offering a double dissociation within animal models. First, she distinguishes between models which are based on fear engendered by secondary aversive stimuli (conditioning models) and those that rely upon reactions to innate fear stimuli (spontaneous models). Second, within each of these categories, she further differentiates those procedures which require *response emission* and those which demand *response suppression*. This revised classification is then used with some success to reconcile the diverse and often contradictory effects of serotonergic manipulations on anxiety. Although a potentially useful development, this classification fails to accommodate those models which comprise a complex interplay between response emission and response suppression, e.g. antipredator defence and, as will be argued later, tests such as the elevated plus-maze.

It is beyond the scope of this chapter to present a detailed review of all animal models of anxiety. Suffice it to say that tests of unconditioned behaviour generally provide much richer behavioural diversity than other procedures (often 'single point' measures) and thereby offer wider scope for defining more precisely their relationship(s) to different forms of human anxiety. It is the aim of the present chapter to contribute to this goal by focusing extensively on one animal model of anxiety, the elevated plus-maze. It is our contention that the inconsistency apparent in the behavioural pharmacology of this test can be attributed to some obvious methodological variations and that its utility, both as a screen and as a simulation, may be enhanced by the adoption of a more ethological perspective.

THE ELEVATED PLUS-MAZE

The elevated plus-maze test of anxiety has acquired considerable popularity in recent years, and is representative of paradigms based on unconditioned responses to potentially dangerous environments. It derives from the work of Montgomery (1955) on the relation between fear and exploratory 'drives' in rats, the basic premise of which was that environmental novelty evokes both fear and curiosity, thereby creating a typical approach–avoid conflict. Using exploration from the home cage, Montgomery found that rats consistently showed higher levels of exploration of enclosed alleys than open alleys and, when faced with a choice of alley type in an elevated Y-maze, consistently preferred the enclosed arms. These data were interpreted as indicating that open arms engender a higher level of fear than enclosed arms, leading to increased avoidance.

This initial work was developed by Handley and Mithani (1984) as a potential animal model of anxiety. They used an X-maze raised 70 cm above floor level, and comprising two (opposite) enclosed and two open arms, each type measuring 45 cm long × 10 cm wide. The enclosed arms had sides and ends 10 cm high and the floor of the maze was lined with wire mesh. Although their pharmacological results are reviewed in greater detail below, they found that anxiolytics (e.g. diazepam) enhanced the ratio of open:total arm entries while anxiogenics (e.g. picrotoxin) diminished this ratio. They concluded that the X-maze may provide a valid model of 'fear-motivated' behaviour. These studies were followed by a more extensive investigation of the rat elevated plus-maze by Pellow and associates (1985), who not only validated the test pharmacologically but also examined its behavioural and physiological validity. It is noteworthy that, while both early studies employed the same rat strain and mazes of roughly comparable dimensions, procedural variations were apparent. Thus, Handley and Mithani employed a 10 min test, whereas Pellow and her colleagues used a 5 min pre-exposure to a hole-board followed by a 5 min test in the maze. Furthermore, the latter authors introduced an open: total time measure as an additional index of anxiety. The species generality of the elevated plus-maze in the measurement of anxiety was subsequently confirmed by Lister (1987) using NIH Swiss mice. Employing a scaled-down version of the maze (arms 30 cm long × 5 cm wide; walls and ends of enclosed arms 15 cm high; raised to 38.5 cm above floor level), prior hole-board exposure and a 5 min test, he found comparable behavioural and pharmaco-logical results to those reported earlier for rats, and concluded that the murine version of the elevated plus-maze also appears to be a useful test with which to study both anxiolytic and anxiogenic agents.

Avoidance of the open arms of the maze is consistent with the view that these areas evoke a stronger fear reaction than the enclosed arms, thereby providing the model with face (and possible construct) validity. But what is it about the open arms that engenders avoidance? In this context, recent studies have (somewhat counter-intuitively) indicated that height is not the key factor (Falter et al., 1992; Treit et al., 1993a). Rather, the main avoidance-promoting feature of the open arms is the lack of side-walls. Thus, in an elegant study, Treit and colleagues (1993a) have demonstrated that varying the height of open arm walls had predictable effects on open arm exploration whereas varying the height of the maze itself had little effect. This finding agrees well with previous research showing that rodents are highly thigmotactic in novel environments.

In the absence of external validation, however, there is a danger of circular-ity in argument regarding interpretation of plus-maze behaviour; thus, (a) animals avoid the open arms because they are anxious, (b) but how do we know they are anxious? (c) because they avoid the open arms! Pellow and colleagues (1985) addressed this problem in two ways: first, they showed that rats displayed more fear-related behaviours (immobility, freezing, defaecation) on the open arms—a behavioural validation; second, they found that confine-ment to the open arms produced a significantly greater ($\times 2$) plasma cortico-sterone response than confinement to the closed arms—a physiological valida-tion. As a further validation, Rodgers and colleagues (Lee and Rodgers, 1990, 1991a, 1991b; Rodgers et al., 1992b) have shown that exposure of mice to the elevated plus-maze produces a non-opioid form of 'stress analgesia', an effect that is prevented by prior treatment with anxiolytic drugs. The general phenomenon of plus-maze antinociception has been independently confirmed in both rats (Taukulis and Goggin, 1990) and mice (Conceicao et al., 1992; Frussa-Filho et al., 1991). Clearly, then, rodents not only avoid the open arms of an elevated plus-maze but also display distinct behavioural and physiological indices of fear in this paradigm.

In considering the general merits of the plus-maze, Pellow and associates (1985) list the following: (1) the test is fast, simple and does not involve expensive equipment; (2) it is based on spontaneous behaviour and thereby avoids lengthy training, the need for food/water deprivation, and the use of noxious stimuli; (3) it is able to identify acute anxiolytic effects of benzodiaze-pine-drugs; (4) it is bidirectionally sensitive to manipulations of anxiety. Given this profile, the elevated plus-maze would seem to offer many advantages over other animal models of anxiety and would be expected to yield consistent and meaningful data. This expectation is challenged in the following section which reviews the behavioural pharmacology of the plus-maze.

THE BEHAVIOURAL PHARMACOLOGY OF THE ELEVATED PLUS-MAZE

In considering the effects of drugs on behaviour in the elevated plus-maze, the obvious starting point is with benzodiazepine receptor ligands. However, in view of problems associated with the benzodiazepine 'gold standard' (criterion drug) approach, it is also essential that the effects of a range of other compounds are considered. This is particularly true of proven/putative anxiolytics and anxiogenics which act via mechanisms unrelated to the benzodiazepine–GABA (γ-aminobutyric acid) receptor complex.

Benzodiazepine receptor ligands

The initial report by Handley and Mithani (1984) that acute diazepam produces an anxiolytic-like profile in the elevated plus-maze has been replicated by numerous authors. As Table 2 illustrates, these findings have been extended to a range of other benzodiazepine receptor full agonists. Although little work has been done on the central sites of action of the benzodiazepines in the plus-maze, anxiolytic-like effects have been reported following microinjection of midazolam into the basolateral amygdala (Green and Vale, 1992), septum (Pesold and Treit, in press) and the dorsal periaqueductal grey matter (Russo et al., 1993). One intriguing finding (to be returned to later) is the observation that the anxiolytic response to benzodiazepines is markedly reduced or even completely abolished in animals with prior plus-maze experience (File, 1990a; File et al., 1990; Lister, 1987; Rodgers et al., 1992b; Rodgers and Shepherd, 1993; Treit et al., 1993a). Chronic treatment with benzodiazepine receptor full agonists also produces anxiolysis in the maze (File and Aranko, 1988; Harro et al., 1990; Johnston and File, 1988b; Pellow et al., 1985; Rodgers et al., 1992b; Rodgers and Shepherd, 1993) and it is interesting to note that these effects appear to generalize to prenatal drug exposure (Kellogg et al., 1991). However, tolerance to benzodiazepine effects occurs with prolonged treatment (File et al., 1987; Ishihara et al., 1993; Pellow et al., 1985), while withdrawal from a period of chronic treatment has been shown to result in an anxiogenic-like profile (Baldwin and File, 1988; File and Andrews, 1991; File et al., 1987; File and Hitchcott, 1990; Harro et al., 1990; Hitchcott et al., 1992). Interestingly, such effects can be reversed not only by the benzodiazepine receptor antagonist, flumazenil (File and Hitchcott, 1990), but also by low doses of buspirone (File and Andrews, 1991).

Table 2 also summarizes the literature on the effects of other benzodiazepine receptor ligands on plus-maze anxiety. Conflicting results have been found with benzodiazepine receptor partial agonists, bretazenil producing a convincing anxioselective profile, CGS 9896 having a weak anxiolytic action and ZK 91296 apparently inactive. However, the benzodiazepine receptor antagonist, flumazenil (formerly Ro15-1788), has consistently been found to have little

Table 2 Acute effects of benzodiazepine receptor ligands on anxiety in the elevated plus-maze test

Drug	Species	Dose range (mg/kg)	Effect	References
Chlordiazepoxide	Rat	0.3–10.0	+	49, 61, 67, 75, 121, 136, 152, 178
	Mouse	0.8–15.0	+	15, 32, 131, 158
Diazepam	Rat	0.5–3.0	+	13, 49, 87, 94, 121, 136, 141, 152, 178, 191, 203
	Mouse	0.1–1.5	+	47, 159
Midazolam	Rat	1.0–10.0	+	143, 175
Lorazepam	Mouse	0.05–0.1	+	47
CL 218,872	Rat	10.0–20.0	+	151
DN-2327	Rat	2.5–5.0	+	203
Bretazenil	Mouse	1.6–15.0	+	32
CGS 9896	Rat	10.0–20.0	+	73
ZK 91296	Rat	5.0–15.0	+	71
Flumazenil	Rat	4.0–20.0	0/–	8, 30, 68, 151, 203
	Mouse	5.0–20.0	0	15, 130
ZK 93426	Rat	5.0–15.0	0	8, 68
CGS 8216	Rat	3.0–10.0	–	152
DMCM	Mouse	0.5–1.5	–	159, 160
FG 7142	Rat	1.0–30.0	–	61, 68, 70, 113, 151, 153
		2.5–20.0	0	136, 185
	Mouse	5.0–10.0	–	131, 132

+, anxiolytic-like; 0, no effect; –, anxiogenic-like.

behavioural activity in the maze, with similar negative results reported for another antagonist, ZK 93426. Although negative and/or unconvincing effects have been reported, the general consensus is that benzodiazepine receptor inverse agonists (e.g. FG 7142, DMCM*, CGS 8216) produce reliable anxiogenic effects in the plus-maze. Compounds acting, not at benzodiazepine receptors, but at non-neuronal benzodiazepine binding sites (e.g. Ro05-4864, PK 11195) have been found to be either ineffective or anxiogenic (Pellow and File, 1986; Rago et al., 1992). Essentially, therefore, the elevated plus-maze is bidirectionally sensitive to changes in anxiety induced by benzodiazepine receptor ligands. The phenomenon of benzodiazepine-withdrawal anxiogenesis further adds to the pharmacological validity of the test for agents of this class.

Other GABA receptor-related compounds

In addition to benzodiazepines, a range of other compounds influence the functioning of the GABA receptor/chloride channel supramolecular complex (Haefely, 1990). These include barbiturates, ethanol, pentylenetetrazol and certain neuroactive steroids, as well as direct/indirect GABA agonists and antagonists. Table 3 presents a summary of the current literature. Barbiturates, as well as progesterone and several pregnane-related steroids (e.g. alphaxalone, allopreganalone and pregnanolone) which exert barbiturate-like effects on the GABA receptor/chloride channel, have also been found to produce anxiolytic effects in this test. As might be predicted, consistent anxiolytic-like actions have also been reported for ethanol, effects that are blocked by benzodiazepine receptor antagonists/inverse agonists such as FG 7142 and Ro15-4513 (Lister, 1988) and by the 5-hydroxytryptamine (5-HT) reuptake inhibitor, fluoxetine (Durcan et al., 1988). Withdrawal from chronic ethanol treatment produces an anxiogenic-like behavioural profile (Baldwin et al., 1991; File et al., 1991, 1992; Rassnick et al., 1993) which can be reversed by chlordiazepoxide, flumazenil and baclofen (File et al., 1991, 1992), α-helical corticotrophin releasing factor (CRF) (Baldwin et al., 1991), buspirone (Lal et al., 1991) and mianserin (Lal et al., 1993).

In contrast, pentylenetetrazol, which inhibits the functioning of the GABA receptor/chloride channel complex, has consistently been reported to produce anxiogenic-like effects. Similarly, picrotoxin, a non-competitive $GABA_A$ receptor antagonist, while ineffective in low doses (0.75 mg/kg), clearly enhances anxiety at higher doses (1–4 mg/kg). Indirect GABA agonists (e.g. vigabatrin, AOAA) have been found to have anxiolytic effects, although the data on sodium valproate are equivocal. Several direct $GABA_A$ and $GABA_B$ agonists (e.g. muscimol, THIP, isoguvacine) have also been reported to have anxiolytic effects, while the $GABA_B$ agonist baclofen, is apparently anxiolytic only in handling-naive rats (Andrews and File, 1993).

*A list of abbreviations is supplied at the end of this chapter.

Table 3 Acute effects of GABA receptor-related compounds on anxiety in the elevated plus-maze test

Drug	Species	Dose range (mg/kg)	Effect	References
Amylobarbitone	Rat	30.0	+	94
	Mouse	7.5–30.0	+	131
Phenobarbitone	Rat	25.0–35.0	+	113, 152
Ethanol	Rat	0.5–1.0 g/kg	+	23, 189
	Mouse	0.8–2.4 g/kg	+	53, 54, 55, 90, 131, 132
Alphaxalone	Rat	6.0–8.0	+	28
Allopregnanolone	Rat	i.c.v.	+	18
Pregnanolone	Rat	i.c.v.	+	18
Progesterone	Rat	1.0–4.0	+	20
Pentylenetetrazol	Rat	10.0–30.0	−	70, 113, 134, 152, 157, 203
	Mouse	12.5	−	15
Picrotoxin	Rat	2.0–4.0	−	94
		0.75	0	18
	Mouse	1.0–2.0	−	131
Sodium valproate	Rat	25–200	0	67
		100–400	+	37
Vigabatrin	Rat	500–1000	+	176
AOAA	Rat	5.0–20.0	+	37
Muscimol		0.5–1.0	+	37
Isoguvacine		25.0	+	37
THIP		2.5–10.0	+	37
Baclofen	Rat	1.25–2.5	0	77, 79
		1.0	+	7
β-(phenyl)GABA	Mouse	12.5	0	160

+, anxiolytic-like; 0, no effect; −, anxiogenic-like; i.c.v., intracerebroventricular injection.

The above review substantiates the conclusion, implicit in the discussion of benzodiazepine receptor ligands, that agents which modulate the functioning of the GABA receptor/chloride ionophore produce predictable effects on anxiety as measured in the elevated plus-maze. Agents which enhance the functioning of this receptor complex (i.e. GABA agonists, barbiturates, ethanol, pregnane-related steroids) reduce anxiety; those which inhibit its function (i.e. pentylenetetrazol, GABA antagonists) increase anxiety. The phenomenon of ethanol-withdrawal anxiogenesis adds yet further weight to the pharmacological validity of the test.

Adrenoceptor ligands

The effects of α-adrenoceptor ligands on anxiety in the elevated plus-maze have been highly variable (Table 4). The α_1-agonist, phenylephrine, has been reported to be inactive or anxiogenic in this test. Similar inconsistency applies

Table 4   Effects of α-adrenoceptor ligands on anxiety in the elevated plus-maze test

Drug	Species	Dose range (mg/kg)	Effect	References
Phenylephrine	Rat	0.25–0.5	0	114
		0.25–2.5	−	94
ST-587	Rat	1.0–2.0	−	94
Prazosin	Rat	0.5–1.0	+	94
		0.1–10.0	0	144, 175
Thymoxamine	Rat	0.5–1.0	+	94
Clonidine	Rat	0.003–0.08	+	58, 94, 136, 183
		0.025–0.5	0	116
Dexmedetomide	Rat	0.001–0.01	0	175
Medetomidine	Rat	0.0005–0.01	0	161
	Mouse	0.0005–0.01	0	161
B-HT 920	Rat	0.025–0.1	0	114
		0.1–2.0	+	58
B-HT 933	Rat	1.0–10.0	0	114
Guanfacine	Rat	0.25–1.0	0	114
		0.125–5.0	−	116
Azepexole	Rat	1.0–2.0	+	94
Guanabenz	Rat	0.1–1.0	+	94
Rimelidine	Rat	1.0–10.0	−	116
Yohimbine	Rat	0.5–5.0	−	11, 44, 58, 70, 94, 114, 152, 153, 192, 203
Piperoxane	Rat	10.0	−	94
RS 21361	Rat	5.0–10.0	−	94
Idazoxan	Rat	0.03–0.25	−	94, 183
	Rat	0.01–10.0	0	100, 141
	Mouse	0.3–6.0	0	55
Atipamezole	Rat	0.01–4.5	0	119, 175
	Mouse	1.0–10.0	0	55

+, anxiolytic-like; 0, no effect; −, anxiogenic-like.

to the α_1-antagonist, prazosin, with non-specific and anxiolytic effects reported. The variability of these limited data does not permit any reliable conclusions regarding the involvement of α_1-adrenoceptor mechanisms in plus-maze anxiety.

Despite a more extensive literature base, the situation is equally confused for α_2-adrenoceptor manipulations (see Table 4). Clonidine has been shown to have anxiolytic effects in most studies to date, although negative findings have also been reported. However, more selective agonists at α_2-receptors have produced variable effects; thus, dexmedetomide, medetomidine and B-HT 933 are reportedly inactive, the effects of B-HT 920 (no effect/anxiolytic) and guanfacine (non-specific/anxiogenic) are equivocal, while azepexole and guanabenz are reported to have anxiolytic effects. In contrast to this variable profile, the α_2-antagonist, yohimbine, has consistently produced anxiogenic-like effects in the elevated plus-maze; similar results have been reported in one study that examined the effects of piperoxane and RS 21361. However, the effects of more selective α_2-antagonists are much less convincing. Thus, idazoxan has been reported to be anxiogenic by some groups but inactive by others, while another highly selective α_2-antagonist, atipamezole, is consistently without effect. It therefore seems more than likely that the anxiogenic effects of yohimbine in the maze are not due to its effects on α_2-adrenoceptor mechanisms.

More clear-cut conclusions are possible with respect to potential β-adrenoceptor involvement in plus-maze anxiety. Thus, isamoltane has no effects in this test (Graeff et al., 1990), whereas the findings with propranolol have been inconsistent (Audi et al., 1991; Johnston and File, 1989b; Njung'e et al., 1993; Pellow et al., 1987). However, it is important to note that several widely used β-blockers also have significant affinity for serotonergic receptors. In this context, a recent and extensive examination of the effects of some 13 non-specific and receptor-selective β-ligands concluded that only those antagonists with additional high affinity for 5-HT$_{1A}$ receptors (e.g. pindolol and alprenolol) exert anxiolytic effects in the elevated plus-maze; other antagonists and a series of agonists were either inactive or had non-specific effects (Njung'e et al., 1993). Interestingly, and in accordance with its mixed agonist–antagonist 5-HT$_{1A}$ actions, pindolol produced anxiolytic effects at low doses and anxiogenic effects at high doses (Critchley et al., 1988; Njung'e et al., 1993). This finding may also help to explain the variable effects of systemic propranolol in the plus-maze. Of potential significance in this context is the finding that direct injection of propranolol into the dorsal periaqueductal grey matter produces an anxiolytic profile in the rat elevated plus-maze test (Audi et al., 1991).

In summary, manipulations of α-adrenoceptor function produce widely inconsistent effects on plus-maze anxiety while β-adrenoceptors appear to have little or no role to play. In view of the putative relationship between α_2-adrenergic function and panic disorder and the involvement of β-adrenoceptors in somatic anxiety (Nutt, 1991), it would appear that these two conditions are not accurately modelled in the plus-maze.

Serotonergic receptor ligands

The discovery of multiple 5-HT receptor subtypes (Hoyer, 1992) has prompted much renewed interest in the involvement of this indoleamine in mechanisms of anxiety. In the plus-maze, PCPA-induced 5-HT depletion has generally been reported to reduce anxiety (Critchley et al., 1992; Moser, 1989; Treit et al., 1993c). However, although similar results have been reported for intracerebroventricular 5,7-dihydroxytryptamine (5,7-DHT)-induced lesions (Briley et al., 1990), the effects of dorsal raphe lesions have been equivocal (Critchley et al., 1992; Treit et al., 1993c). The latter discrepancy may, however, be due to variations in lesioning technique. As might be predicted from this general pattern of results, systemic administration of the 5-HT precursor, L-5-HTP, is reported to exert anxiogenic-like effects in the maze (Soderpalm et al., 1989). Over the past decade, an increasingly large number of 5-HT receptor-selective compounds have become available, as have a range of 5-HT-selective reuptake inhibitors. An extremely wide range of such compounds has been studied in the plus-maze and, for convenience, these will be considered under four major subheadings. Table 5 summarizes the main findings.

Table 5   Effects of 5-HT receptor ligands on anxiety in the elevated plus-maze test

Drug	Species	Dose range (mg/kg)	Effect	References
8-OH-DPAT	Rat	0.01–1.0	−	42, 44, 121, 123, 141, 200
		0.06–0.25	0	153
		0.03–3.0	+	49, 135, 184
	Mouse	0.01–1.0	+	170
Buspirone	Rat	0.06–8.0	−	7, 66, 121, 123, 124, 141, 153
		0.25–20.0	0	44, 66, 151, 203
		0.01–4.0	+	49, 123, 135, 184
	Mouse	0.1–10.0	+	33, 129
Gepirone	Rat	1.0–10.0	−	144
		0.001–3.0	0	44
		0.1–5.0	+	49, 135, 184
Ipsapirone	Rat	1.25–10.0	−	111, 141, 153
		0.001–5.0	+	5, 44, 82, 135, 184
Ritanserin	Rat	0.05–10.0	−	111, 153
		0.5–1.0	0	82
		0.05–5.0	+	5, 42, 193
Ketanserin	Rat	0.1–0.5	+	42, 144
Seganserin	Rat	0.5	+	42
Metergoline	Rat	4.0	+	153
Amperozide	Rat	0.05–0.1	+	56
DOI	Rat	0.1–0.64	0	125, 193
Ondansetron	Rat	0.005–1.0	0	24, 111, 156
		0.001–0.1	+	38, 51, 157, 179
	Mouse	0.001–0.1	0	172
MDL 72222	Rat	0.1–10.0	+	38, 51
ICS 205-930	Rat	0.01–10.0	0	111
		0.001–0.5	+	38, 51
BRL 43694	Rat	0.005–1.0	0	38, 111, 156
BRL 46470A		0.0001–0.1	+	21
Zacopride	Rat	0.01–1.0	0	71
		0.05–0.1	+	7, 38, 51
DAU 6215	Rat	0.008–0.15	0	24
WAY 100,289	Mouse	0.01–10.0	0	172
RS-42358-197	Rat	0.1–100 ng/kg	+	41
mCPB	Rat	1.0–10.0	−	6

+, anxiolytic-like; 0, no effect; −, anxiogenic-like.

5-HT₁ receptor ligands

In view of the clinical success of buspirone, most research has been conducted on the effects of $5\text{-}HT_{1A}$ receptor agonists and partial agonists (Dourish, 1987; Traber and Glaser, 1987). Generally speaking, however, the results have been disappointingly inconsistent. 8-Hydroxy-2-(di-n-propylamino)tetralin (8-OH-DPAT), the prototypical agonist at these sites, has been found to exert anxiogenic effects, no effect and anxiolytic-like effects. Of potential relevance to this contradictory pattern is the finding that the same dose of 8-OH-DPAT can be anxiolytic (high light) or anxiogenic (low light) depending upon the level of test illumination (Handley and McBlane, 1993). Similar highly variable results have been obtained with buspirone itself, although its profile tends to be confounded by behavioural suppressant actions possibly related to its additional dopamine antagonist properties (Cole and Rodgers, 1994). Nevertheless, plus-maze effects ranging from anxiolysis through no effect to anxiogenesis have been reported. Interestingly, the one study to report on the effects of centrally administered buspirone found anxiolytic-like effects following injection into hippocampal sites (Kostowski *et al.*, 1989). Although the general inconsistency concerning the effects of systemically administered buspirone has often been attributed to dose ranges employed (anxiolysis at low doses; anxiogenesis at high doses; e.g. Soderpalm *et al.*, 1989), direct comparison between studies would not support this proposal (Table 5). Of potentially greater relevance is the issue of acute versus chronic treatment; even here, however, the two studies to report such contrasts arrive at opposing conclusions (Cole and Rodgers, 1994; Moser, 1989). Recent work by Andrews and File (1993) may have relevance to this pattern of inconsistency in that they report that buspirone produces anxiogenic-like effects only in handling-habituated rats.

The effects of the closely related analogues, gepirone and ipsapirone, are equally confusing. Acute administration of gepirone has been reported to enhance, have no effect upon or to reduce anxiety in the plus-maze. However, one study has reported that an acute anxiogenic-like profile of gepirone reverses to an anxiolytic profile following a period of chronic treatment (Motta *et al.*, 1992). The situation is no clearer for ipsapirone, with both anxiogenic and anxiolytic effects reported. While both enantiomers of MDL 72832 have been found to have anxiogenic effects in the maze (Moser, 1989), the related compound, MDL 73005EF, produces a convincing anxiolytic profile (Moser *et al.*, 1990). Other compounds which possess $5\text{-}HT_{1A}$ antagonist or mixed agonist–antagonist effects (e.g. spiroxatrine, LY165,163, NAN-190, BP 554, (S)-UH-301) have all been reported to exert anxiolytic profiles in the maze (Luscombe *et al.*, 1992; Moreau *et al.*, 1992; Moser, 1989; Soderpalm *et al.*, 1989). Although inconsistent effects have been found with propranolol, a range of β-blockers which possess significant $5\text{-}HT_{1A}$ antagonist properties have also been reported to evidence anxiolytic profiles in this test. Finally, although fewer data are available, compounds with mixed $5\text{-}HT_{1A/1B/1C}$ agonist effects (fluprazine, eltoprazine, TFMPP, mCPP, RU24969, quipazine, 5-MeODMT) have consistently been found to produce increases in anxiety in the plus-maze (Benjamin *et al.*, 1990; Blackburn *et al.*, 1993; Critchley and Handley, 1987; Critchley *et al.*, 1992; Pellow *et al.*, 1987; Rodgers *et al.*, 1992a).

$5\text{-}HT_2$ receptor ligands

$5\text{-}HT_2$ receptor antagonists have also yielded somewhat inconsistent results in the plus-maze. Ritanserin has been found to have anxiolytic effects, no effect or anxiogenic effects. However, metergoline, ketanserin, seganserin and amperozide have all been reported to have anxiolytic-like effects. Somewhat surprisingly, therefore, the $5\text{-}HT_2$ agonist, DOI, is inactive in this model. Acute administration of the atypical antidepressant, mianserin, has been found to produce either no effect or non-specific effects in the plus-maze (Benjamin *et al.*, 1992; Briley *et al.*, 1986; Pellow *et al.*, 1987). However, if administered 48 h prior to test, an anxiolytic action is seen which has been related to the compound's ability to down-regulate $5\text{-}HT_2$ receptors (Benjamin *et al.*, 1992). These data suggest that more research is needed on the potential involvement of $5\text{-}HT_2$ receptors in plus-maze anxiety.

$5\text{-}HT_3$ receptor ligands

Again the picture is one of confusion and one that cannot simply be attributed to dose range differences. Stemming from initial reports of antianxiety effects in social interaction and light/dark exploration tests (Jones *et al.*, 1988), many laboratories have found very potent anxiolytic effects with a range of $5\text{-}HT_3$ receptor antagonists, including ondansetron, zacopride, MDL 72222, ICS 205930, BRL 46470A and RS-42358-197. Furthermore, the $5\text{-}HT_3$ receptor agonist, mCPB, has been found to have an anxiogenic action in the maze. However, an equally large number of studies have reported negative results for ondansetron, MDL 72222, ICS 205-930, BRL 43694 and DAU 6215. These discrepancies are as enigmatic as those observed with $5\text{-}HT_{1A}$ receptor agonists and, as Table 5 indicates, cannot be simply attributed to dose levels employed. Interestingly, however, recent data suggest that zacopride may only exert anxiolytic-like effects in handling-naive rats (Andrews and File, 1993), again introducing general methodology as a significant variable in the behavioural pharmacology of the plus-maze.

5-HT reuptake inhibitors

A number of research groups have examined the effects of antidepressant drugs on plus-maze behaviour; some of these compounds are more selective than others in their effects on 5-HT function. Imipramine, given either acutely or chronically, has been found not to significantly alter anxiety in the plus-maze (Briley *et al.*, 1986; File and Johnston, 1987; Pellow *et al.*, 1985; Vasar *et al.*, 1993). Similar negative results have been obtained with acutely administered desipramine, amitriptyline and citalopram (Briley *et al.*, 1986; Durcan *et al.*, 1988). The atypical antidepressant, tianeptine, which (somewhat paradoxically) increases 5-HT reuptake, also fails to affect plus-maze behaviour (File and Mabbutt, 1991). However, the effects of acute fluoxetine are equivocal with both anxiogenic activity (Handley and McBlane, 1992) and no effect (Durcan *et al.*, 1988) reported. Similarly, acute fluvoxamine has an inconsistent profile with, on this occasion, both anxiolytic (Alder and Morinan, 1992) and no effect (Durcan *et al.*, 1988) documented. Interestingly, chronic paroxetine has been shown to have an anxiolytic profile in the test (Cadogen *et al.*, 1992), suggesting that further study of chronically administered 5-HT-selective reuptake inhibitors is warranted.

In overall summary, manipulations of 5-HT function produce highly inconsistent effects on anxiety in the elevated plus-maze. Clearly, one methodological issue which may contribute to this inconsistency is the tendency for researchers to employ acute treatment regimens whereas, clinically, both 5-HT$_{1A}$ anxiolytics and 5-HT reuptake inhibitors are effective only following a period of chronic treatment. A related issue is the degree to which the 5-HT system is activated by plus-maze exposure. Presumably this will depend, among other factors, upon endogenous tone in the system (e.g. genetic strain, housing conditions, handling experience) and the specific conditions under which the test is conducted. In this context, it is pertinent to recall that (a) 8-OH-DPAT can be either anxiogenic or anxiolytic depending on light level used, (b) buspirone may only be anxiogenic in handling-habituated animals and (c) zacopride may be anxiolytic only in handling-naive animals.

CCK receptor ligands

Recent interest has been expressed in the potential involvement of the neuropeptide, cholecystokinin (CCK), in mechanisms of anxiety (Harro *et al.*, 1993; Ravard and Dourish, 1990). In an early report, rats classed as behaviourally non-anxious in the plus-maze were found to have reduced cortical CCK density compared with animals rated as anxious (Harro *et al.*, 1990). Since then, systemic and/or central injection studies have revealed anxiogenic-like effects of a variety of CCK-related peptides (CCK-4, CCK-8 unsulphated; caerulein; pentagastrin, BC-264) (Chopin and Briley, 1993; Dauge *et al.*, 1992; Harro *et al.*, 1990; Harro and Vasar, 1991a; Singh *et al.*, 1991a, 1991b). Of particular interest is the question of the relative importance of CCK$_A$ and CCK$_B$ receptors in these effects. Although anxiolytic-like profiles have been reported for the CCK$_A$ antagonist, devazepide, negative results have also been obtained (Chopin and Briley, 1993; Rataud *et al.*, 1991; Singh *et al.*, 1991b; Vasar *et al.*, 1993). The more likely involvement of CCK$_B$ receptors in plus-maze anxiety has been suggested by the consistent and very much more potent anxiolytic-like effects of selective antagonists of these sites, including L 365,260, CI-988 (formerly PD 134308) and PD 135158 (Chopin and Briley, 1993; Costall *et al.*, 1991; Hughes *et al.*, 1990; Rataud *et al.*, 1991; Singh *et al.*, 1991a, 1991b; Vasar *et al.*, 1993). Most intriguing is the recent finding that the benzodiazepine receptor antagonist, flumazenil, can block the anxiogenic effects of CCK-8 unsulphated as well as the anxiolytic effects of devazepide and L 365,260 (Chopin and Briley, 1993). This result potentially implicates benzodiazepine receptor mechanisms in the influence of CCK-related agents on anxiety expressed in the plus-maze. Finally, of direct relevance to the whole question of CCK involvement in anxiety expressed in rodent exploration models (including the plus-maze) is the suggestion that CCK receptor antagonism may directly enhance exploration rather than reduce anxiety (Harro and Vasar, 1991b; Harro *et al.*, 1993).

NMDA receptor ligands

Recent research has pointed to the potential involvement of excitatory amino acids (EAA) in anxiety, and in particular the role of N-methyl-D-aspartate (NMDA) receptor-related mechanisms. In both rat and mouse elevated plus-maze, injection of NMDA produces an enhancement of anxiety (Dunn *et al.*, 1989; Vasar *et al.*, 1993) while, reciprocally, anxiolytic-like effects have generally been reported for a range of competitive and non-competitive NMDA receptor antagonists (Corbett and Dunn, 1991, 1993; Dunn *et al.*, 1989, 1990, 1992; Guimaraes *et al.*, 1991; Schmitt *et al.*, 1990; Stephens *et al.*, 1986; Vasar *et al.*, 1993). Further studies in this area are clearly warranted.

Miscellaneous

Table 6 summarizes the effects of a range of other manipulations which have been studied for their effects in the elevated plus-maze. Many of these are 'one-off' findings, the true significance of which remains to be determined. In other cases, however, a more definitive picture is emerging. Examples of the latter include the anxiogenic-like effects of cocaine, caffeine and intraventricularly administered CRF, and the anxiolytic-like effects of lesions of the posterior septum. It is pertinent to note that a large number of other compounds do not appear to alter anxiety in the maze; these include calcium channel antagonists, dopaminergics, monoamine oxidase inhibitors and nootropics.

PLUS-MAZE: METHODOLOGICAL ISSUES

It is clear from the above review that, with the exception of the effects of benzodiazepine–GABA receptor/chloride channel manipulations, the literature on the behavioural pharmacology of the plus-maze is rife with inconsistency

Table 6   Effects of miscellaneous treatments on anxiety in the elevated plus-maze test

Anxiolytic effects (refs)	No effect/inconsistent (refs)	Anxiogenic effects (refs)
AF64A (127)	α-Helical CRF (1, 101, 163)	Aminophylline (208)
Casein diet (5, 149)	ACTH (60, 94)	Amygdala kindling (146)
Cannabidol (87)	Amineptine (26)	Antisense NPY (204)
Carbamazepine (208)	Amphetamine (131, 152)	Caffeine (11, 131, 152)
DUP 753 (118)	Apomorphine (114)	Cocaine (173, 190, 205)
F 2692 (8, 31)	Clorgyline (26)	CRF (2, 12)
Morphine (143)	DFP (145)	Imidazole (59)
Neuropeptide Y (100)	Diltiazem (110, 190)	Lindane (134)
Papaverine (208)	Haloperidol (33, 152)	Nitrendipine (79)
Phenelzine (112)	Indomethacin (90)	
Scopolamine (178)	Nicotine (13)	*Lesions*
	Nifedipine (190)	Dorsomedial thalamus (17)
Lesions	Nomifensine (26)	
Septum (154, 197, 199)	Oxiracetam (47)	
Mammillary body (17)	Pargyline (26)	
	Piracetam (47)	
	PK 8165 (151)	
	Quinpirole (114)	
	SKF 38393 (114)	
	Tofisopam (151)	
	Tracazolate (151)	
	Verapamil (106, 110, 190)	
	Lesions	
	Amygdala (199)	

and contradiction. Despite general opinion to the contrary, these problems (e.g. the effects of 5-HT receptor manipulations) cannot readily be attributed to the obvious variable of drug dose. As such, we must look to organismic and procedural variables for potential sources of confound. Table 7 lists the major variables of interest.

Table 7   Major organismic and procedural variables which influence behaviour and/or drug response in the elevated plus-maze test

Organismic variables	Procedural variables
Species	Housing conditions
Genetic strain	Prior handling
Age	Pretesting in hole-board
Gender	Prior stress
	Level of illumination at test
	Time of day at test
	Prior maze experience

Organismic variables

Species, strain, age and gender are the main organismic variables that have been studied in the context of the elevated plus-maze. Although the majority of studies have involved rats, close examination of Tables 3–6 indicates that the inconsistency observed in pharmacological studies cannot be ascribed to species differences. However, behavioural research suggesting major strain differences in basal levels of plus-maze anxiety could have an important bearing upon this issue. Such differences have been reported both for rats (Costall *et al.*, 1989a; Mangiafico *et al.*, 1989; Pare, 1992; Pellow *et al.*, 1985; Soderpalm, 1989) and mice (Alder and Morinan, 1992; Miyamoto *et al.*, 1992; Rodgers and Cole, 1993b). Indeed, a very recent and comprehensive analysis of 16 inbred mouse strains has confirmed major strain differences in plus-maze anxiety measures, at least 70% of which can be attributed to genetic factors (Trullas and Skolnick, 1993).

Age at testing also appears to be an important factor in baseline levels of plus-maze behaviour, with anxiety measures reported to increase with age in both species (File, 1990b; Frussa-Filho *et al.*, 1992; Lamberty and Gower, 1990). In contrast, the influence of gender on plus-maze behaviour is more equivocal, with some studies showing no effect (Alder and Morinan, 1992; Steenbergen *et al.*, 1990), others indicating that females are less anxious than males (Johnston and File, 1991; Rodgers and Cole, 1993b; Steenbergen *et al.*, 1991), and yet others suggesting that males are less anxious than females (Kellogg *et al.*, 1991). There is also one report that lactating females are less anxious than females at different stages of the oestrous cycle (Bitran *et al.*, 1991b), a finding which appears to link well with the anxiolytic-like effects of progesterone-related steroids reviewed above.

Clearly, then, the choice of strain, age and gender can all be important determinants of basal levels of anxiety in the plus-maze and, hence, of drug response: low basal anxiety levels will reduce the chances of detecting anxiolytic agents, while a high basal anxiety level will make difficult the task of identifying compounds with anxiogenic action.

Procedural variables

Housing, prior handling, pretesting, prior stress, lighting levels and prior maze experience have all been shown to have significant effects on basal anxiety. In rats, individual housing has been reported to have either no effect (Frussa-Filho *et al.*, 1991) or to increase anxiety (Janowska *et al.*, 1991). In contrast, individual housing for periods of longer than one week has been found to decrease plus-maze anxiety in mice (Hilakivi *et al.*, 1989a; Rodgers and Cole, 1993b). Although these species differences may relate to the different social organization of the two species (colonial versus territorial), no apparent differences have been noted in the behavioural profiles of socially dominant and socially subordinate male mice (Hilakivi *et al.*, 1989b). Furthermore, behavioural profiles in the elevated plus-maze do not predict future dominant or subordinate social status in male mice (Hilakivi-Clarke and Lister, 1992).

While the effects of prior handling have not been studied extensively, this procedure has been reported to either increase (Andrews and File, 1993) or have no effect upon (Brett and Pratt, 1990) basal levels of open arm exploration in rats. Very significantly, however, and irrespective of effects on basal anxiety, handling history has been found to significantly alter responses to certain drugs, including diazepam, cocaine, zacopride and buspirone (Andrews and File, 1993; Brett and Pratt, 1990; File and Andrews, 1991; Rogerio and Takahashi, 1992). Several laboratories routinely expose their test animals to a novel environment (e.g. hole board) prior to plus-maze testing. This is often done to provide additional measures of drug effects on locomotor activity and exploration. However, pretesting of this type has been found to reduce basal anxiety levels in both rats (Pellow *et al.*, 1985; Soderpalm *et al.*, 1989) and mice (Lister, 1987; Rodgers and Cole, 1993b). In this context, it is important to note that prior novelty can interact with genetic strain to produce diametrically opposite behavioural outcomes: thus, whereas T1 mice show reduced anxiety in response to prior novelty, DBA/2 mice show increased anxiety (Rodgers and Cole, 1993b).

The above findings indicate that, under certain circumstances, prior exposure to a novel arena can produce anxiogenic-like effects on plus-maze behaviour in mice. Similar effects of prior novelty have also been reported in rats (DaCunha *et al.*, 1992). Furthermore, a very wide range of other stressors have been found to enhance anxiety in rats and mice tested on the elevated plus-maze: these include immobilization (Albonetti and Farabollini, 1992; Handley and McBlane, 1993; but see also Falter *et al.*, 1992), forced swim (Britton *et al.*, 1991), electric shock (Steenbergen *et al.*, 1990; but see also Falter *et al.*, 1992 and Steenbergen *et al.*, 1991), surgical stress (Adamec *et al.*, 1991), saline injection (Adamec *et al.*, 1991), social defeat (Heinrichs *et al.*, 1992; Rodgers and Cole, 1993a), conspecific scent (Rodgers and Cole, 1993a), cat odour (Zangrossi and File, 1992a, 1992b) and cat exposure (Adamec and Shallow, 1993).

At present, opinion is divided concerning the influence of level of illumination on plus-maze performance, with several groups reporting no effect (Falter *et al.*, 1992; Handley and McBlane, 1993; Pellow *et al.*, 1985) and others finding significant reductions in open arm exploration (Benjamin *et al.*, 1990; Lee and Rodgers, 1990; Morato and Castrechini, 1989). However, it is worth re-emphasizing that even in the absence of a basal effect on plus-maze anxiety, lighting level can produce exactly opposite profiles for certain drugs (e.g. 8-OH-DPAT) (Handley and McBlane, 1993). Very recently, it has been found that rats tested (normal light cycle) between 08.00 and 12.00 h are less anxious than those tested between 14.00 and 17.00 h (Griebel *et al.*, 1993). Clearly, then, level of illumination at testing, circadian factors and their possible interaction may be important methodological factors to be considered with respect to basal anxiety and drug response in the elevated plus-maze.

Finally, although some laboratories report stable test–retest behavioural profiles in the elevated plus-maze (File, 1990a; Lister, 1987; Pellow et al., 1985; Taukulis and McKay, 1992), the majority of studies which have examined this variable have found reduced open arm exploration on retesting (Griebel et al., 1993; Lee and Rodgers, 1990; Rodgers et al., 1992b; Rodgers and Shepherd, 1993; Shepherd, 1992; Treit et al., 1993a). Given that exposure to the maze elevates plasma corticosterone levels (Pellow et al., 1985), it may be relevant to note that repeated exposure to a novel environment has been shown to sensitize the plasma corticosterone response in both rats and mice (Hennessy, 1991). As already noted in the above discussion of benzodiazepine effects, prior maze experience markedly attenuates or even abolishes the anxiolytic effects of chlordiazepoxide and diazepam in the maze (so-called 'one trial tolerance' (File, 1990a)). Such effects are seen with intertest intervals of up to 21 days, are not dependent on drug state on trial 1 or the construction details of the maze but do appear to critically depend upon initial experience of the open arms (File, 1993; File et al., 1990; File and Zangrossi, 1993). Furthermore, in relation to the earlier discussion of the effects of handling, the phenomenon of 'one trial tolerance' is not seen in unhandled rats (File et al., 1992). Overall, these findings (altered baselines and drug response) combine to suggest that naive subjects should be used when this test is employed either for screening purposes or for studies on the mechanisms underlying certain forms of anxiety. However, as it would appear that the nature of the anxiety provoked on maze retest is different from that provoked by initial exposure (File, 1993; Rodgers et al., 1992b), it has been suggested that the behaviour of maze-experienced animals may provide a useful animal model for the study of phobias and their treatment (File, 1993). Importantly, however, the effects of prior maze experience on the efficacy of non-benzodiazepine anxiolytics has not as yet been studied.

It is clear from the above review that multiple organismic and procedural variables can influence basal levels of anxiety and drug response in the elevated plus-maze. Furthermore, even those variables which do not always affect behavioural baselines (e.g. handling, level of illumination, prior maze experience) can quite dramatically modify drug response. As such, the general inconsistency in the behavioural pharmacology of the plus-maze becomes more understandable. While it has been argued that such inconsistency and contradiction actually undermine the use of the plus-maze as a valid model of anxiety (Moser, 1989), the above methodological analysis together with issues related to dosing regimen (acute versus chronic) suggest that this conclusion may be somewhat premature (see also Treit, 1991). What does appear to be required at this stage in the evolution of the plus-maze test of anxiety is a comprehensive analysis of its behavioural pharmacology under *standardized* test conditions, preferably using a more sophisticated approach to behavioural analysis.

ETHOLOGY AND THE PLUS-MAZE

Traditionally, the basic parameters scored in plus-maze studies comprise total arm entries, the percentage/proportion of open arm entries relative to the total, and the percentage of time that animals spend in the open arms. The former measure is often considered as an index of general activity, while the latter two measures are the primary indices of anxiety. In an important factor-analytic study, Lister (1987) reported that measures of anxiety (per cent open arm entries and per cent open arm time) loaded heavily on one factor while total arm entries loaded heavily upon another. While this profile might suggest the potential utility of total arm entries as a measure of general locomotor activity, it is worth emphasizing that total entries also loaded, albeit less strongly, on the 'anxiety' factor. As such, total entries cannot be viewed as reflecting locomotor activity independent of anxiety state (see also Harro, 1993; Rodgers and Cole, 1993a). Other behavioural measures are therefore required to facilitate interpretation of drug profiles. While one approach has been to employ pretesting in a hole board (see above), the direct relevance of these data to the interpretation of plus-maze profiles remains uncertain and may be analogous to the dubious relevance of rota-rod data in assessing the behavioural specificity of drugs which reduce aggression in social interaction tests.

The previous section on methodology pointed to a range of organismic and procedural factors which contribute multiple sources of confound to the literature on the elevated plus-maze. In this context, variation within and between laboratories is also readily apparent with respect to the key definition of 'arm entry'. Most research groups, including our own, employ a definition of 'whole body entry/all four paws entry' as their test criterion. However, analysis of the literature reveals that many studies on the plus-maze fail to provide this critical information, others employ a very liberal criterion of two paws only, while yet others appear to employ a 'sliding' criterion. In addition, many papers report only the per cent open arm measures (entries and time), without providing any information on absolute values for open, closed and total entry scores. These differences in scoring and/or data-reporting represent further sources of contamination in research on the behavioural pharmacology of the plus-maze. Thus, if absolute measures are low, the percentage calculations and, hence, interpretations, can be severely compromised (Harro, 1993). Furthermore, given the approach/avoidance conflict engendered by the maze configuration (Montgomery, 1955), it is rather extraordinary that the classical plus-maze scoring method does not include measures related to the central platform area. Thus, very few laboratories routinely measure time spent on the central platform which might be assumed to reflect relevant processes related to decision-making (Lee and Rodgers, 1990; Rodgers et al., 1992b; Trullas and Skolnick, 1993).

In view of these considerations, the influence of behavioural baselines (rate dependency) in behavioural pharmacology and the fact that standard plus-maze scoring actually pays minimal attention to actual *behaviour*, we (Rodgers,

1991; Rodgers *et al.*, 1992a) and others (Adamec and Shallow, 1993; Falter *et al.*, 1992; Moser, 1989; Shepherd, 1992) have argued that the utility/sensitivity of the plus-maze might be improved by adopting a more ethological approach to data collection. Early (though limited) examples include the work of (a) Pellow and colleagues (1985) who incorporated measures of freezing, immobility and defaecation, (b) Rodgers and associates (Lee and Rodgers, 1990) who included measures of total rearing and time spent on the central platform, and (c) Moser (1989) who recorded rearing, stretch attend postures, doubling back into closed arms and defaecation/urination.

On the basis of extensive observations on the behaviour of intact mice, we have developed a plus-maze *ethogram* representing a catalogue of high-probability behaviours displayed on the maze (Rodgers *et al.*, 1992a). As Table 8 illustrates, this ethogram includes both traditional and novel measures; the latter comprise time spent on the centre platform, total rearing, entry latency (equates with emergence latency, a measure that has previously been used as an index of initial tendency to explore a potentially dangerous environment), non-exploratory behaviour (a composite measure of movement arrest and grooming) and a group of behaviours which are believed to reflect *risk assessment*. This concept derives from the work of Blanchard and colleagues on the antipredator defensive repertoire of wild and laboratory rats and subsumes information-gathering behaviours which function to permit frightened/anxious animals to return to non-defensive (i.e. normal) behaviour. These behaviours have proven very sensitive in the analysis of drug effects on antipredator defence (Blanchard *et al.*, 1991). In the murine plus-maze, head-dipping, stretch attend postures and closed arm returns appear to fulfil the requirements of risk assessment. Thus, having entered a closed arm, more 'cautious'

Table 8 Ethogram for the murine elevated plus-maze test. All measures listed are recorded, with those described as 'risk assessment' particularly sensitive to anxiety-related manipulations. See original sources (Cole and Rodgers, 1994; Rodgers and Cole, 1993a, 1993b; Rodgers *et al.*, 1993) for full detail

Classical measures	Ethologically derived measures
Total arm entries	Entry latency (s)
Open arm entries	Non-exploratory behaviour (s)
Closed arm entries	% central platform time $[C/T \times 100]$
% open arm entries $[O/T \times 100]$	% closed arm time $[C/T \times 100]$
% open arm time $[O/T \times 100]$	Rearing
	Risk assessment behaviours
	Closed arm returns
	Head-dipping
	Stretch attend postures (SAP)
	% protected dipping $[P/T \times 100]$
	% protected SAP $[P/T \times 100]$

subjects will only slowly approach the exit to the centre platform, exhibit high levels of stretch attend and head-dipping, and then double back into the same closed arm (closed arm return). Although head-dipping and stretch attend can and do occur on the open arms, by far the highest frequency of such behaviour is seen in and around the centre platform area. Thus, as a further refinement, the head-dipping and stretch attend measures are also classified on the basis of whereabouts on the maze they occur: as such, the 'per cent protected' score for each of these measures reflects occurrence on or from the relatively secure central platform and closed sections of the maze.

This novel scoring method has been used in a series of studies in which we have examined the effects of social stress (Rodgers and Cole, 1993a), organismic and procedural variables (Rodgers and Cole, 1993b), and pharmacological manipulations (Cole and Rodgers, 1993, 1994; Rodgers et al., 1992a, 1993) on the behaviour of mice in the plus maze. As the specific results of these studies have already been incorporated in earlier sections of this chapter, only the general principles to emerge from this work will now be discussed.

First, from our studies on social stressors (Rodgers and Cole, 1993a), it is clear that anxious mice will not only show reductions in open arm measures but also display depressed levels of general activity and rearing in the maze. As no drugs were involved in these studies, the generally held view that reductions in total entries and/or rearing reflects non-specificity is undermined. Second, from the same experiments, the observation that prior stress actually *increases* risk assessment measures while depressing other behaviours indicates that the former can be usefully employed in differentiating anxiogenic from non-specific behavioural profiles. Third, in the same studies, and other work on mixed 5-HT$_1$ receptor agonists (Rodgers et al., 1992a), we have shown that anxiogenic effects can be revealed through increases in risk assessment measures *in the absence of* significant changes in per cent open arm entries and time. Finally, in our recent examination of a variety of anxiolytic (benzodiazepine and non-benzodiazepine) compounds (Cole and Rodgers, 1993, 1994; Rodgers et al., 1993), we have repeatedly observed that risk assessment measures are generally *more sensitive* to drug action than are the traditional indices of anxiety in this test. This finding has particular importance for those agents which may have a rather small dose differential between anxiolytic and non-specific actions. Significantly, similar conclusions are beginning to appear from parallel work on the rat elevated plus-maze (Adamec and Shallow, 1993; Shepherd, 1992; Shepherd et al., 1993).

In summary, the use of ethologically derived behavioural measures alongside traditional spatiotemporal indices appears to greatly enhance the utility and sensitivity of the plus-maze model of anxiety. As ethologically based animal models are becoming ever more popular in this field of research (Green and Hodges, 1991; Lister, 1990; Treit, 1991), it is to be hoped that researchers will not only continue to use and develop paradigms based on spontaneous behaviour, but also employ behavioural scoring techniques which are congruent with this approach. The richness of the resulting database will undoubtedly facilitate interpretation of drug effects and should also help to resolve the existing confusion in the preclinical pharmacology of anxiety.

CONCLUSIONS

Handley and McBlane (1993) have recently commented that 'research into animal models of anxiety is at an exciting crossroads'. It is clearly no longer appropriate to view behavioural models as mere bioassays, as simple procedures designed to detect certain drugs but about which little is otherwise known. Sole reliance on pharmacological validation of animal models of anxiety has backfired on researchers with the growing appreciation of the problems associated with classical benzodiazepine therapy, the multifaceted nature of anxiety and the inability of many tests to detect compounds other than those which interact with the benzodiazepine–GABA receptor complex.

It is hoped that this review of the elevated plus-maze will draw the attention of research groups both to the importance of subtle (and not so subtle) methodological factors and to the utility of a more ethological approach in the interpretation and recording of behaviours displayed in this test. In their work on antipredator behaviour, Blanchard and colleagues (1991) have emphasized the Darwinian view that an understanding of defence is crucial to an understanding of human fear and anxiety reactions. They have clearly shown that the defensive repertoire extends well beyond the classical indices of freezing, flight and defensive attack, and that risk assessment behaviours are exquisitely sensitive to both traditional and novel antianxiety agents. This principle appears to generalize to the elevated plus-maze test, and may well be applicable to a much wider range of existing animal models of anxiety. Thus, while new tests are to be welcomed, behavioural refinement of existing models offers an exciting challenge to those frustrated by the inconsistencies and contradictions which currently plague the preclinical behavioural pharmacology of anxiety.

ACKNOWLEDGEMENT

J.C.C. is supported by the Medical Research Council.

REFERENCES

1. Adamec, R.E. and Shallow, T. (1993) Lasting effects on rodent anxiety of a single exposure to a cat. *Physiol. Behav.*, **54**, 101–109.
2. Adamec, R.E., Sayin, U. and Brown, A. (1991) The effects of corticotropin releasing factor (CRF) and handling stress on behavior in the elevated plus-maze test of anxiety. *J. Psychopharmacol.*, **5**, 175–186.

3. Albonetti, M.E. and Farabollini, F. (1992) Behavioural responses to single and repeated restraint in male and female rats. *Behav. Proc.*, **28**, 97–110.

4. Alder, T. and Morinan, A. (1992) Strain differences in behavioural responses in murine models of anxiety. *Br. J. Pharmacol.*, **106**, 45P.

5. Almeida, S.S., de Oliveira, L.M. and Graeff, F.G. (1991) Early life protein malnutrition changes exploration of the elevated plus-maze and reactivity to anxiolytics. *Psychopharmacology*, **103**, 513–518.

6. Andrews, N. and File, S.E. (1992) Are there changes in the sensitivity to 5-HT$_3$ receptor ligands following chronic diazepam treatment? *Psychopharmacology*, **108**, 333–337.

7. Andrews, N. and File, S.E. (1993) Handling history of rats modifies behavioural effects of drugs in the elevated plus-maze test of anxiety. *Eur. J. Pharmacol.*, **235**, 109–112.

8. Assie, M.-B., Chopin, P., Stenger, A. *et al.* (1993) Neuropharmacology of a new potential anxiolytic compound, F-2692, 1-(3′-trifluoromethyl phenyl) 1,4-dihydro 3-amino 4-oxo 6 methyl pyrdiazine. I. Acute and in vitro effects. *Psychopharmacology*, **110**, 13–18.

9. Audi, E.A., De-Oliviera, C.E. and Graeff, F.G. (1991) Microinjection of propranolol into the dorsal periaqueductal gray causes an anxiolytic effect in the elevated plus-maze antagonized by ritanserin. *Psychopharmacology*, **105**, 553–557.

10. Baldwin, A.A. and File, S.E. (1988) Reversal of increased anxiety during benzodiazepine withdrawal: evidence for an anxiogenic endogenous ligand for the benzodiazepine receptor. *Brain Res. Bull.*, **20**, 603–606.

11. Baldwin, H.A., Johnston, A.L. and File, S.E. (1989) Antagonistic effects of caffeine and yohimbine in animal tests of anxiety. *Eur. J. Pharmacol.*, **159**, 211–215.

12. Baldwin, H.A., Rassnick, S., Rivier, J. *et al.* (1991) CRF antagonist reverses the 'anxiogenic' response to ethanol withdrawal in the rat. *Psychopharmacology*, **103**, 227–232.

13. Balfour, D.J.K., Graham, C.A. and Vale, A.L. (1986) Studies on the possible role of brain 5-HT systems and adrenocortical activity in behavioural responses to nicotine and diazepam in an elevated plus-maze. *Psychopharmacology*, **90**, 528–532.

14. Barrett, J.E. (1991) Animal behaviour models in the analysis and understanding of anxiolytic drugs acting at serotonin receptors. In: *Animal Models in Psychopharmacology* (eds B. Olivier, J. Mos and J.L. Slangen). Birkhauser, Basle, pp. 37–52.

15. Benjamin, D., Lal, H. and Meyerson, L.R. (1990) The effects of 5-HT$_{1B}$ characterizing agents in the mouse elevated plus-maze. *Life Sci.*, **47**, 195–203.

16. Benjamin, D., Saiff, E.I., Nevins, T. and Lal, H. (1992) Mianserin-induced 5-HT$_2$ receptor downregulation results in anxiolytic effects in the elevated plus-maze test. *Drug Dev. Res.*, **26**, 287–297.

17. Beracocchea, D.J. and Krazem, A. (1991) Effects of mammiliary body and mediodorsal thalamic lesions on elevated plus maze exploration. *NeuroReport*, **2**, 793–796.

18. Bitran, D., Hilvers, R.J. and Kellogg, C.K. (1991a) Anxiolytic effects of 3α-hydroxy-5α[β]-pregan-20-one: endogenous metabolites of progesterone that are active at the GABA$_A$ receptor. *Brain Res.*, **561**, 157–161.

19. Bitran, D., Hilvers, R.J. and Kellogg, C.K. (1991b) Ovarian endocrine status modulates the anxiolytic potency of diazepam and the efficacy of gamma-aminobutyric acid–benzodiazepine receptor-mediated chloride ion transport. *Behav. Neurosci.*, **105**, 653–662.

20. Bitran, D., Purdy, R.H. and Kellogg, C.K. (1993) Anxiolytic effect of progesterone is associated with increases in cortical allopregnanolone and GABA$_A$ receptor function. *Pharmacol. Biochem. Behav.*, **45**, 423–428.

21. Blackburn, T.P., Baxter, G.S., Kennett, G.A. *et al.* (1993) BRL 46470A: a highly potent, selective and long-acting 5-HT$_3$ receptor antagonist with anxiolytic-like properties. *Psychopharmacology*, **110**, 257–264.

22. Blanchard, D.C., Blanchard, R.J. and Rodgers, R.J. (1991) Risk assessment and animal models of anxiety. In: *Animal Models in Psychopharmacology* (eds B. Olivier, J. Mos and J.L. Slangen). Birkhauser, Basle, pp. 117–134.

23. Blokland, A., Prickaerts, J. and Raaijmakers, W. (1992) Reduced level of anxiety in adult Lewis rats after chronic ethanol consumption. *Physiol. Behav.*, **51**, 245–248.

24. Borsini, F., Brambilla, A., Cesana, R. and Donetti, A. (1993) The effect of DAU 6215, a novel 5HT-3 antagonist in animal models of anxiety. *Pharmacol. Res.*, **27**, 151–164.

25. Brett, R.R. and Pratt, J.A. (1990) Chronic handling modifies the anxiolytic effect of diazepam in the elevated plus-maze. *Eur. J. Pharmacol.*, **178**, 135–138.

26. Briley, M., Chopin, P. and Veigner, M. (1986) The 'plus-maze test of anxiety': validation in different rat strains and effect of a wide variety of antidepressants. *Br. J. Pharmacol.*, **87**, 217P.

27. Briley, M., Chopin, M. and Moret, C. (1990) Effect of serotonergic lesion on 'anxious' behaviour measured in the elevated plus-maze test in the rat. *Psychopharmacology*, **101**, 187–189.

28. Britton, K.T., Page, M., Baldwin, H.A. and Koob, G.F. (1991) Anxiolytic activity of steroid anesthetic alphaxalone. *J. Pharmacol. Exp. Ther.*, **258**, 124–129.

29. Cadogan, A.K., Wright, I.K., Coombs, I. *et al.* (1992) Repeated paroxetine administration in the rat produces an anxiolytic profile in the elevated X-maze and a decreased [^{3}H]-ketanserin binding. *Neurosci. Lett.*, **42**, S8.

30. Chopin, P. and Briley, M. (1993) The benzodiazepine antagonist, flumazenil blocks the effects of CCK receptor agonists and antagonists in the elevated plus-maze. *Psychopharmacology*, **110**, 409–414.

31. Chopin, P., Assie, M.-B. and Briley, M. (1993) Neuropharmacology of a new potential anxiolytic compound, F 2692, 1-(3'-trifluoromethyl phenyl) 1,4-dihydro 3-amino 4-oxo 6-methyl pyridazine. 2. Evaluation of its tolerance and dependence producing potential and of its effects on benzodiazepine withdrawal in the elevated plus-maze test in rats. *Psychopharmacology*, **110**, 19–26.

32. Cole, J.C. and Rodgers, R.J. (1993) An ethological analysis of the effects of chlordiazepoxide and bretazenil (Ro16-6028) in the murine elevated plus-maze. *Behav. Pharmacol.*, **4**, 573–580.

33. Cole, J.C. and Rodgers, R.J. (1994) Ethological evaluation of the effects of acute and chronic buspirone treatment in the murine elevated plus-maze test: comparison with haloperidol. *Psychopharmacology*, **114**, 288–296.

34. Conceicao, I.M., Maiolini, M., Mattia, N. *et al.* (1992) Anxiety-induced antinociception in the mouse. *Brazilian J. Med. Biol. Res.*, **25**, 831–834.

35. Corbett, R. and Dunn, R.W. (1991) Effects of HA-966 on conflict, social interaction, and plus maze behaviors. *Drug Dev. Res.*, **24**, 201–205.

36. Corbett, R. and Dunn, R.W. (1993) Effects of 5,7 dichlorokynurenic acid on conflict, social interaction and plus-maze behaviors. *Neuropharmacology*, **32**, 461–466.

37. Corbett, R., Fielding, S., Cornfeldt, M. and Dunn, R.W. (1991) GABAmimetic agents display anxiolytic-like effects in the social interaction and elevated plus-maze procedures. *Psychopharmacology*, **104**, 312–316.

38. Costall, B., Kelly, M.E. and Tomkins, D.M. (1989a) Use of the elevated plus-maze to assess anxiolytic potential in the rat. *Br. J. Pharmacol.*, **96**, 312P.

39. Costall, B., Kelly, M.E., Tomkins, D.M. and Tyers, M.B. (1989b) Profile of action of diazepam and 5-HT₃ receptor antagonists in the elevated plus-maze. *J. Psychopharmacol.*, **3**, 10P.

40. Costall, B., Domeney, A.M., Hughes, J. *et al.* (1991) Anxiolytic effects of CCK-B antagonists. *Neuropeptides*, **19** (suppl.), 65–73.

41. Costall, B., Domeney, A.M., Kelly, M.E. *et al.* (1993) The effect of 5-HT₃ receptor antagonist, RS-42358-197, in animal models of anxiety. *Eur. J. Pharmacol.*, **234**, 91–99.

42. Critchley, M.A.E. and Handley, S.L. (1987) Effects in the X-maze anxiety model of agents acting at 5-HT₁ and 5-HT₂ receptors. *Psychopharmacology*, **93**, 502–506.

43. Critchley, M.A.E., Njung'e, K. and Handley, S.L. (1988) Prevention of 8-OH-DPAT anxiogenic effect by ipsapirone and 5-HT₁ antagonist beta-blockers. *Br. J. Pharmacol.*, **94**, 389P.

44. Critchley, M.A.E., Njung'e, K. and Handley, S.L. (1992) Actions and some interactions of 5-HT₁A ligands in the elevated X-maze and effects of dorsal raphe lesions. *Psychopharmacology*, **106**, 484–490.

45. DaCunha, C., Levi de Stein, M., Wolfman, C. *et al.* (1992) Effects of various training procedures on performance in an elevated plus-maze: possible relation with brain regional levels of benzodiazepine-like molecules. *Pharmacol. Biochem. Behav.*, **43**, 677–681.

46. Dauge, V., Derrien, M., Durieux, C. *et al.* (1992) Etude des effets induits par les agonistes selectifs CCK-B de la cholecystokinine dans la nociception et le comportement des rongeurs. *Therapie*, **47**, 531–539.

47. DeAngelis, L. (1992) The nootropic drugs piracetam and oxiracetam do not induce anxiety in mice during elevated plus-maze. *Curr. Ther. Res.*, **52**, 230–237.

48. Dourish, C.T. (1987) Brain 5-HT₁A receptors and anxiety. In: *Brain 5-HT₁A Receptors* (eds C.T. Dourish, S. Ahlenius and J.P. Hutson). Horwood, Chichester, pp. 261–277.

49. Dunn, R.W., Corbett, R. and Fielding, S. (1989) Effects of 5-HT₁A receptor agonists and NMDA receptor antagonists in the social interaction test and the elevated plus maze. *Eur. J. Pharmacol.*, **169**, 1–10.

50. Dunn, R.W., Corbett, R., Martin, L.L. *et al.* (1990) Preclinical anxiolytic profiles of 7189 and 8319, novel non-competitive NMDA antagonists. In: *Current and Future Trends in Anticonvulsant, Anxiety and Stroke Therapy.* Wiley–Liss, New York, pp. 495–512.

51. Dunn, R.W., Carlezon, W.A. and Corbett, R. (1991) Preclinical anxiolytic versus antipsychotic profiles of the 5-HT₃ antagonists ondansetron, zacopride, 3α-tropanyl-1*H*-indole-3-carboxylic acid ester and 1α*H*,3α,5α*H*-tropan-3-yl-3,5-dichlorobenzoate. *Drug Dev. Res.*, **23**, 289–300.

52. Dunn, R.W., Flanagan, D.M., Martin, L.L. *et al.* (1992) Stereoselective *R*-(+) enantiomer of HA-966 displays anxiolytic effects in rodents. *Eur. J. Pharmacol.*, **214**, 207–214.

53. Durcan, M.J. and Lister, R.G. (1988) Time course of ethanol's effects on locomotor activity, exploration and anxiety in mice. *Psychopharmacology*, **96**, 67–72.

54. Durcan, M.J., Lister, R.G., Eckardt, M.J. and Linnoila, M. (1988) Behavioral interactions of fluoxetine and other 5-hydroxytryptamine uptake inhibitors with ethanol in tests of anxiety, locomotion and exploration. *Psychopharmacology*, **96**, 528–533.

55. Durcan, M.J., Lister, R.G. and Linnoila, M. (1989) Behavioral effects of α_2

adrenoceptor antagonists and their interactions with ethanol in tests of locomotion, exploration and anxiety in mice. *Psychopharmacology*, **97**, 189–193.

56. Engel, J.A., Egbe, P., Liljequist, S. and Soderpalm, B. (1989) Effects of
amperozide in two animal models of anxiety. *Pharmacol. Toxicol.*, **64**, 429–433.

57. Falter, U., Gower, A.J. and Gobert, J. (1992) Resistance of baseline activity in
the elevated plus-maze to exogenous influences. *Behav. Pharmacol.*, **3**, 123–128.

58. Ferrari, F., Tartoni, P.L. and Mangiafico, V. (1989a) B-HT 920 antagonizes rat
neophobia in the X-maze test: a comparative study with other drugs active on
adrenergic and dopaminergic receptors. *Arch Int. Pharmacodyn. Ther.*, **298**,
7–14.

59. Ferrari, F., Tartoni, P.G., Monti, A. and Mangiafico, V. (1989b) Does anxiety
underlie imidazole-induced behavioural effects in the rat? *Psychopharmacology*,
99, 345–351.

60. Ferrari, F., Pelloni, F. and Gilliani, D. (1992) B-HT 920 stimulates feeding and
antagonizes anorexia indiced by ACTH and immobilisation. *Eur. J. Pharmacol.*,
210, 17–22.

61. Field, M.J., Lewis, A.S., Lloyd, C. and Singh, L. (1991) Automation of the rat
elevated X-maze test of anxiety. *Br. J. Pharmacol.*, **102**, 304P.

62. File, S.E. (1990a) One-trial tolerance to the anxiolytic effects of chlordiazepoxide
in the plus-maze. *Psychopharmacology*, **100**, 281–282.

63. File, S.E. (1990b) Age and anxiety: increased anxiety, decreased anxiolytic,
but enhanced sedative, response to chlordiazepoxide in old rats. *Hum. Psychopharmacol.*, **5**, 169–173.

64. File, S.E. (1992) Behavioural detection of anxiolytic action. In: *Experimental
Approaches to Anxiety and Depression*. Wiley, Chichester, pp. 25–44.

65. File, S.E. (1993) The interplay of learning and anxiety in the elevated plus-maze.
Brain Res. Bull., *Behav.*, **58**, 119–202.

66. File, S.E. and Andrews, N. (1991) Low but not high doses of buspirone reduce
the anxiogenic effects of diazepam withdrawal. *Psychopharmacology*, **105**,
578–582.

67. File, S.E. and Aranko, K. (1988) Sodium valproate and chlordiazepoxide in the
elevated plus-maze test of anxiety in the rat. *Neuropsychobiology*, **20**, 82–86.

68. File, S.E. and Baldwin, H.A. (1987) Effects of β-carbolines in animal models of
anxiety. *Brain Res. Bull.*, **19**, 293–299.

69. File, S.E. and Hitchcott, P.K. (1990) A theory of benzodiazepine dependence
that can explain whether fumazenil will enhance or reverse the phenomena.
Psychopharmacology, **101**, 525–532.

70. File, S.E. and Johnston, A.L. (1987) Chronic treatment with imipramine does
not reverse the effects of 3 anxiogenic compounds in a test of anxiety in the rat.
Neuropsychobiology, **17**, 187–192.

71. File, S.E. and Johnston, A.L. (1989) Lack of effects of 5-HT₃ receptor antagonists in the social interaction and elevated plus-maze tests of anxiety in the rat.
Psychopharmacology, **99**, 248–251.

72. File, S.E. and Mabbutt, P.S. (1991) Effects of tianeptine in animal models of
anxiety and on learning and memory. *Drug Dev. Res.*, **23**, 47–56.

73. File, S.E. and Pellow, S. (1986) Behavioural pharmacology of the pyrazoloquino-
line CGS 9896, a novel putative anxiolytic. *Drug Dev. Res.*, **7**, 245–253.

74. File, S.E. and Zangrossi, H. (1993) 'One-trial tolerance' to the anxiolytic actions
of benzodiazepines in the elevated plus-maze, or the development of a phobic
state? *Psychopharmacology*, **110**, 240–244.

75. File, S.E., Baldwin, H.A. and Aranko, K. (1987) Anxiogenic effects in benzodiazepine withdrawal are linked to the development of tolerance. *Brain Res.
Bull.*, **19**, 607–610.

76. File, S.E., Mabbutt, P.S. and Hitchcott, P.K. (1990) Characterisation of the phenomenon of 'one trial tolerance' to the anxiolytic effect of chlordiazepoxide in the elevated plus-maze. *Psychopharmacology*, 102, 98–101.

77. File, S.E., Zharkovsky, A. and Gulati, K. (1991) Effects of baclofen and nitrendipine on ethanol withdrawal responses in the rat. *Neuropharmacology*, 30, 183–190.

78. File, S.E., Andrews, N., Wu, P.Y. *et al.* (1992a) Modification of chlordiazepoxide's behavioural and neurochemical effects by handling and plus-maze experience. *Eur. J. Pharmacol.*, 218, 9–14.

79. File, S.E., Zharkovsky, A. and Hitchcott, P.K. (1992b) Effects of nitrendipine, chlordiazepoxide, flumazenil and baclofen on the increased anxiety resulting from alcohol withdrawal. *Prog. Neuro-Psychopharmacol. Biol. Psychiatry*, 16, 87–93.

80. Frussa-Filho, R., Otoboni, J.R., Uema, F.T. and Sa-Rocha, L.C. (1991) Evaluation of memory and anxiety in rats observed in the elevated plus-maze: effects of age and isolation. *Brazilian J. Med. Biol. Res.*, 24, 725–728.

81. Frussa-Filho, R., Otoboni, J.R., Giannotti, A.D. *et al.* (1992) Effect of age on antinociceptive effects of elevated plus-maze exposure. *Brazilian J. Med. Biol. Res.*, 25, 827–829.

82. Graeff, F.G., Audi, E.A., Almeida, S.S. *et al.* (1990) Behavioral effects of 5-HT receptor ligands in the aversive brain stimulation, elevated plus-maze and learned helplessness tests. *Neurosci. Biobehav. Rev.*, 14, 501–506.

83. Green, S. (1991) Benzodiazepines, putative anxiolytics and animal models of anxiety. *Trends Pharmacol. Sci.*, 14, 101–104.

84. Green, S. and Hodges, H. (1991) Animal models of anxiety. In: *Behavioural Models in Psychopharmacology* (ed. P. Willner), Cambridge University Press, pp. 21–49.

85. Green, S. and Vale, A.L. (1992) Role of amygdaloid nuclei in the anxiolytic effects of benzodiazepines in rats. *Behav. Pharmacol.*, 3, 261–264.

86. Griebel, G., Moreau, J-L., Jenck, F. *et al.* (1993) Some critical determinants of the behaviour of rats in the elevated plus-maze. *Behav. Proc.*, 29, 37–48.

87. Guimaraes, F.S., Chiaretti, T.M., Graeff, F.G. and Zuardi, A.W. (1990) Antianxiety effect of cannabidol in the elevated plus-maze. *Psychopharmacology*, 100, 558–559.

88. Guimaraes, F.S., Carobrez, A.P., De Aguiar, J.C. and Graeff, F.G. (1991) Anxiolytic effect in the elevated plus-maze of the NMDA receptor antagonist AP7 microinjected into the dorsal periaqueductal grey. *Psychopharmacology*, 103, 91–94.

89. Haefely, W. (1990) The GABA$_A$–benzodiazepine receptor: biology and pharmacology. In: *Handbook of Anxiety Vol. 3: The Neurobiology of Anxiety* (eds G.D. Burrows, M. Roth and R. Noyes). Elsevier, Amsterdam, pp. 165–188.

90. Hale, R.L., Johnston, A.L. and Becker, H.C. (1990) Indomethacin does not antagonize the anxiolytic action of ethanol in the elevated plus-maze. *Psychopharmacology*, 101, 203–207.

91. Handley, S.L. (1991) Serotonin in animal models of anxiety: the importance of stimulus and response. In: *Serotonin, Sleep and Mental Disorder* (eds C. Idzikowski and P.J. Cowen). Wrightson Biomedical, Petersfield, pp. 89–115.

92. Handley, S.L. and McBlane, J.W. (1992) Opposite effects of fluoxetine in two animal models of anxiety. *Br. J. Pharmacol.*, 107, 446P.

93. Handley, S.L. and McBlane, J.W. (1993) 5HT drugs in animal models of anxiety. *Psychopharmacology*, 112, 13–20.

94. Handley, S.L. and Mithani, S. (1984) Effects of alpha-adrenoceptor agonists and antagonists in a maze-exploration model of 'fear'-motivated behaviour. *Naunyn-*

Schmiedeberg's Arch. Pharmacol., **327**, 1–5.
95. Harro, J. (1993) Measurement of exploratory behavior in rodents. In: *Methods in Neurosciences* (ed. P.M. Conn). Academic Press, New York, pp. 359–377.
96. Harro, J. and Vasar, E. (1991a) Evidence that CCK$_B$ receptors mediate the regulation of exploratory behaviour in the rat. *Eur. J. Pharmacol.*, **193**, 379–381.
97. Harro, J. and Vasar, E. (1991b) Cholecystokinin-induced anxiety: how is it reflected in studies on exploratory behaviour? *Neurosci. Biobehav. Rev.*, **15**, 473–477.
98. Harro, J., Pold, M. and Vasar, E. (1990) Anxiogenic-like action of caerulein, a CCK-8 receptor agonist, in the mouse: influence of acute and subchronic diazepam treatment. *Naunyn-Schmeidebergs Arch. Pharmacol.*, **341**, 62–67.
99. Harro, J., Vasar, E. and Bradwejn, J. (1993) Cholecystokinin in animal and human research on anxiety and panic. *Trends Pharmacol. Sci.*, **14**, 244–249.
100. Heilig, M., Soderpalm, B., Engel, J.A. and Widerlow, E. (1989) Centrally administered neuropeptide Y (NPY) produces anxiolytic-like effects in animal anxiety models. *Psychopharmacology*, **98**, 524–529.
101. Heinrichs, S.C., Pich, E.M., Miczek, K.A. *et al.* (1992) Corticotropin-releasing factor antagonist reduces emotionality in socially defeated rats via direct neurotropic action. *Brain Res.*, **581**, 190–197.
102. Hennessy, M.B. (1991) Sensitization of the plasma corticosterone response to novel environments. *Physiol. Behav.*, **50**, 1175–1179.
103. Hilakivi, L.A., Lister, R.G., Durcan, M.J. *et al.* (1989a) Behavioral, hormonal and neurochemical characteristics of aggressive α-mice. *Brain Res.*, **502**, 158–166.
104. Hilakivi, L.A., Ota, M. and Lister, R.G. (1989b) Effect of isolation on brain monoamines and the behavior of mice in tests of exploration, locomotion, anxiety and behavioral 'despair'. *Pharmacol. Biochem. Behav.*, **33**, 371–374.
105. Hilakivi-Clarke, L.A. and Lister, R.G. (1992) Are there preexisting behavioral characteristics that predict the dominant status of male NIH Swiss mice (*Mus musculus*)? *J. Comp. Psychol.*, **106**, 184–189.
106. Hitchcott, P.K., Zharkovsky, A. and File, S.E. (1992) Concurrent treatment with verapamil prevents diazepam withdrawal-induced anxiety, in the absence of altered calcium flux in cortical synaptosomes. *Neuropharmacology*, **31**, 55–60.
107. Hoyer, D. (1992) Agonists and antagonists at 5-HT receptor subtypes. In: *Serotonin, CNS Receptors and Brain Function* (eds P.B. Bradley, S.L. Handley, S.J. Cooper *et al.*). Pergamon, Oxford, pp. 29–47.
108. Hughes, J., Boden, P., Costall, B. *et al.* (1990) Development of a class of selective cholecystokinin type B receptor antagonists having potent anxiolytic activity. *Proc. Natl Acad. Sci. USA*, **87**, 6728–6733.
109. Ishihara, S., Hiramatsu, M., Kameyama, T. and Nabeshima, T. (1993) Development of tolerance to anxiolytic effects of chlordiazepoxide in elevated plus-maze and decrease of GABAA receptors. *J. Neural. Transm. (Gen. Sect.)*, **91**, 27–37.
110. Janowska, E., Pucilowski, O. and Kostowski, W. (1991) Chronic oral treatment with diltiazem or verapamil decreases isolation-induced activity impairment in elevated plus-maze. *Behav. Brain Res.*, **43**, 155–158.
111. Johnston, A.L. and File, S.E. (1988a) Effects of ligands for specific 5-HT receptor sub-types in two animal tests of anxiety. In: *Buspirone: A New Introduction to the Treatment of Anxiety* (ed. M. Lader). Royal Society, London, pp. 31–41.
112. Johnston, A.L. and File, S.E. (1988b) Profiles of the antipanic compounds, triazolobenzodiazepines and phenelzine, in two animal tests of anxiety. *Psychiatr. Res.*, **25**, 81–90.

113. Johnston, A.L. and File, S.E. (1989a) Sodium phenobarbitone reverses the anxiogenic effects of compounds acting at three different central sites. *Neuropharmacology*, **28**, 83–88.

114. Johnston, A.L. and File, S.E. (1989b) Yohimbine's anxiogenic action: evidence for noradrenergic and dopaminergic sites. *Pharmacol. Biochem. Behav.*, **32**, 151–156.

115. Johnston, A.L. and File, S.E. (1991) Sex differences in animal tests of anxiety. *Physiol. Behav.*, **49**, 245–250.

116. Johnston, A.L., Koening-Berard, E., Cooper, T.A. and File, S.E. (1988) Comparison of the effects of clonidine, rimelidine and guanfacine in the holeboard and elevated plus-maze. *Drug Dev. Res.*, **15**, 405–414.

117. Jones, B.J., Costall, B., Domeney, A.M. *et al.* (1988) The potential anxiolytic activity of GR 38032F, a 5-HT₃ receptor antagonist. *Br. J. Pharmacol.*, **93**, 985–993.

118. Kaiser, F.C., Palmer, G.C., Wallace, A.V. *et al.* (1992) Antianxiety properties of the angiotensin II antagonist, DUP 753, in the rat using the elevated plus-maze. *NeuroReport*, **3**, 922–924.

119. Kauppila, T., Tanila, H., Carlson, S. and Taira, T. (1991) Effects of atipamezole, a novel α_2-adrenoceptor antagonist, in open-field, plus-maze, two compartment exploratory, and forced swimming tests in the rat. *Eur. J. Pharmacol.*, **205**, 177–182.

120. Kellogg, C.K., Primus, R.J. and Bitran, D. (1991) Sexually-dimorphic influence of prenatal exposure to diazepam on behavioral responses to environmental challenge and on gamma-aminobutyric acid (GABA)-stimulated chloride uptake in the brain. *J. Pharmacol. Exp. Ther.*, **256**, 259–265.

121. Klint, T. (1991) Effects of 8-OH-DPAT and buspirone in a passive avoidance test and in the elevated plus-maze test in rats. *Behav. Pharmacol.*, **2**, 481–489.

122. Kostowski, W., Plaznik, A. and Stefanski, R. (1989) Intra-hippocampal buspirone in animal models of anxiety. *Eur. J. Pharmacol.*, **168**, 393–396.

123. Kostowski, W., Dyr, W., Krzascik, P. *et al.* (1992) 5-Hydroxytryptamine₁ₐ receptor agonists in animal models of depression and anxiety. *Pharmacol. Toxicol.*, **71**, 24–30.

124. Lal, H., Prather, P.L. and Rezazadeh, S.M. (1991) Anxiogenic behavior in rats during acute and protracted ethanol withdrawal: reversal by buspirone. *Alcohol*, **8**, 467–471.

125. Lal, H., Prather, P.L. and Rezazadeh, S.M. (1993) Potential role of 5HT₁C and/or 5HT₂ receptors in the mianserin-induced prevention of anxiogenic behaviors occurring during ethanol withdrawal. *Alcoholism: Clin. Exp. Res.*, **17**, 411–417.

126. Lamberty, Y. and Gower, A.J. (1990) Age-related changes in spontaneous behavior and learning in NMRI mice from maturity to middle age. *Physiol. Behav.*, **47**, 1137–1144.

127. Lamberty, Y., Gower, A.J., Gobert, J. *et al.* (1992) Behavioural, biochemical and histological effects of AF64A following injection into the third ventricle of the mouse. *Behav. Brain Res.*, **51**, 165–177.

128. Lee, C. and Rodgers, R.J. (1990) Antinociceptive effects of elevated plus-maze exposure: influence of opiate receptor manipulations. *Psychopharmacology*, **102**, 507–513.

129. Lee, C. and Rodgers, R.J. (1991a) Effects of buspirone on antinociceptive and behavioural responses to the elevated plus-maze in mice. *Behav. Pharmacol.*, **2**, 491–496.

130. Lee, C. and Rodgers, R.J. (1991b) Effects of benzodiazepine receptor antagonist, flumazenil, on murine antinociceptive and behavioural responses to the elevated

plus-maze. *Neuropharmacology*, **30**, 1263–1267.
131. Lister, R.G. (1987) The use of a plus-maze to measure anxiety in the mouse. *Psychopharmacology*, **92**, 180–185.
132. Lister, R.G. (1988) Interactions of three benzodiazepine receptor inverse agonists with ethanol in a plus-maze test of anxiety. *Pharmacol. Biochem. Behav.*, **30**, 701–706.
133. Lister, R.G. (1990) Ethologically-based animal models of anxiety disorders. *Pharmacol. Ther.*, **46**, 321–340.
134. Llorens, J., Tusell, J.P., Sunol, C. and Rodriguez-Farre, E. (1990) On the effects of lindane on the plus-maze model of anxiety. *Neurotoxicol. Teratol.*, **12**, 643–647.
135. Luscombe, G.P., Mazurkiewicz, S.E. and Heal, D.J. (1992) The 5-HT$_{1A}$ ligand BP 554 mimics the anxiolytic activity of buspirone, gepirone and ipsapirone in the elevated plus-maze in rats. *Br. J. Pharmacol.*, **108**, 130P.
136. Mangiafico, V., Cassetti, G. and Ferrari, F. (1989) Effect of putative anxiolytics and anxiogenics on a modified X-maze apparatus. *Pharmacol. Res.*, **21**, 469–470.
137. Miyamoto, M., Kiyota, Y., Nishiyama, M. and Nagaoka, A. (1992) Senescence-accelerated mouse (SAM): age-related reduced anxiety-like behavior in the SAM-P/8 strain. *Physiol. Behav.*, **51**, 979–985.
138. Montgomery, K.C. (1955) The relation between fear induced by novelty stimulation and exploratory behaviour. *J. Comp. Physiol. Psychol.*, **48**, 254–260.
139. Morato, S. and Castrechini, P. (1989) Effects of floor surface and environmental illumination on exploratory activity in the elevated plus-maze. *Brazilian J. Med. Biol. Res.*, **22**, 707–710.
140. Moreau, J.-L., Griebel, G., Jenck, F. *et al.* (1992) Behavioral profile of the 5-HT$_{1A}$ receptor antagonist (S)-UH-301 in rodents and monkeys. *Brain Res. Bull.*, **29**, 901–904.
141. Moser, P.C. (1989) An evaluation of the elevated plus-maze test using the novel anxiolytic buspirone. *Psychopharmacology*, **99**, 48–53.
142. Moser, P.C., Tricklebank, M.D., Middlemiss, D.N. *et al.* (1990) Characterization of MDL 73005EF as a 5-HT$_{1A}$ selective ligand and its effects in animal models of anxiety: comparison with buspirone, 8-OH-DPAT and diazepam. *Br. J. Pharmacol.*, **99**, 343–349.
143. Motta, V. and Brandao, M.L. (1993) Aversive and antiaversive effects of morphine in the dorsal periaqueductal gray of rats submitted to the elevated plus-maze. *Pharmacol. Biochem. Behav.*, **44**, 119–125.
144. Motta, V., Maisonette, S., Morato, S. *et al.* (1992) Effects of blockade of 5-HT$_2$ receptors and activation of 5-HT$_{1A}$ receptors on the exploratory activity of rats in the elevated plus-maze. *Psychopharmacology*, **107**, 135–139.
145. Neiminen, S.A., Sirkka, U., Lecklin, A., Heikkinen, O. and Ylitalo, P. (1991) Assessment of acute behavioral toxicity of low doses of disopropylfluorophosphate (DFP) in rats. *Methods Find. Exp. Clin. Pharmacol.*, **13**, 617–623.
146. Nieminen, S.A., Sirvio, J., Teittinen, K. *et al.* (1992) Amygdala kindling increased fear-response, but did not impair spatial memory in rats. *Physiol. Behav.*, **51**, 845–849.
147. Njung'e, K., Critchley, M.A.E. and Handley, S.L. (1993) Effects of β-adrenoceptor ligands in the elevated X-maze 'anxiety' model and antagonism of the 'anxiogenic' response to 8-OH-DPAT. *J. Psychopharmacol.*, **7**, 173–180.
148. Nutt, D.J. (1991) Anxiety and its therapy: today and tommorrow. In: *New Concepts in Anxiety* (eds M. Briley and S.E. File). Macmillan, London, pp. 1–12.
149. Onaivi, E.S., Brock, J.W. and Prasad, C. (1992) Dietary protein levels alter rat behavior. *Nutrition Res.*, **12**, 1025–1039.
150. Pare, W.P. (1992) The performance of WKY rats on three tests of emotional

behavior. *Physiol. Behav.*, 51, 1051–1056.
151. Pellow, S. and File, S.E. (1986) Anxiolytic and anxiogenic drug effects on exploratory activity in an elevated plus-maze: a novel test of anxiety in the rat. *Pharmacol. Biochem. Behav.*, 24, 525–529.
152. Pellow, S., Chopin, P., File, S.E. and Briley, M. (1985) Validation of open: closed arm entries in an elevated plus-maze as a measure of anxiety in the rat. *J. Neurosci. Methods*, 14, 149–167.
153. Pellow, S., Johnston, A.L. and File, S.E. (1987) Selective agonists and antagonists for 5-hydroxytryptamine receptor subtypes, and interactions with yohimbine and FG 7142 using the elevated plus-maze test in the rat. *J. Pharm. Pharmacol.*, 39, 917–928.
154. Pesold, C. and Treit, D. (1992) Excitotoxic lesions of the septum produce anxiolytic effects in the elevated plus-maze and shock-probe burying tests. *Physiol. Behav.*, 52, 37–47.
155. Pesold, C. and Treit, D. (1994). The septum and amygdala differentially mediate the anxiolytic effects of benzodiazepines *Brain Res.*, 638, 295–301.
156. Piper, D., Upton, N., Thomas, D. and Nicholass, J. (1988) The effects of 5-HT$_3$ receptor antagonists BRL 43694 and GR 38032F in animal behavioural models of anxiety. *Br. J. Pharmacol.*, 94, 314P.
157. Prather, P.L., Rezazadeh, S.M., Lane, J.D. *et al.* (1993) Conflicting evidence regarding the efficacy of ondansetron in benzodiazepine withdrawal. *J. Pharmacol. Exp. Ther.*, 264, 622–630.
158. Quock, R.M. and Nguyen, E. (1992) Possible involvement of nitric oxide in chlordiazepoxide-induced anxiolysis in mice. *Life Sci.*, 51, PL 255–260.
159. Rago, L., Kiivet, R.-A., Harro, J. and Pold, M. (1988) Behavioral differences in an elevated plus-maze: correlation between anxiety and decreased number of GABA and benzodiazepine receptors in mouse cerebral cortex. *Naunyn-Schmeidebergs Arch. Pharmacol.*, 337, 675–678.
160. Rago, L., Kiivet, R.-A., Adojaan, A. *et al.* (1990) Stress-protective effects of β-phenyl(GABA): involvement of central and peripheral type benzodiazepine binding sites. *Pharmacol. Toxicol.*, 66, 41–44.
161. Rago, L., MacDonald, E., Saano, V. and Airaksinen, M.M. (1991) The effect of medetomidine on GABA and benzodiazepine receptors *in vivo*: lack of anxiolytic but some evidence of possible stress-protective activity. *Pharmacol. Toxicol.*, 69, 81–86.
162. Rago, L., Saano, V., Auvinen, T. *et al.* (1992) The effect of chronic treatment with peripheral benzodiazepine receptor ligands on behavior and GABA$_A$/benzodiazepine receptors in rat. *Naunyn-Schmeidebergs Arch. Pharmacol.*, 346, 432–436.
163. Rassnick, S., Heinrichs, S.C., Britton, K.T. and Koob, G.F. (1993) Microinjection of a corticotropin-releasing factor antagonist into the central nucleus of the amygdala reverses anxiogenic-like effects of ethanol withdrawal. *Brain Res.*, 605, 25–32.
164. Rataud, J., Darche, F., Piot, O. *et al.* (1991) 'Anxiolytic' effect of CCK-antagonists on plus-maze behavior in mice. *Brain Res.*, 548, 315–317.
165. Ravard, S. and Dourish, C.T. (1990) Cholecystokinin and anxiety. *Trends Pharmacol. Sci.*, 11, 271–273.
166. Rodgers, R.J. (1991) A step in the right direction. *J. Psychopharmacol.*, 5, 316–319.
167. Rodgers, R.J. and Cole, J.C. (1993a) Anxiety enhancement in the murine elevated plus maze by immediate prior exposure to social stressors. *Physiol. Behav.*, 53, 383–388.
168. Rodgers, R.J. and Cole, J.C. (1993b) Influence of social isolation, gender, strain

and prior novelty on plus-maze behaviour in mice. *Physiol. Behav.*, **54**, 729–736.

169. Rodgers, R.J. and Shepherd, J.K. (1993) Influence of prior maze experience on behaviour and response to diazepam in the elevated plus-maze and light/dark tests of anxiety in mice. *Psychopharmacology*, **113**, 237–242.

170. Rodgers, R.J., Cole, J.C., Cobain, M.R. *et al.* (1992a) Anxiogenic-like effects of fluprazine and eltoprazine in the mouse elevated plus-maze: profile comparisons with 8-OH-DPAT, CGS 12066B, TFMPP and mCPP. *Behav. Pharmacol.*, **3**, 621–634.

171. Rodgers, R.J., Lee, C. and Shepherd, J.K. (1992b) Effects of diazepam on behavioural and antinociceptive responses to the elevated plus-maze in male mice depend upon treatment regimen and prior maze experience. *Psychopharmacology*, **106**, 102–110.

172. Rodgers, R.J., Cole, J.C. and Tredwell, J. (1993) Ethological analysis fails to reveal anxiolytic effects of 5-HT$_3$ receptor antagonists, ondansetron and WAY 100,289, in the murine plus-maze. *Br. J. Pharmacol.*, **110**, 12P.

173. Rogerio, R. and Takahashi, R.N. (1992) Anxiogenic action of acute but not repeated cocaine administration in handling-habituated mice in the plus-maze test. *Brazilian J. Med. Biol. Res.*, **25**, 713–716.

174. Russo, A.S., Guimaraes, F.S., De Aguiar, J.C. and Graeff, F.G. (1993) Role of benzodiazepine receptors located in the dorsal periaqueductal grey of rats in anxiety. *Psychopharmacology*, **110**, 198–202.

175. Salonen, M., Onaivi, E.S. and Maze, M. (1992) Dexmedetomidine synergism with midazolam in the elevated plus-maze test in rats. *Psychopharmacology*, **108**, 229–234.

176. Sayin, U., Purali, N., Ozkan, T. *et al.* (1992) Vigabatrin has an anxiolytic effect in the elevated plus-maze test of anxiety. *Pharmacol. Biochem. Behav.*, **43**, 529–535.

177. Schmitt, M.L., Graeff, F.G. and Carobrez, A.P. (1990) Anxiolytic effect of kynurenic acid microinjected into the dorsal periaqueductal gray matter of rats placed in the elevated plus-maze test. *Brazilian J. Med. Biol. Res.*, **23**, 677–679.

178. Shepherd, J.K. (1992) Preliminary evaluation of an elevated 'zero-maze' as a model of anxiety in laboratory rats. *J. Psychopharmacol.*, Abstract Book 1992, A56.

179. Shepherd, J.K., Grewal, S.S., Fletcher, A. *et al.* (1993) Pharmacological evaluation of the elevated 'zero-maze' as a model of anxiety in rats. *Br. J. Pharmacol.*, **110**, 13P.

180. Singh, L., Field, M.J., Hughes, J. *et al.* (1991a) The behavioural properties of CI-988, a selective cholecystokinin$_B$ receptor antagonist. *Br. J. Pharmacol.*, **104**, 239–245.

181. Singh, L., Lewis, A.S., Field, M.J. *et al.* (1991b) Evidence for an involvement of the brain cholecystokinin B receptor in anxiety. *Proc. Natl Acad. Sci. USA*, **88**, 1130–1133.

182. Soderpalm, B. (1989) The SHR exhibits less 'anxiety' but increased sensitivity to the anticonflict effect of clonidine compared to normotensive rats. *Pharmacol. Toxicol.*, **65**, 381–386.

183. Soderpalm, B. and Engel, J.A. (1989) Alpha$_2$-adrenoceptor antagonists potentiate the anticonflict and the rotarod impairing effects of benzodiazepines. *J. Neural. Transm.*, **76**, 191–204.

184. Soderpalm, B., Hjorth, S. and Engel, J.A. (1989) Effects of 5-HT$_{1A}$ receptor agonists and L-5-HTP in Montgomery's conflict test. *Pharmacol. Biochem. Behav.*, **32**, 259–265.

185. Stanford, S.C., Baldwin, H.A. and File, S.E. (1989) Effects of a single or

repeated administration of the benzodiazepine inverse agonist FG 7142 on behaviour and cortical adrenoceptor binding in the rat. *Psychopharmacology*, **98**, 417–424.

186. Steenbergen, H.L., Heinsbroek, R.P.W., van Hest, A. and van de Poll, N.E. (1990) Sex-dependent effects of inescapable shock administration on shuttlebox-escape performance and elevated plus-maze behavior. *Physiol. Behav.*, **48**, 571–576.

187. Steenbergen, H.L., Farabollini, F., Heinsbroek, R.P.W. and van de Poll, N.E. (1991) Sex-dependent effects of aversive stimulation on holeboard and elevated plus-maze behavior. *Behav. Brain Res.*, **43**, 159–165.

188. Stephens, D.N., Meldrum, B.S., Weidmann, R. *et al.*, (1986) Does the excitatory amino acid receptor antagonist 2-APH exhibit anxiolytic activity? *Psychopharmacology*, **90**, 166–169.

189. Stewart, R.B., Gatto, G.J., Lumeng, L. *et al.* (1993) Comparison or alcohol-preferring (P) and nonpreferring (NP) rats on tests of anxiety and for the anxiolytic effects of ethanol. *Alcohol*, **10**, 1–10.

190. Takahashi, R.N. and Rogerio, R. (1991) Nifedipine interacts with cocaine in the elevated plus-maze in rats. *Res. Commun. Subst. Abuse*, **12**, 19–25.

191. Taukulis, H.K. and Goggin, C.E. (1990) Diazepam–stress interactions in the rat: effects on autoanalgesia and a plus-maze model of anxiety. *Behav. Neural. Biol.*, **53**, 205–216.

192. Taukulis, H.K. and McKay, R.W. (1992) Postdrug retention of diazepam's effects on habituation to a novel environment in an animal model of anxiety. *Psychobiology*, **20**, 286–293.

193. Tomkins, D.M., Costall, B. and Naylor, R.J. (1990) Action of ritanserin and DOI on the elevated plus-maze. *Psychopharmacology*, **101** (Suppl.), 219P.

194. Traber, J. and Glaser, T. (1987) 5-HT$_{1A}$ receptor-related anxiolytics. *Trends Pharmacol. Sci.*, **8**, 432–437.

195. Treit, D. (1985) Animal models for the study of anti-anxiety agents: a review. *Neurosci. Biobehav. Rev.*, **9**, 203–222.

196. Treit, D. (1991) Anxiolytic effects of benzodiazepines, and 5-HT$_{1A}$ agonists: animal models. In: *5-HT$_{1A}$ Agonists, 5-HT$_3$ Antagonists and Benzodiazepines: Their Comparative Behavioural Pharmacology* (eds R.J. Rodgers and S.J. Cooper). Wiley, Chichester, pp. 107–131.

197. Treit, D. and Pesold, C. (1990) Septal lesions inhibit fear reactions in two animal models of anxiolytic drug action. *Physiol. Behav.*, **47**, 365–370.

198. Treit, D., Menard, J. and Royan, C. (1993a) Anxiogenic stimuli in the elevated plus-maze. *Pharmacol. Biochem. Behav.*, **44**, 463–469.

199. Treit, D., Pesold, C. and Rotzinger S. (1993b) Dissociating the anti-fear effects of septal and amygdala lesions using two pharmacologically validated models of rat anxiety. *Behav. Neurosci.*, **107**, 770–785.

200. Treit, D., Robinson, A., Rotzinger, S. and Pesold, C. (1993c) Anxiolytic effects of serotonergic interventions in the shock-probe burying test and the elevated plus-maze test. *Brain Res.*, **544**, 23–34.

201. Trullas, R. and Skolnick, P. (1993) Differences in fear motivated behaviors among inbred mouse strains. *Psychopharmacology*, **111**, 323–331.

202. Vasar, E., Harro, J., Lang, A. *et al.* (1993) Anti-exploratory effect of *N*-methyl-D-aspartate in elevated plus-maze: involvement of NMDA and CCK receptors. *Eur. Neuropsychopharmacol.*, **3**, 63–73.

203. Wada, T. and Fukuda, N. (1991) Effects of DN-2327, a new anxiolytic, diazepam and buspirone on exploratory activity of the rat in an elevated plus-maze. *Psychopharmacology*, **104**, 444–450.

204. Wahlestedt, C., Pich, E.M., Koob, G.F. *et al.* (1993) Modulation of anxiety and neuropeptide Y-Y1 receptors by antisense oligodeoxynucleotides. *Science*, **259**, 528–531.
205. Yang, X.-M., Gorman, A.L., Dunn, A.J. and Goeders, N.E. (1992) Anxiogenic effects of acute and chronic cocaine administration: neurochemical and behavioral studies. *Pharmacol. Biochem. Behav.*, **41**, 643–650.
206. Zangrossi, H. and File, S.E. (1992a) Behavioral consequences in animal tests of anxiety and exploration of exposure to cat odor. *Brain Res. Bull.*, **29**, 381–388.
207. Zangrossi, H. and File, S.E. (1992b) Chlordiazepoxide reduces the generalised anxiety, but not the direct responses, of rats exposed to cat odor. *Pharmacol. Biochem. Behav.*, **43**, 1195–1200.
208. Zangrossi, H., Leite, J.R. and Graeff, F.G. (1992) Anxiolytic effect of carbamazepine in the elevated plus-maze: possible role of adenosine. *Psychopharmacology*, **106**, 85–89.

ABBREVIATIONS

AOAA   aminoxyacetic acid

DMCM   methyl 6,7-dimethoxy-4-ethyl-β-carboline-3-carboxylate

5,7-DHT   5,7-dihydroxytryptamine

DOI   1-(2,5-dimethoxy-4-iodophenyl)-2-aminopropane

L-5-HTP   L-5-hydroxytryptophan

mCPB   1-(3-chlorophenyl)-biguanide

mCPP   1-(3-chlorophenyl)piperazine

5-MeODMT 5-methoxy-dimethyltryptamine

TFMPP N-(3-trifluomethylphenyl)piperazine

THIP   4,5,6,7-tetrahydroisoxazolo[5,4-c]pyridin-3-ol

PCPA   parachlorophenylalanine

3 Anxiolytic Drugs: Does Ethopharmacological Analysis Indicate Commonalities in their Mode of Action?

M.G. CUTLER

Department of Biological Sciences, Glasgow Caledonian University, UK

INTRODUCTION

The unambiguous description and classification of the naturally occurring social behaviour of several rodent species by Grant and Mackintosh (1963) in Birmingham has been used by several subsequent workers in ethology and ethopharmacology (Dixon *et al.*, 1990; Brain *et al.*, 1989). Early studies had demonstrated that behavioural activities are distributed in time in the form of clusters of associated acts and postures (Mackintosh *et al.*, 1977). These clusters of behavioural elements, or categories of behaviour, are thought to have causal factors in common and provide the basic structure of behaviour. Four major categories which have been identified include non-social behaviour, social and sexual investigation, aggression and flight. It has repeatedly been shown that the recording of drug-induced changes to the categories and elements of the naturally occurring behaviour of rodents provides a highly sensitive and quantitative evaluation of psychopharmacological actions (Cutler *et al.*, 1975; Dixon *et al.*, 1990). Accordingly, these ethopharmacological methods have been employed in the present series of studies to examine the behavioural actions of conventional and novel anxiolytic compounds.

The tests for detecting anxiolytic efficacy of novel compounds in animal models were for many years based on the properties of benzodiazepine agonists which release behaviour from the suppression produced by punishment. As new classes of anxiolytic agents, acting at different receptors and receptor subtypes, were introduced and subjected to preclinical screening, it became apparent that previous concepts on the mode of action of anxiolytic agents may have been unduly simplistic. The traditional tests for detecting anxiolytic efficacy were found frequently to be inappropriate for the novel compounds (Gardner, 1988; Sanger *et al.*, 1991). They yielded conflicting results in tests such as responsiveness of the animals to such aversive stimuli as electric

Ethology and Psychopharmacology. Edited by S.J. Cooper and C.A. Hendrie
© 1994 John Wiley & Sons Ltd

shocks, aggression from conspecifics or the fear-inducing effects of unfamiliar and brightly lit environments (Lader, 1989; Lal and Emmett-Ogglesby, 1983). Middleton (1991) is one of those who, after considering the recent evidence, has suggested that there is a need to revise basic approaches to further our understanding of anxiety and of the mode of action of anxiolytic agents. Use of ethopharmacological methods in testing a wide range of anxiolytic agents should illuminate the changes in behavioural responsiveness induced by anxiolytic agents within each pharmacological 'class', and show whether there are effects on social behaviour which are common to the substances examined.

For example, effective anxiolytic agents may influence the characteristics of an animal's social interaction, not only by releasing suppressed behaviour but also by altering the intensity of the stress-orientated responses of flight, aggression and ambivalent behaviour. Anxiolytic compounds may also increase the occurrence of behavioural activities which had not previously been considered to be aversive.

The studies reported in this chapter provide some preliminary data. Behavioural effects of acute and subchronic administration of anxiolytic agents representative of five different pharmacological classes have been observed in mice. Chlordiazepoxide has been employed as a representative benzodiazepine agonist. Buspirone, known to be as effective clinically as the benzodiazepines in controlling anxiety (Goa and Ward, 1986), has been employed as an agent whose main effect is at the 5-HT_{1A} receptor site. A long-acting 5-HT_3 receptor antagonist (BRL 46470A; SmithKline Beecham) has also been tested, since compounds of this class show anxiolytic potential at extremely small dose levels in certain animal models and appear also to be effective clinically (Jones et al., 1988; Lecrubier et al., 1990; Upton and Blackburn, 1991). The other compounds tested were dl-propranolol, a β-adrenoceptor antagonist, found to be effective in the treatment of generalized anxiety disorder and in the treatment of acute stress reactions and performance anxiety (Meibach et al., 1987), and ritanserin, a $5\text{-HT}_2/5\text{-HT}_{2C}$ receptor antagonist, which is effective clinically in the treatment of several syndromes related to anxiety and depressive illness (Bersani et al., 1991; Ceulemans et al., 1985), although it fails to show positive effects in several of the traditional animal models for detecting anxiolytic potential (Gardner, 1985, 1988). I shall now describe the methods that have been employed in these behavioural assessments.

METHODS

Buspirone hydrochloride, chlordiazepoxide hydrochloride and dl-propranolol were obtained from Sigma, ritanserin was purchased from Research Biochemicals Ltd and the 5-HT_3 receptor antagonist, BRL 46470A, was a gift from SmithKline Beecham, Harlow. All drugs were tested in adult male CD1 mice. These had been previously pair-housed for a period of 10–14 days. All mice received an ad libitum supply of pelleted stock cubes (RM3 expanded diet,

SDS, Wetham, Essex) and drinking fluid. Ambient temperature was maintained at $21 \pm 2\,°C$, and animals were kept under a 24 h cycle of reversed lighting (lights on from 18.00 to 06.00 h).

Effects of each of the compounds on behaviour were examined in both acute and subchronic experiments. In the acute studies, each compound was given by a single intraperitoneal (i.p.) injection at two to three dose levels, and effects on behaviour of the mice during social encounters were examined for a 5 min period, commencing at 30 min after injection. The dose levels employed are summarized in Table 1, these being within the ranges reported to be behaviourally effective. All drugs had been dissolved in physiological saline, with ritanserin, which was less soluble than the other compounds, having been sonicated prior to injections. All control mice received i.p. injections of physiological saline, at a similar volume.

In the subchronic studies, each compound was administered in the drinking fluid at a single 'effective' dose level for a 12–15-day period before behavioural testing. Mice of the control group received tap water to drink. Fluid intake of the mice was monitored throughout the experiments, and Table 2 summarizes the concentrations of each compound in drinking fluid together with the mean daily intake in milligrams per kilogram.

Table 1 Compounds tested and their dose levels: acute studies

Compounds and abbreviated names used	Dose levels (mg/kg)		
	LD (smallest dose level tested)	MD (middle dose level tested)	HD (greatest dose level tested)
Chlordiazepoxide (CDP)	1	4	8
Buspirone (BUS)	1	5	10
BRL 46470A (BRL)	0.0025	0.025	2.5
Propranolol (PROP)	1.5	6.0	–
Ritanserin (RIT)	0.1	0.3	0.6

Table 2 Compounds tested and their dose levels: subchronic studies

Compounds tested and abbreviated names used	Concentration in drinking fluid (mg/l)	Mean daily intake (mg/kg)
Chlordiazepoxide (CDP)	21.5	5
Buspirone (BUS)	12.8	3.4
BRL 46470A (BRL)	0.04	0.01
Propranolol (PROP)	12.4	1.9
Ritanserin (RIT)	1.6	0.3

Effects on behaviour were assessed in two test situations, when each mouse was resident in its home cage (33 × 15 × 13 cm) and encountering an unfamiliar untreated male partner for a 5 min period and when each mouse had been placed in an unfamiliar neutral cage (60 × 25 × 25 cm; light intensity 38 cd/m²) and again encountering an unfamiliar partner male for a period of 5 min. The situation of testing in the neutral cage resembles that of the rat social interaction test described by File (1980).

Behaviour of each of the mice during the social encounters was recorded by videotape, and the acts and postures shown by each animal were recorded as a spoken commentary by tape recorder using the ethogram of behavioural elements listed by Gao and Cutler (1992). These are derived from the ethological profile described by Mackintosh *et al.* (1977), with elements of behaviour being grouped within each of the major behavioural categories of non-social activity, immobility, social investigation and sexual behaviour, aggression and flight. Data from the spoken commentaries were transcribed onto a floppy disc for analysis by computer of the frequency and duration of each behavioural category and element.

Data were recorded as the means for each group, and the significance of the differences between mean values from the treated and control groups was estimated by the non-parametric Mann–Whitney U test and the Kruskal–Wallis one-way analysis of variance (ANOVA), as in previous ethopharmacological studies (Cutler and Dixon, 1988; Cutler and Piper, 1990).

RESULTS AND DISCUSSION

Acute studies

Each of the tested anxiolytic compounds significantly increased social investigation of an introduced partner mouse placed within the home cage (Figure 1). Chlordiazepoxide (CDP) enhanced social investigation most markedly at the smallest dose tested, 1 mg/kg. This was associated with the appearance of sedative effects from CDP at the greater dose levels of 4 and 8 mg/kg (drug-induced increase in the duration of immobility (s), mean ± s.e.m.; LD − 0.7 ± 1.6, MD 24.8 ± 17.1, HD 49.3 ± 20.5*; *$P < 0.05$). This type of sedative action did not occur in the mice treated with buspirone (BUS), BRL 46470A (BRL), propranolol (PROP) or ritanserin (RIT). Social investigation was most markedly increased at intermediate dose levels by BUS (5 mg/kg), BRL (0.025 mg/kg) and RIT (0.3 mg/kg), and by PROP at 6 mg/kg. The enhancement of social investigation by BRL at 0.025 mg/kg was accompanied by an increase of aggressive behaviour (increase in duration (s), mean ± s.e.m., 19.8 ± 6.3; $P < 0.05$). The observed increase of social and sometimes of aggressive behaviour in the home cage may well arise from an increase of territorial dominance induced by the anxiolytic compounds, and further studies examining effects on behaviour of the mice in territories are needed to investigate this (Mackintosh, 1970).

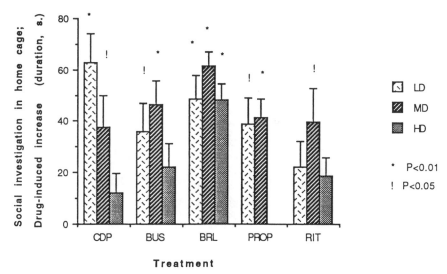

Figure 1 Increase of social investigation by mice in their home cage (duration, s; mean ± s.e.m.) after acute administration of each dose of the anxiolytic compounds tested (CDP = chlordiazepoxide; BUS = buspirone; BRL = BRL 46470A; PROP = propranolol, RIT = ritanserin).

The only other significant effect of the anxiolytic compounds on behaviour in the home cage was to reduce the amount of time spent by the mice in non-social activity. As shown in Figure 2, the duration of non-social activity was significantly decreased by CDP and by BRL at all dose levels tested, by BUS at 1 and 5 mg/kg, by PROP at 6 mg/kg and by RIT at 0.3 mg/kg. Such a decrease in non-social activity may arise from a significant change in behavioural motivation from non-social towards social activities, although the possibility of sedative actions cannot be ruled out until behavioural effects have been re-examined in non-social situations of testing.

Figure 3 shows that in the unfamiliar neutral cage each of the anxiolytic compounds again increased social investigation. The increase of social investigation by CDP was most marked at 1 and 4 mg/kg ($P < 0.01$), since CDP induced significant sedative effects at 8 mg/kg (increase in the duration of immobility (s), mean ± s.e.m.; LD − 0.7 ± 1.5, MD 27 ± 17, HD 49 ± 22*; *$P < 0.05$). The enhancement of social investigation by BRL and RIT was most pronounced at the intermediate dose levels, whereas BUS increased social investigation most markedly at the smallest dose tested, 1 mg/kg, and PROP increased social investigation at the greatest dose, 6 mg/kg.

The increase of social investigation by CDP was accompanied by a dose-related increase of aggressive behaviour (increase in duration (s), mean ± s.e.m.; LD 0, MD 7.6 ± 5.0, HD 16.7 ± 9.6), which was close to statistical significance. The 5-HT$_3$ receptor antagonist BRL, at the intermediate dose of 0.025 mg/kg also increased aggressive behaviour during the social encounters

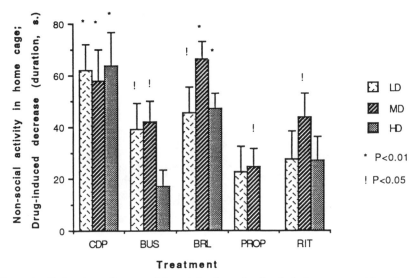

Figure 2 Reduction of non-social activity by mice in their home cage (duration, s; mean ± s.e.m.) after acute administration of each dose of the anxiolytic compounds tested (CDP = chlordiazepoxide; BUS = buspirone; BRL = BRL 46470A; PROP = propanolol; RIT = ritanserin).

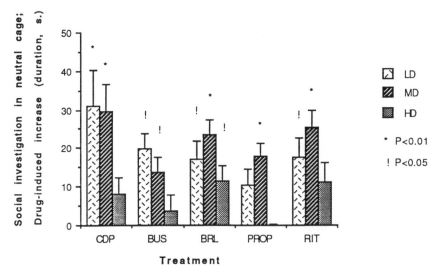

Figure 3 Increase of social investigation by mice in the neutral cage (duration, s; mean ± s.e.m.) after acute administration of each dose of the anxiolytic compounds tested (CDP = chlordiazepoxide; BUS = buspirone, BRL = BRL 46470A; PROP = propranolol; RIT = ritanserin).

in a neutral cage (increase in the duration of aggression (s), mean ± s.e.m.; LD 8.5 ± 5.0, MD 19.8 ± 5.2*, HD 11.5 ± 8.0; *$P < 0.05$), while RIT at the two higher dose levels increased the duration of aggression to a level which was close to statistical significance (increase in the duration of aggression (s), mean ± s.e.m.; LD 1.6 ± 7.8, MD 11.2 ± 5.0, HD 11.2 ± 5.2). On the other hand, there was no increase of aggression in the neutral cage among the mice treated with BUS or PROP, indicating that enhancement of aggression in this test situation is not an essential correlate of anxiolytic drug action.

Figure 4 shows that 'digging' of the unfamiliar sawdust in the neutral cage was significantly increased by three of the anxiolytic compounds tested (BRL and PROP at all dose levels, and BUS at 1 and 5 mg/kg). The dose-related effects associated with the enhancement of digging differed from those associated with the enhancement of social investigation by these compounds, indicating that the stimulus for digging operates via a different mechanism. The smallest dose levels of BUS and PROP tested (1 and 1.5 mg/kg respectively) elicited the greatest amount of digging, whereas in mice treated with BRL the duration of digging increased progressively with increase of dose.

It is possible that novel sawdust may be mildly stressful to mice; D'Amato and Cabib (1987) have demonstrated that the unfamiliar odour of clean bedding enhances stress-mediated ultrasonic calling in mouse pups when subjected to short periods of maternal separation. Thus, further studies are needed to assess the possibility that odours in unfamiliar sawdust are aversive

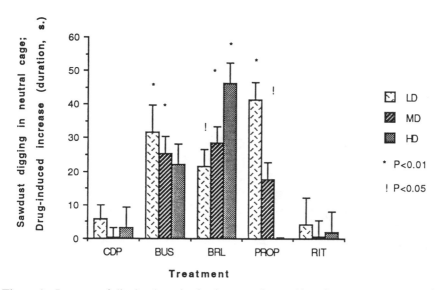

Figure 4 Increase of digging by mice in the neutral cage (duration, s; mean ± s.e.m.) after acute administration of each dose of the anxiolytic compounds tested (CDP = chlordiazepoxide; BUS = buspirone; BRL = BRL 46470A; PROP = propranolol; RIT = ritanserin).

to mice, and whether this may underlie the increased digging of unfamiliar sawdust by mice treated with anxiolytic agents.

Figure 5 shows that mice of all the drug-treated groups spent significantly less time in other non-social activity than their control counterparts. This effect was most probably due to the increased time spent by the drug-treated mice in social investigation, digging and sometimes in aggressive behaviour. A detectable sedative effect was seen only in the mice given CDP at the higher dose levels.

In conclusion, it can be seen that after acute administration, each of the anxiolytic compounds significantly increased social investigation in both the home cage and the unfamiliar neutral cage. In the neutral cage, other effects of the anxiolytic compounds became evident. BUS, BRL and PROP increased digging of the sawdust in the neutral cage, while CDP, BRL and RIT induced some increase of aggressive behaviour. Sedative effects occurred only in mice treated with the higher dose levels of CDP.

Subchronic studies

Figure 6 shows that in these subchronic experiments each of the anxiolytic compounds increased social investigation of an unfamiliar mouse introduced into the home cage. At the dose levels employed, the enhancement of social investigation by PROP and BRL was significant at 99% confidence limits,

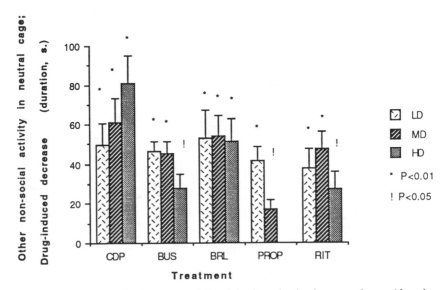

Figure 5 Reduction of other non-social activity by mice in the neutral cage (duration, s; mean ± s.e.m.) after acute administration of each dose of the anxiolytic compounds tested (CDP = chlordiazepoxide; BUS = buspirone, BRL = BRL 46470A; PROP = propranolol; RIT = ritanserin).

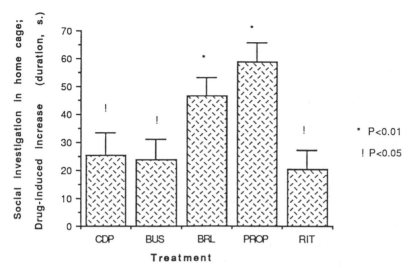

Figure 6 Increase of social investigation by mice in their home cage (duration, s; mean ± s.e.m.) after subchronic administration of each of the anxiolytic compounds tested (CDP = chlordiazepoxide; BUS = buspirone; BRL = BRL 46470A; PROP = propranolol; RIT = ritanserin).

being somewhat more marked than the increase of social investigation induced by CDP, BUS and RIT. The only other significant change to behaviour of these mice was a corresponding reduction in the duration of their non-social activity. As in the acute studies, this probably reflects a change in behavioural motivation towards social from non-social activities.

Figure 7 illustrates the major effects produced by each of the anxiolytic compounds on behaviour of the mice during social encounters in the more aversive circumstances of an unfamiliar neutral cage. In this situation, each of the anxiolytic compounds significantly increased digging. Aggression was significantly increased by PROP and RIT, and was raised to a level close to statistical significance by BRL and CDP. In contrast, enhancement of social investigation was less marked than in the home cage. As shown in Figure 7, PROP was the only compound which significantly increased overall social investigation in the neutral cage. Nonetheless, CDP, BUS and BRL did significantly raise duration of the specific social element 'nose' (increase in duration (s), mean ± s.e.m.; CDP $4.8 \pm 1.6^*$; BUS $3.8 \pm 1.3^*$; BRL $2.3 \pm 1.1^*$; $^*P < 0.05$) and RIT significantly increased the duration of the social element 'attend' (increase in duration (s), mean ± s.e.m., 8.5 ± 2.3, $P < 0.01$). Thus, in the neutral cage after subchronic treatment, enhancement of digging was more pronounced than after acute administration, whereas the converse was true for the drug-induced enhancement of social investigation. PROP increased aggressive behaviour only after subchronic and not after acute administration.

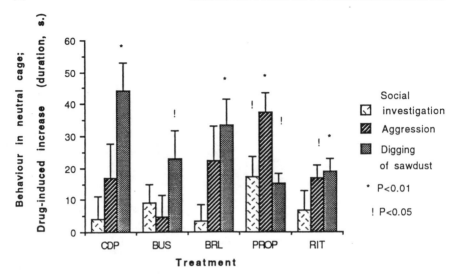

Figure 7   Increase of social investigation, aggression and digging by mice in the neutral cage (duration, s; mean ± s.e.m.) after subchronic administration of each of the anxiolytic compounds tested (CDP = chlordiazepoxide; BUS = buspirone; BRL = BRL 46470A; PROP = propranolol; RIT = ritanserin).

The time spent in other non-social activity was significantly decreased by all of the anxiolytic compounds other than BUS. There were, however, no significant changes to the frequency of other non-social activity by the drug treatments, and thus no evidence of sedative effects.

In conclusion, it can be seen that in the home cage behavioural changes after subchronic treatment of the mice were similar to the effects induced by acute administration. Each of the compounds significantly increased social investigation and reduced time spent by the mice in non-social activity. In the neutral cage following subchronic treatment, all of the compounds increased social investigation or some of its elements, but these effects were less marked than after acute treatment of the mice with these compounds. Digging of the sawdust was increased by all compounds in the subchronic studies, and aggression was significantly increased by PROP and RIT.

GENERAL DISCUSSION

From these ethopharmacological studies it can be seen that anxiolytic compounds representative of five different pharmacological classes did induce a range of common effects on the behavioural responsiveness of mice during social encounters. These behavioural changes appeared to be situation specific.

During encounters in the home cage, in which an unfamiliar animal had been used to provide a social stimulus, each of the compounds significantly increased social investigation and reduced the duration of non-social activity both after acute and subchronic administration.

When tested under the more aversive conditions of encounters in an unfamiliar illuminated neutral cage, the changes to behaviour were more complex. Tests in the neutral cage also revealed differences between the effects of acute and subchronic drug treatments. Social investigation, or some of its elements, continued to be increased in the neutral cage (as in the home cage), and yet this effect was much less marked in the subchronic than in the acute experiments. Increased digging of the sawdust appeared as an additional behavioural effect produced by the anxiolytic compounds in the neutral cage. This increase of digging was shown by all of the anxiolytic compounds in the subchronic studies, but only by buspirone, BRL 46470A and propranolol after acute administration. A further effect which became evident during tests in the neutral cage was enhancement of aggressive behaviour after subchronic and not after acute treatment of the animals with propranolol. Ritanserin also increased aggression in the neutral cage following subchronic administration, but its effects differed from those of propranolol in that it induced some increase of aggressive behaviour when given acutely.

The release of behaviour suppressed by 'fear' of an unfamiliar animal or by environmental constraints has been a major criterion in the development of anxiolytic drugs (e.g. Lader, 1989). Enhancement of social investigation during encounters in an unfamiliar neutral cage represents such an anxiolytic effect, and this was found to be a common behavioural action of the anxiolytic compounds in the present studies. Increased digging of the sawdust in the neutral cage, which was another 'common' behavioural action of subchronically administered anxiolytic compounds, is more difficult to interpret. This may arise either because novel sawdust is mildly aversive (D'Amato and Cabib, 1987) or merely represent an increased reactivity of the drug-treated mice to non-aversive unfamiliar odours from the bedding. Olfactory stimuli are known to play an important part in regulating the behaviour of rodents, and the major sources of unfamiliar odour in the present experiments arose from the partner animal and from the substrate. However, in the acute experiments, the dose–response relationships for enhancement of social investigation by each of the anxiolytic compounds differed from those for enhancement of sawdust-digging. It thus appears probable that the stimulus for increased digging may involve different neurochemical mechanisms from those associated with the drug-induced enhancement of social investigation.

Further study of the factors underlying the drug-induced enhancement of aggressive behaviour is needed. In particular, it appears appropriate to examine the possibility that propranolol may have antidepressant potential. Many antidepressant agents decrease aggression in rodents when given acutely and increase aggression after chronic treatment (Mitchell *et al.*, 1992; Willner *et al.*, 1981). In the present studies, propranolol increased aggression in the neutral cage after subchronic administration and yet induced a slight decrease of aggressive behaviour when it had been given acutely. When given by acute administration at a greater dose level than that employed in the present experiments, propranolol is known to decrease aggression in mice significantly (Yoshimura et al., 1987).

In conclusion, it can be seen that results from the present ethopharmacological studies have added to our existing knowledge of the behavioural actions of this range of anxiolytic compounds. These findings provide confirmatory support for the suggestion that several anxiolytic agents act not merely to release suppressed behaviour but also to enhance responsiveness to naturally occurring social and environmental stimuli. It is thus possible that these compounds may act through common mechanisms, perhaps influencing the gating of incoming sensory stimuli as suggested by Gray (1984).

Previous studies have already shown that benzodiazepine agonists release behaviour from the suppression produced by punishment (Geller et al., 1962), to reduce escape and submissive reactions in the presence of aversive stimuli (Krsiak, 1975) and to increase social interaction (File, 1980). Partial agonists at the 5-HT$_{1A}$ receptor site reduce aggression and ambivalent behaviour in mice alongside their enhancement of social interest (Cutler and Dixon, 1988; Olivier et al., 1989); they are effective in several, although not all of the currently used preclinical models of anxiety (Chopin and Briley, 1987; Gardner, 1988). The 5-HT$_3$ receptor antagonists, likewise, are effective in several of the preclinical models of anxiety (Costall and Naylor, 1991), although they also show a wide range of other therapeutic applications. Propranolol induces a range of behavioural modifications which are associated with anxiolytic activity. For example, it reduces arousal (Redmond, 1987), decreases defensive withdrawal behaviour (Yang et al., 1990) and after chronic administration induces some release of punished responding in certain paradigms (Salmon and Gray, 1986). Ritanserin, in contrast, fails to show positive effects in several of the animal models for detecting anxiolytic potential (Gardner, 1988), although it does show mild anxiolytic effects in a punished responding paradigm in the pigeon (Gleeson et al., 1989). In view of the diversity of these reported effects, the present findings of commonalities in the behavioural actions of these anxiolytic agents are of particular interest.

This observation that anxiolytic agents from different pharmacological 'classes' can induce similar effects on the behavioural responsiveness of rodents is a new finding, and provides evidence of the value of ethopharmacological methods of behavioural analysis for furthering our understanding of psychopharmacological effects. It appears that ethopharmacological methods should be employed more widely in all studies which require detailed analysis of the effects of drugs upon behaviour.

ACKNOWLEDGEMENTS

These findings arise from collaborative work with Mrs Beirong Gao. I wish to express my thanks to Mrs Veronic Graham and Mr Brian Leiper for technical assistance, and I am grateful to SmithKline Beecham, Harlow, for the gift of BRL 46470A.

REFERENCES

Bersani, G., Pozzi, F., Marini, S. *et al.* (1991) 5-HT$_2$ receptor antagonism in dysthymic disorder: a double blind placebo-controlled study with ritanserin. *Acta Physiol. Scand.*, **83**, 244–248.

Brain, P.F., McAllister, K.H. and Walmsley, S.V. (1989) Drug effects on social behaviour. In: *Methods in Ethopharmacology: Neuromethods*, Vol. 13 (A.A. Boulton, G.B. Baker and A.J. Greenshaw). Humana, Clifton, NJ, pp. 687–739.

Ceulemans, D.L., Hoppenbouwers, M.L., Gelders, Y.G. and Reynjens, A.J. (1985) The influence of ritanserin, a serotonin antagonist, in anxiety disorders: a double-blind placebo-controlled study versus lorazepam. *Pharmacopsychiatry*, **18**, 303–305.

Chopin, P. and Briley, M. (1987) Animal models of anxiety: the effect of compounds that modify 5-HT neurotransmission. *Trends Pharmacol. Sci.*, **8**, 383–388.

Costall, B. and Naylor, R.J. (1991) Anxiolytic effects of 5-HT$_3$ receptor antagonists in animals. In: *5-HT$_{1A}$ Agonists, 5-HT$_3$ Antagonists and Benzodiazepines: Their Comparative Behavioural Pharmacology* (eds R.J. Rodgers and S.J. Cooper). Wiley, Chichester, pp. 133–158.

Cutler, M.G. and Dixon, A.K. (1988) Effects of ipsapirone on the behaviour of mice during social encounters. *Neuropharmacology*, **27**, 1039–1044.

Cutler, M.G. and Piper, D.C. (1990) Chronic administration of the 5-HT$_3$ receptor antagonist BRL 43694; effects on reflex epilepsy and social behaviour of the Mongolian gerbil. *Psychopharmacology*, **101**, 244–249.

Cutler, M.G., Mackintosh, J.H. and Chance, M.R.A. (1975) Effects of cannabis resin on social behaviour in the laboratory mouse. *Psychopharmacologia*, **41**, 271–276.

D'Amato, F.R. and Cabib, S. (1987) Chronic exposure to a novel odor increases pups vocalizations, maternal care and alters dopaminergic functioning in developing mice. *Behav. Neural Biol.*, **48**, 197–205.

Dixon, A.K., Fisch, H.U. and McAllister, K.H. (1990) Ethopharmacology: a biological approach to the study of drug-induced changes in behavior. *Adv. Stud. Behav.*, **19**, 171–204.

File, S.E. (1980) The use of social interaction as a method for detecting anxiolytic-like activity of chlordiazepoxide-like drugs. *J. Neurosci. Methods*, **2**, 219–238.

Gao, B. and Cutler, M.G. (1992) Effects of subchronic treatment with chlordiazepoxide, buspirone and the 5-HT$_3$ receptor antagonist, BRL 46470, on the social behaviour of mice. *Neuropharmacology*, **31**, 207–213.

Gardner, C.R. (1985) Pharmacological studies of the role of serotonin in animal models of anxiety. In: *The Neuropharmacology of Serotonin* (ed. A.R. Green), Oxford University Press, Oxford, pp. 281–325.

Gardner, C.R. (1988) Potential use of drugs modulating 5-HT activity in the treatment of anxiety. *Gen. Pharmacol.*, **19**, 347–356.

Geller, I., Kulak, J.T. and Seifter, J. (1962) The effects of chlordiazepoxide and chlorpromazine on a punishment discrimination task. *Psychopharmacologia*, **3**, 374–385.

Gleeson, S., Ahlers, S.T., Mansbach, R.S. *et al.* (1989) Behavioral studies with anxiolytic drugs. VI. Effects on punished responding of drugs interacting with serotonin receptor subtypes. *J. Pharmac. Exp. Ther.*, **250**, 809–817.

Goa, K.L. and Ward, A. (1986) Buspirone: a preliminary review of its pharmacological properties and therapeutic efficacy as an anxiolytic. *Drugs*, **32**, 114–129.

Grant, E.C. and Mackintosh, J.H. (1963) A comparison of the social postures of some common laboratory rodents. *Behaviour*, **21**, 246–259.

Gray, J.A. (1984) *The Neuropsychology of Anxiety: an Enquiry into the Functions of the Septo-hippocampal System.* Oxford University Press, Oxford.

Jones, B.J., Costall, B., Domeney, A.M. *et al.* (1988) The potential anxiolytic activity of GR 38032F, a 5-HT$_3$ receptor antagonist. *Br. J. Pharmacol.*, **93**, 985–993.

Krsiak, M. (1975) Timid singly housed mice: their value in predictions of psychotropic activity of drugs. *Br. J. Pharmacol.*, **55**, 141–150.

Lader, M. (1989) Drug treatment of anxiety: implications for animal models. *Behav. Pharmacol.*, **1**, 95–100.

Lal, H. and Emmett-Oglesby, M.W. (1983) Behavioural analogues of anxiety: animal models. *Neuropharmacology*, **22**, 1423–1441.

Lecrubier, Y., Puech, A.J. and Azoona, A. (1990) 5-HT$_3$ receptors in anxiety disorders. *J. Psychopharmacol. Proc. BAP Meeting*, 19p.

Mackintosh, J.H. (1970) Territory formation in laboratory mice. *Anim. Behav.*, **18**, 177–183.

Mackintosh, J.H., Chance, M.R.A. and Silverman, A.P. (1977) The contribution of ethological techniques to the study of drug effects. In: *Handbook of Psychopharmacology*, Vol. 7 (eds L.L. Iversen, S.D. Iversen and S.H. Snyder). Plenum Press, London, pp. 3–35.

Meibach, R.C., Mullain, J.F. and Binstok, G. (1987) A placebo-controlled multicenter trial of propranolol and chlordiazepoxide in the treatment of anxiety. *Curr. Ther. Res.*, **41**, 65–76.

Middleton, H.C. (1991) Psychology and pharmacology in the treatment of anxiety disorders: a cooperation or confrontation. *J. Psychopharmacol.*, **5**, 281–285.

Mitchell, P.J., Fletcher, A. and Redfern, P.H. (1992) Is antidepressant efficacy revealed by drug-induced changes in rat behaviour exhibited during social interactions? *Neurosci. Biobehav. Rev.*, **15**, 539–544.

Olivier, B., Mos, J., van der Heyden, J. and Hartog, J. (1989) Serotonergic modulations of social interactions in isolated male mice. *Psychopharmacology*, **97**, 154–156.

Redmond, D.E. (1987) Studies of the nucleus locus coeruleus in monkeys and hypotheses for neuopharmacology. In: *Psychopharmacology: The Third Generation of Progress* (ed. H.Y. Meltzer). Raven Press, New York, pp. 967–973.

Salmon, P. and Gray, J.A. (1986) Effects of propranolol on conditioned suppression, discriminated punishment and discriminated non-reward in the rat. *Psychopharmacology*, **88**, 252–257.

Sanger, D.J., Perrault, G., Morel, E. *et al.* (1991) Animal models of anxiety and the development of novel anxiolytic drugs. *Prog. Neuropsychopharmacol. Biol. Psychiatry*, **15**, 205–212.

Upton, N. and Blackburn, T.P. (1991) Anxiolytic-like activity of the selective 5-HT$_3$ receptor antagonist, BRL 46470A, in the rat elevated X-maze test. *Br. J. Pharmacol.*, **102**, 253p.

Willner, P., Theodorou, R. and Montgomery, A. (1981) Subchronic treatment with the tricyclic antidepressant DMI increases isolation-induced fighting in rats. *Pharmacol. Biochem. Behav.*, **14**, 475–479.

Yang, X.M., Gorman, A.L. and Dunn, A.J. (1990) The involvement of central noradrenergic systems and corticotropin-releasing factor in defensive-withdrawal behavior in rats. *J. Pharmacol. Exp. Ther.*, **255**, 1064–1070.

Yoshimura, H., Kihara, Y. and Ogawa, N. (1987) Psychotropic effects of adrenergic β-blockers on agonistic behavior between resident and intruder mice. *Psychopharmacology*, **91**, 445–450.

4 Novel Ethological Models of Anxiety in the Rat and Ferret

JON SHEPHERD, SAVRAJ GREWAL AND MARK COBAIN
Department of Neuropharmacology, Wyeth Research (UK) Ltd, Taplow,
Maidenhead, UK

The aim of this chapter is to illustrate the utility of the ethological approach in the development of two novel animal models of anxiety. The first of these to be discussed is the elevated 'zero-maze', a modification of the traditional elevated plus-maze design which is now proving to be a sensitive screen for traditional and novel anxiolytic compounds. The second section provides an overview of the rationale and preliminary findings in the development of an animal model of anxiety in the ferret.

CHARACTERIZATION OF THE ELEVATED 'ZERO-MAZE': A NOVEL MODEL OF ANXIETY IN RATS

Introduction

In a classic series of experiments, Montgomery (1955) attempted to investigate the relationships between novelty, fear and exploratory behaviour. Montgomery observed that rats allowed to explore either an elevated, open or an enclosed alley, from the relative safety of their home cage, exhibited an approach–avoidance conflict which was determined by the relative strengths of the exploratory and fear drives evoked by the novel situations. Therefore, due to the greater aversiveness of the open elevated alley, rats tended to exhibit more avoidance behaviour (i.e. less exploration and a greater number of retreats to the rear of the cage and looks away from the open cage door) than they did with the enclosed alley. This work by Montgomery has been widely accepted as providing evidence for the 'two-factor theory' of the dynamic relationship between exploratory behaviour and 'anxiety/fear' (Russell, 1973).

Over the last 15 years, a number of rodent models of anxiety have been derived from ethological studies which centre around unconditioned or 'spontaneous' behaviours (e.g. see Lister, 1990). Many of these utilize the 'two-factor theory' by measuring the extent to which exploratory behaviour is suppressed by 'fear-provoking' stimuli intrinsic to the experimental situation.

Ethology and Psychopharmacology. Edited by S.J. Cooper and C.A. Hendrie
© 1994 John Wiley & Sons Ltd

One such model is the elevated plus-maze (Handley and Mithani, 1984; Pellow *et al.*, 1985). It consists of an elevated platform in the shape of a cross, with two opposite pairs of enclosed and open arms. Rats forced to stay on the open arms show classic fear reactions such as freezing, defaecation and increased levels of plasma corticosteroids (Pellow *et al.*, 1985), and recently Treit *et al.* (1993) have shown that a major contributory factor to this unconditioned, innate fear reaction is thigmotaxis, a natural defensive response in which rats remain close to vertical surfaces in order to avoid detection by predators (Barnett, 1966; Grossen and Kelley, 1973; Treit and Fundytus, 1988). As a consequence of the aversive properties of the open arms, subjects spend a greater proportion of the test period exploring the closed arms, and subsequently any drug-induced increase in the percentage time spent on the open arms and/or percentage open-arm entries is considered to reflect a decrease in anxiety. The plus-maze has been pharmacologically validated for both rats (Pellow *et al.*, 1985) and mice (Lister, 1987) and has proved sensitive to both anxiolytic and anxiogenic drug action (e.g. Pellow and File, 1986).

The elevated zero-maze provides a modified version of the traditional plus-maze design. In addition, the current procedure incorporates a detailed behavioural analysis in order to improve the sensitivity to, and facilitate the interpretation of, drug action.

Design modifications

Empirical evidence indicates that mice (Lee and Rodgers, 1990; Rodgers *et al.*, 1992b) and rats (Pellow *et al.*, 1985; Soderpalm *et al.*, 1989) spend a high proportion (20–30%) of the test period on the central square of the traditional elevated plus-maze. Lee and Rodgers (1990) discussed the potential significance of this in the interpretation of more subtle drug effects. Thus, in the murine elevated plus-maze, low doses of the opioid antagonist, naltrexone, induced a reliable shift in behavioural distribution away from the open arms to the central platform, whilst at higher doses there was an increase in time spent on the combined central/closed regions, suggesting that an increase in time on the central square may be associated with a transition towards open arm avoidance, i.e. anxiogenesis. Similarly, Vasar *et al.* (1993) suggested that observed anxiogenic effects of the cholecystokinin (CCK) agonist, caerulein, in the rat elevated plus-maze reflected a shift in what they termed the 'central platform behaviour' of control animals to 'anxious' behaviour of drug-treated rats who made virtually no entries onto the open areas (central square + open arms) of the plus-maze.

Following the same line of reasoning, an increase in time spent on the central square at the expense of time on the closed arms could reflect mild anxiolytic activity—an effect that cannot be detected if, as is very often the case, the percentage time spent on the open arms is expressed as a proportion of the total time spent on the maze, i.e. total test time. This suggests that a more comprehensive analysis of behaviour on the different sections of the plus-maze may aid interpretation of drug effects.

However, the central square may also be seen as a potential experimental confound. Therefore, removal of the central area entirely may be a simpler alternative method of detecting more subtle drug effects on exploration of the open areas. In this context, the present design (Shepherd, 1992; Shepherd *et al.*, 1993; Shepherd *et al.*, in press) comprises an elevated annular platform with two opposite open/closed quadrants (i.e. no 'dead area'). This has the additional advantage of allowing uninterrupted exploration, since it lacks the closed arm 'boxed ends' which are integral to the conventional plus-maze configuration (see Figure 1 and Figure 2, left panel).

Behavioural analysis

The search for novel classes of anxiolytics which are free from the numerous problems associated with chronic benzodiazepine use is clearly an important task. It has been generally accepted that animal models of anxiety should be validated with benzodiazepines. However, because of this approach, one criticism that has often been levelled at current animal models of anxiety is that they provide a reference behavioural profile which may be specific to 'benzodiazepine-like' activity (a self-fulfilling prophecy). Since a major requirement of a novel model is the ability to detect anxiolytics which produce their effects in a manner which is different from that of the benzodiazepines, it

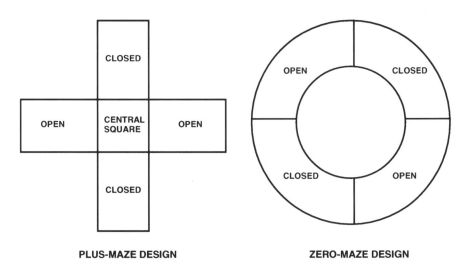

Figure 1 Diagram showing plan views of the open and closed areas of the traditional plus-maze and the novel zero-maze designs.

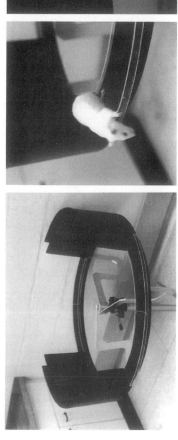
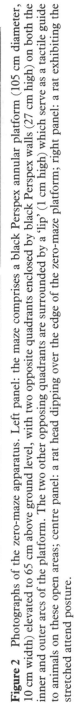

Figure 2 Photographs of the zero-maze apparatus. Left panel: the maze comprises a black Perspex annular platform (105 cm diameter, 10 cm width) elevated to 65 cm above ground level, with two opposite quadrants enclosed by black Perspex walls (27 cm high) on both the inner and outer arcs of the platform. The two other opposing quadrants are surrounded by a 'lip' (1 cm high) which serve as a tactile guide to animals on these open areas; centre panel: a rat head dipping over the edge of the zero-maze platform; right panel: a rat exhibiting the stretched attend posture.

would be counter-intuitive to predict that an exact duplication of the benzo-diazepine behavioural profile would be achieved using novel compounds such as $5\text{-}HT_{1A}$ receptor agonists and $5\text{-}HT_3$ receptor antagonists. Thus, in the present context, whilst traditional measures on the elevated plus-maze have provided consistent behavioural profiles with benzodiazepines, they have proved somewhat inconsistent in the detection of anxiolytic effects of novel drugs. Additionally, it has been suggested that the utility of measures of open arm activity on the elevated plus-maze can be compromised by shifts in baseline behaviour. Consequently, a number of workers have proposed that a more ethological approach should be incorporated into the analysis of behavi-our in order to enhance the sensitivity of the model (e.g. Moser, 1989; Rodgers, 1991; Falter et al., 1992).

Several ethological studies have identified a collection of behaviours which appear to be an important and integral part of an animal's defensive repertoire. These behaviours have been catagorized within the collective term 'risk assessment'. In a recent review Blanchard and Blanchard (1988) noted that these behaviours occur 'in situations involving any considerable degree of unfamiliarity or unpredictability, in addition to danger from predation, con-specific attack or natural hazard' where they play a role in information gathering about potential threat. As such, they regard risk assessment as 'a central element in the behavioural expression of anxiety' (Blanchard et al., 1989). In view of this, we decided that analysis of risk assessment behaviours on the zero-maze, in addition to the more traditional measure of percentage time spent on the open quadrants, could provide a sensitive measure of the approach–avoidance conflict. This suggestion was strengthened by the obser-vation that rats spent in the region of 30% of the time on the zero-maze at the open/closed quadrant divides, i.e. the locations at which an approach–avoidance conflict might be experienced. Preliminary studies revealed that time spent at these divides (at least one paw over the dividing line) alone was not a sensitive measure of anxiety. However, it was observed that rats on the zero-maze exhibited a number of 'stretched attention postures' (Grant and Mackintosh, 1963)—a behaviour associated with risk assessment (Kaesermann, 1986; Blanchard et al., 1989)—and that the majority of these postures oc-curred at the open/closed divide with the rats, in the closed quadrants, investigating the open areas. Frequency of stretched attend postures from the closed to the open quadrants was therefore incorporated into the behavioural analysis. Pilot studies also revealed that rats frequently exhibited head-dipping behaviour over the edge of the open platform (HDIPS). This measure closely resembles head-dipping observed in the hole board test (e.g. Suzuki et al., 1990) and is believed to provide a further index of exploratory behaviour. Thus, in the context of Montgomery's (1955) approach–avoidance conflict, pretreatment with benzodiazepines would be expected to increase the explora-tory drive by reducing fear and, subsequently, increase frequency of HDIPS. This measure has also proved to be a useful tool in a more detailed behavioural analysis of the murine elevated plus-maze (see Rodgers and Cole, this volume) and as such was included in our studies with the elevated zero-maze.

Drug studies

Two series of experiments were initially carried out with the elevated zero-maze to evaluate the utility of the new design and novel behavioural analysis in determining drug effects. In the first series of experiments, the effects of the benzodiazepines, diazepam and chlordiazepoxide, were investigated to provide behavioural profiles for two clinically efficacious anxiolytics. In a second series of experiments, the effects of manipulation of serotonergic function on behaviour on the zero-maze was investigated.

5-HT$_{1A}$ receptor agonists and 5-HT$_3$ receptor antagonists are generally considered putative anxiolytics, but have previously been shown to produce inconsistent results across a range of animal models of anxiety, including the traditional elevated plus-maze paradigm (for reviews see Dourish, 1987; Barrett and Gleeson, 1991; Costall and Naylor, 1991; Treit, 1991; Wilkinson and Dourish, 1991). For this reason the effects of the prototypical 5-HT$_{1A}$ receptor agonist 8-hydroxy-2-(di-n-propylamino)tetralin (8-OH-DPAT) and the 5-HT$_3$ receptor antagonist ondansetron were assessed. In addition, the 5-HT$_{1B/2C}$ receptor agonist mCPP (1-(m-chlorophenyl)piperazine), which has been shown to have anxiogenic activity in both animals and man (for review see Kahn and Wetzler, 1991), was included to assess the 'bidirectional sensitivity' of the model, i.e. detection of both anxiogenic and anxiolytic effects by behavioural analysis.

Methods

Group-housed (four per cage) male Sprague–Dawley rats (285–430 g) were injected subcutaneously with either drug or vehicle (10% polyethylene glycol/physiological saline). Thirty minutes later subjects were placed onto a closed quadrant of the zero-maze and a 5 min test period was recorded on video for subsequent analysis. The apparatus was illuminated by dim lighting arranged in such a manner as to provide similar lux levels in open and closed quadrants (40–60 lux). Behavioural measures included percentage time spent on the open areas (%TO), frequency of head dips over the edge of the platform (HDIPS: see Figure 2, centre panel), and frequency of stretched attend postures (SAP: see Figure 2, right panel) from closed to open quadrants, determined when the subject, on a closed quadrant, exhibited an elongated body posture stretched forwards with at least the snout passing over the closed–open divide. All testing was carried out between 13.00 and 17.00 h. A diazepam treatment group (0.5 or 0.75 mg/kg) was included as a positive control in all studies with the serotonergic compounds. Data were analysed by Kruskal–Wallis one-way analysis of variance. Planned comparisons between vehicle-treated controls and drug-treated groups were performed using the Mann–Whitney U-test.

Effect of diazepam and chlordiazepoxide in the rat elevated zero-maze

The preliminary data demonstrated that the reference benzodiazepine anxiolytics, diazepam and chlordiazepoxide, produced a consistent behavioural profile in the rat zero-maze (Figures 3 and 4). The proportion of time spent on

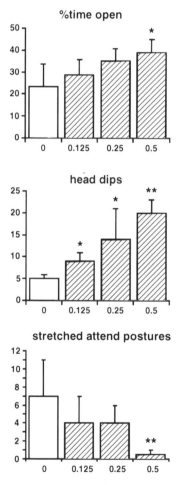

Figure 3 Effect of diazepam (0.125–0.5 mg/kg) on percentage time open, head dips and stretched attend postures in rats tested on the elevated zero-maze. Data are expressed as median values ± median absolute deviations (m.a.d.; calculated as the median of the set of differences between each data point and the median of the data). $^\star p < 0.05$, $^{\star\star} p < 0.01$ versus vehicle-treated group.

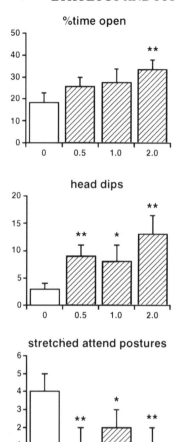

Figure 4 Effect of chlordiazepoxide (0.5–2.0 mg/kg) on percentage time open, head dips and stretched attend postures in rats tested on the elevated zero-maze. Data are expressed as median values ± m.a.d. $*p < 0.05$, $**p < 0.01$ versus vehicle-treated group.

the open quadrants—one of the traditional measures employed in the elevated plus-maze procedure—was increased dose-dependently by both compounds. Follow-up comparisons revealed that these effects were significant at doses of 0.5 mg/kg with diazepam and at 2.0 mg/kg with chlordiazepoxide, whilst the effects at both 0.5 and 1.0 mg/kg chlordiazepoxide approached but failed to reach statistical significance ($p = 0.052$ in each case). The inclusion of more detailed ethological analysis revealed significant increases in exploratory head-dipping over the edges of the platform at all doses tested with both compounds. In addition, significant decreases in stretched attend postures from the closed to the open quadrants were observed at a dose of 0.5 mg/kg with diazepam and at all doses tested with chlordiazepoxide.

Interestingly, the observed effects on HDIPS and SAP were generally evident at lower doses than those required to significantly affect time spent on the open quadrants. Thus, it can be postulated that a more detailed behavioural analysis appears to increase the sensitivity of the elevated zero-maze to benzodiazepine anxiolytic activity. This finding is entirely in keeping with recent studies employing the mouse elevated plus-maze, in which chlordiazepoxide increased %TO at a higher dose (15 mg/kg) than that (10 mg/kg) required to produce a significant reduction in SAP (Cole and Rodgers, 1994).

Effects of 5-HT receptor ligands in the rat elevated zero-maze

mCPP (0.25–1.0 mg/kg; Figure 5) dose-dependently decreased both %TO (vehicle versus 0.5 mg/kg, $p < 0.05$; 1.0 mg/kg, $p < 0.01$) and HDIPS (vehicle versus 1.0 mg/kg, $p < 0.01$). SAP was significantly increased at 0.5 mg/kg ($p < 0.05$) and 1.0 mg/kg ($p < 0.01$). These findings illustrate further the utility of the behavioural profile, as opposed to models employing a single measure. Specifically, mCPP has been found to increase behavioural indices of anxiogenesis in several animal models including the rat social interaction and light/dark exploration models (Kennett *et al.*, 1989), mouse elevated plus-maze (Benjamin *et al.*, 1990; Rodgers *et al* 1992a) and free exploration and light–dark exploration (Griebel *et al.*, 1991) tests. However, a potential confound exists in view of the reported general reduction in activity with higher doses of mCPP (Kennett and Curzon, 1988; Kennett *et al.*, 1989) which may produce apparent 'anxiogenic' observations in many behavioural models. In this context, the bidirectional nature of the behavioural profile obtained in the present studies using the zero-maze appears to resolve this problem as our findings indicate a reduction in %TO and HDIPS and a concomitant increase in SAP which, as would be predicted with an anxiogenic drug, is diametrically opposite to the behavioural changes induced by the benzodiazepines. While the observed reductions in the former two behaviours could be equivocal in terms of anxiogenesis and/or a non-specific reduction in locomotor activity, the *increase* in SAP would suggest a specific influence of mCPP on anxiety.

The observed effects of the two putative 5-HT anxiolytics, 8-OH-DPAT and ondansetron, in the zero-maze are of considerable importance in view of the many inconsistent findings reported in the literature with both compounds. Thus, the 5-HT$_{1A}$ receptor agonist 8-OH-DPAT has been shown to produce a range of effects in elevated plus-maze experiments which include anxiolytic (Dunn *et al.*, 1989; Soderpalm *et al.*, 1989), no effect (Pellow *et al.*, 1987) and anxiogenic profiles (Critchley and Handley, 1987; Moser *et al.*, 1990; Klint, 1991; Critchley *et al.*, 1992). Similarly, ondansetron has proved anxiolytic in the rodent elevated plus-maze in some laboratories (Costall *et al.*, 1989; Upton

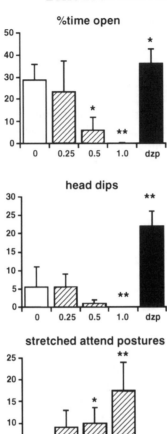

Figure 5 Effect of mCPP (0.25–1.0 mg/kg; hatched bars) and diazepam (dzp; 0.75 mg/kg; black bars) on percentage time open, head dips and stretched attend postures in rats tested on the elevated zero-maze. Data are expressed as median values ± m.a.d. $^*p < 0.05$, $^{**}p < 0.01$ versus vehicle-treated group.

and Blackburn, 1991; Tomkins *et al.*, 1990), while others have failed to find any significant effects (File and Johnston, 1989; Wright *et al.*, 1992).

In this series of studies, the data failed to indicate any significant effects of 8-OH-DPAT on %TO or HDIPS (Figure 6). However, at one dose only (0.01 mg/kg), consistent with recent findings in the mouse elevated plus-maze (Rodgers *et al.*, 1992a), SAP was significantly reduced, indicating some anxiolytic activity. A similar behavioural profile was evoked by the 5-HT$_3$ receptor antagonist ondansetron (Figure 7), which produced a reduction in SAP, an effect which was again limited to one dose (0.01 mg/kg). In addition,

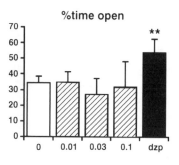

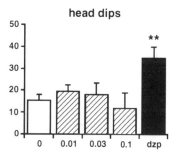

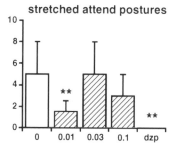

Figure 6 Effect of 8-OH-DPAT (0.01–1.0 mg/kg; hatched bars) and diazepam (dzp; 0.75 mg/kg; black bars) on percentage time open, head dips and stretched attend postures in rats tested on the elevated zero-maze. Data are expressed as median values ± m.a.d. $*p < 0.05$, $**p < 0.01$ versus vehicle-treated group.

at the same dose ondansetron produced a marked trend toward an increase in %TO and, to a lesser extent, HDIPS, consistent with anxiolysis.

Discussion

Montgomery's (1955) original observations of an approach–avoidance conflict in rats between exploratory drive and the natural aversion to an unprotected elevated open environment provided the basis for the elevated plus-maze—an animal model of anxiety which is now a well-established screen for compounds

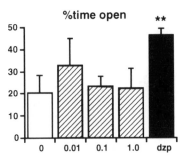

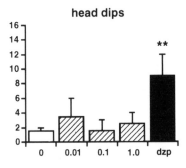

Figure 7 Effect of ondansetron (0.01–1.0 mg/kg; hatched bars) and diazepam (dzp; 0.5 mg/kg; black bars) on percentage time open, head dips and stretched attend postures in rats tested on the elevated zero-maze. Data are expressed as median values ± m.a.d. *$p < 0.05$, **$p < 0.01$ versus vehicle-treated group.

affecting anxiety (e.g. Pellow and File, 1986). The annular design resolves the potential ambiguity associated with the central square of the traditional apparatus, thereby providing a direct inverse relationship between time spent on the open and closed quadrants. In addition, the zero-maze design removes the 'boxed ends' associated with the closed arms of the plus-maze, thereby promoting uninterrupted exploration. This therefore increases the number of locations (i.e. probability of occurrence) on the apparatus in which an approach–avoidance conflict might be experienced; the very phenomenon it is intended to measure.

As discussed previously, it would be counter-intuitive to predict that an exact duplication of the benzodiazepine behavioural profile would be achieved using novel compounds such as $5-HT_{1A}$ and $5-HT_3$ receptor ligands. In the present context, the behavioural measures of HDIPS and %TO, although sensitive to the anxiogenic mCPP, proved more useful in the detection of benzodiazepine anxiolysis than the effects induced by the putative 5-HT anxiolytics. The observed increase in HDIPS is consistent with an increase in both frequency and duration of exploratory head-dipping exhibited by rats on a hole board following the adminstration of non-sedative doses of diazepam— an effect which was reversed at high doses of diazepam which induced sedation (Suzuki et al., 1990).

However, a common feature of the behavioural profile of all the anxiolytics tested to date appears to be a reduction in SAP. The behavioural element 'stretched attend posture' was originally described in the context of social interaction and classified as an ambivalent element reflecting an approach– avoidance tendency (Grant and Mackintosh, 1963). Subsequent studies have shown that SAP occurs in non-social aversive situations in both rats (Van der Poel, 1979; Blanchard et al., 1990, 1991) and mice (Kaesermann, 1986) and there is now a body of empirical evidence to support the view that SAP provides a reliable index of anxiety. This notion is supported by ethological studies carried out by Blanchard and Blanchard on anxiety-related defensive behaviour in rats. They have consistently observed that presentation of a cat odour stimulus to rats (i.e. potential threat) increases the frequency of SAP, suggesting that this behaviour is an ethologically valid and naturalistic corre- late of anxiety/fear-related behaviour. Moreover, anxiolytic compounds, such as diazepam and ethanol (Blanchard et al., 1990), and putative anxiolytics such as ritanserin (Shepherd et al., 1992), reduce the frequency of SAP. Similarly, investigations in mice demonstrate a reduction in SAP (to conspecific urine and faeces spread over a platform) following administration of diazepam, chlordiazepoxide, clobazam, alprazolam, buspirone, phenobarbitone and pentobarbitone (Kaesermann, 1986; Kaesermann and Dixon, 1986; Pollard and Howard, 1988). While interpretation of the murine SAP response was questioned due to the potential confound of sedative drug activity (Pollard and Howard, 1988, the bidirectional nature of the changes in HDIPS and SAP described above enables the assessment of behavioural specificity using the present design. This is an important point since, as a typical anxiolytic/ anxiogenic profile involves both increases and decreases in the relevant behavi- oural elements, this removes any confound due to baseline levels.

For example, if %TO were the only measure employed then a potential anxiogenic drug effect may be masked by a 'floor effect' produced by a low baseline level, a problem which is resolved by the potential for an increase in SAP. This issue is illustrated by the effects of 0.5 mg/kg mCPP which did not significantly reduce HDIPS, probably as a consequence of the low baseline level of this response, but which significantly increased SAP (and in this case decreased %TO). Thus, while other workers have manipulated environmental variables such as illumination in order to provide a baseline level of %TO more appropriate for the detection of anxiolytic or anxiogenic effects (e.g. Handley and McBlane, 1993), the current protocol eliminates the requirement for any ad hoc methodological changes.

In conclusion, preliminary evidence suggests that the zero-maze design, combined with a detailed behavioural analysis, represents a new and reliable animal model of anxiety which will prove useful in the detection of novel non-benzodiazepine anxiolytics.

PRELIMINARY EVALUATION OF A MODEL OF ANXIETY BASED ON TERRITORIAL BEHAVIOUR IN THE FERRET (*MUSTELA FURO*)

Introduction

This series of studies was initiated with the primary objective of developing a non-rodent model of anxiety. The development of novel potential anxiolytics, particularly in an industrial context, requires empirical evidence from animal studies before the decision can be made to proceed with clinical trials. Thus, the rationale for the present work is unequivocal; the use of a wider range of animal species in preclinical research should enable greater confidence that observed anxiolytic effects will generalize to human trials. In addition, the inclusion of a non-rodent species would resolve any ambiguities in drug activity which may arise from the present emphasis on rats and mice as research subjects. Finally, there is evidence from binding studies to suggest that in ferret brain, as in human brain, the 5-HT_{1D} receptor is more common than the 5-HT_{1B} receptor while the opposite case is true in rodents (Brammer *et al.*, 1993). Therefore, data derived from serotonergic manipulations in the ferret may provide a closer parallel to the potential outcome in humans.

Having determined the rationale for the development of a ferret model of anxiety, the problem was to identify any 'fear-provoking' stimuli which might be effective with this animal. In general terms, the aim was to apply our knowledge of ethology in the introduction and measurement of natural behavioural responses within a laboratory setting. The 'aversive' stimuli presented to rodents in similar 'ethological models' can be broadly categorized as non-social (e.g. elevated open spaces), full or partial predator stimuli (e.g. cat or cat odour, respectively) and social conspecific (e.g. social interaction). The non-social stimulus category is indirectly related to predator stimuli as such paradigms frequently incorporate behavioural responses which can be considered as adaptive strategies for predator avoidance, e.g. avoidance of brightly lit or open elevated areas. The feral ferret (and close relation, the polecat) has few natural predators, and those that are known, such as raptors (Powell, 1979), would not provide a particularly accessible stimulus for laboratory manipulation. Thus, the focus of the current model was directed toward the investigation of social conspecific stimuli.

Ferrets are solitary-dwelling territorial animals with an organized pattern of spacing between individuals of the same gender, referred to as 'intrasexual territoriality' (Powell, 1979). Scent-marking, dominance relationships and food supply are the principal mechanisms which affect the maintenance and stability of these territorial spacing patterns in mustelids (Powell, 1979; Moors and Lavers, 1981). Support for a 'territorial defence' role of scent-marking comes from a variety of ethological studies. For example, Poole (1967) observed that following agonistic encounters between pairs of male mustelids the victor extensively scent-marked the neutral arena, particularly the area previously occupied by the loser. Similarly, when two male ferrets were placed in a neutral arena in the presence of fresh scent samples, aggression was increased in animals with their own odour present and decreased in the presence of opponent odour (Clapperton et al., 1988), supporting the territorial defence hypothesis and scent-matching mechanism by which an association between a resident and its defended area could be maintained (Gosling, 1982). Interestingly, Clapperton and colleagues (1988) observed no scent-marking behaviour over female-scented sites in a T-maze test utilizing female and male scents, suggesting that the scent-mark behaviour performed by male ferrets is specific to situations of territorial defence and aggression directed towards other male ferrets. Chemical analysis indicated clear sexual and individual differences in the major chemical components of anal sac secretions, supporting the suggestion that odours provide an important source of information as an individual recognition system, subsequently mediating social organization (Clapperton et al., 1988).

The most commonly observed scent-marking behaviour in ferrets kept in an outdoor enclosure was described as the 'belly crawl', characterized by lowering the chest onto the ground and pushing forward with the back legs until all the ventral body surface was flattened to the ground, and the back legs were splayed out either side; the animal would then slide further forwards using wriggling movements, and paddling with the front legs (Clapperton, 1989). In a quasi-natural situation, Clapperton (1989) first determined dominance relationships by allowing contact between male ferrets in neighbouring outdoor enclosures. Subsequently, when the ferrets were allowed access to the same neighbouring compounds, dominant animals briefly investigated, then scent-marked over the subordinate's home marking sites, whilst subordinates investigated, but did not exhibit any scent-marking behaviour around dominant home sites. These findings again provide evidence for an important role of scent-marking in territorial defence and perhaps in the consolidation of dominance hierarchies.

The present studies were designed in order to model these territorial phenomena in laboratory context with the hope that a quantifiable index of anxiety may emerge.

Procedural details

Subjects

Twelve sexually mature adult male ferrets were singly housed, and a felt-covered wood block was kept permanently in each cage in order to enable individuals to saturate it with scent. In the second experiment, singly housed sexually mature female ferrets were employed as stimulus animals where appropriate.

Apparatus design

The test apparatus (see Figure 8) comprised a black Perspex chamber (240 × 80 × 70 cm) divided into two halves with a connecting door. A clear Perspex side wall was fitted to permit video-recording of behaviour for subsequent analysis.

General protocol

Experiments 1 and 3: the procedure comprised an initial 5 min habituation period with the experimental subject (male ferret) placed in one side of the chamber, with its own scent block connected to the end wall and either (1) a control (non-scented) block or (2) a stimulus animal (Experiments 1 and 3: male ferret; Experiment 2: male or female ferret) with its own scent block in the opposite side of the chamber. During the habituation period each animal

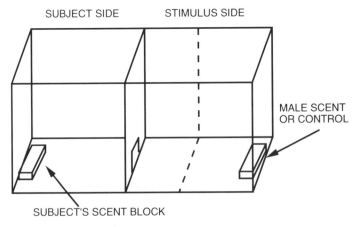

Figure 8 Diagram showing the ferret territorial avoidance apparatus.

was allowed to freely explore and scent-mark their respective compartment. The stimulus ferret was then removed to its home cage, leaving the stimulus scent block in position in the chamber. The dividing door was then removed, allowing the test subject free access to both sides of the apparatus during a 5 min observation period. The apparatus was thoroughly cleaned with a deodorizing solution between trials.

Behavioural analysis

Behavioural measures scored from videotape included time spent in the quarter of the chamber containing the stimulus block, time spent in contact with the stimulus block, and frequency of scent-marking in which the ventral body surface is dragged over the stimulus block (wipe/belly crawl described by Clapperton, 1989). All studies employed repeated-measures designs such that each subject was exposed to all conditions, counterbalanced for order of stimulus presentation and drug treatment where appropriate.

Drug administration (Experiment 3)

Diazepam (0.1–1.0 mg/kg) was administered subcutaneously in a 10% poly-ethylene glycol/90% physiological saline vehicle, in an injection volume of 0.5 ml/kg, 30 min prior to behavioural testing.

Experiment 1: Male scent versus unscented control

Figure 9 shows that presentation of unfamiliar male scent produced a signifi-cant ($p < 0.05$) decrease in time spent in the quarter of the test chamber containing the stimulus block, and in time spent in physical contact with the scent block, when compared with responding in the presence of an unscented control block. This profile would suggest that the stimulus side of the test chamber and the stimulus block is more aversive to the subject when another male's scent is present, and such a difference in response could well represent a laboratory model of the phenomenon of territorial avoidance previously observed in the feral animal (Powell, 1979; Moors and Lavers, 1981). The baseline level of scent-marking over the stimulus block was very low, produ-cing a floor effect such that no significant difference could be observed when subjects were exposed to an unfamiliar male scent.

While the above profile does provide preliminary evidence for a model of territorial avoidance (NB: this response profile was replicated several times; unpublished data), there is an alternative explanation for these findings. Thus, on the basis of this data alone, the possibility cannot be ruled out that the presence of any odour would have the same effect, i.e. that the observed avoidance of the stimulus block is not directly associated with intrasexual territoriality, but may simply reflect aversion to a non-specific unfamiliar

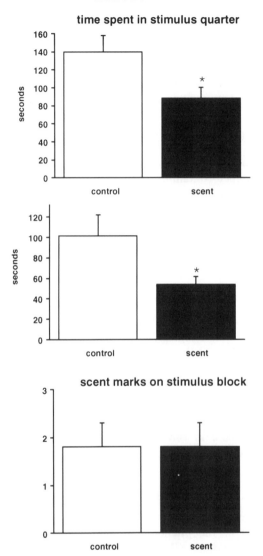

Figure 9 Effect of unfamiliar male scent presentation on behaviour in the territorial avoidance apparatus. Data are expressed as mean values ($\pm$ standard error). $^{*}p < 0.05$ versus control (no scent).

odour. The following experiment was designed to investigate this hypothesis by replacing the male stimulus ferret with a female and assessing any difference in the response. If the behavioural profile obtained with a female (non-threatening) stimulus is equivalent to that of the male stimulus, it might be inferred that the procedure simply reflects a non-specific avoidance of novel unfamiliar odour. Clearly, if the response to a female stimulus does not differ from control then it would support the notion that the male scent stimulus provides a biologically relevant cue to the subject.

Experiment 2: Male and female scent versus unscented control

Figure 10 shows that presentation of unfamiliar male scent produced a very similar profile to that of Experiment 1, i.e. a consistent significant decrease in time spent in the stimulus quarter and time spent in physical contact with the stimulus block, compared with responding in the presence of an unscented control block ($p < 0.05$). The response profile obtained with presentation of an unfamiliar female scent did not significantly differ from that of the unscented control condition. Frequency of scent-marking was again at a low level in all three scent conditions, and analysis failed to indicate any significant differences between control and male or female stimulus groups.

These data suggest that in the present context unfamiliar male ferret odour is likely to reflect a specific and ecologically relevant stimulus to the male subject, and the response profile obtained is not simply an artifact of novelty *per se*. The following study was designed to assess the effects of a reference benzodiazepine anxiolytic, diazepam, on behaviour in the territorial avoidance apparatus.

Experiment 3: Effects of diazepam on responding to male scent versus unscented control

Figure 11 shows that presentation of unfamiliar male scent again produced a significant ($p < 0.05$) decrease in time spent in the stimulus quarter and time in contact with the stimulus block in vehicle-treated control animals. However, there was no significant difference in responding, for both of these measures, between scent and unscented control conditions when subjects were pretreated with diazepam (all doses). These findings may suggest that pretreatment with diazepam attenuates the anxiety-provoking properties of the unfamiliar scent presentation. However, the generally lower baselines for each of these behavioural measures with drug treatment would question the specificity of this effect. Further investigation would certainly be required prior to forming any more confident conclusion.

In contrast to the previous two studies, assessment of scent-marking frequencies in this experiment provided the most interesting data. First, it is clear from Figure 11 that the baseline level (vehicle-treated, control block condition) of scent-marking was about two-fold higher than that observed in the previous studies. One reason for this could be the time of testing as only the final experiment was carried out within the breeding season (late spring). This would be consistent with the highest levels of scent-marking having been

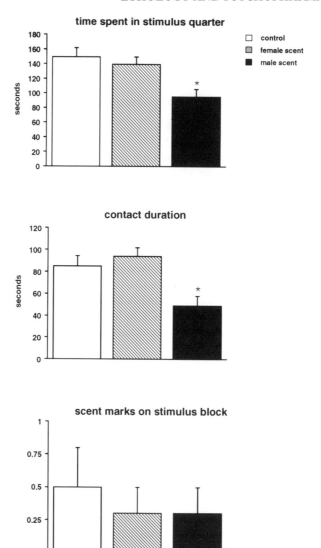

Figure 10 Comparison of the effects of male and female scent on behaviour in the territorial avoidance apparatus. Data are expressed as mean values (± standard error). *$p < 0.05$ versus control (no scent).

reported for male ferrets in a semi-natural outdoor enclosure during springtime (Clapperton, 1989).

While frequency of scent marks did not differ significantly for vehicle-treated groups exposed to control or male scent conditions (again possibly due to a floor effect), frequency of scent-marking was dose-dependently increased

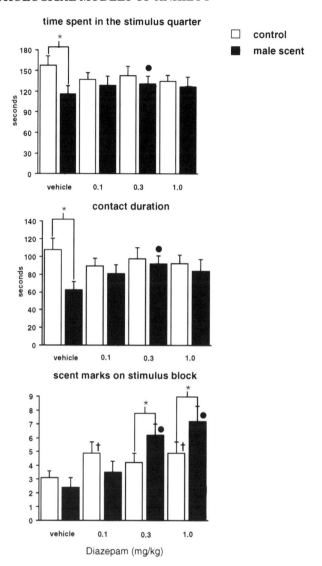

Figure 11 Effect of diazepam on behavioural response to unfamiliar male scent in the territorial avoidance apparatus. Data are expressed as mean values (± standard error). $*p < 0.05$ versus control (no scent); $\bullet p < 0.05$ versus vehicle scent-exposed; $\dagger p < 0.05$ versus vehicle control (no scent).

by diazepam pretreatment (0.3 and 1.0 mg/kg: $p < 0.05$ or less, versus vehicle) in the presence of an unfamiliar male scent. Although scent-marking on the control block was also significantly increased at 0.1 and 1.0 mg/kg diazepam, perhaps suggesting a non-specific increase in activity, it should be noted that there was a significant increase in scent-marking between scent-exposed and unscented control conditions at 1.0 mg/kg. Thus, the fact that a higher level of scent-marking was induced following diazepam pretreatment when the subject was confronted with another male's 'territory' would support the validity and social/ecological relevance of this measure as an index of anxiolysis. Alternatively, it may have been the case that the control condition was not completely free of odour from a previous trial, despite attempts to clean and deodorize the apparatus. Further studies will again assist to elucidate this point.

Discussion

These studies have attempted to model the phenomenon of territorial avoidance previously observed in natural and quasi-natural situations (Powell, 1979; Moors and Lavers, 1981; Clapperton, 1989). The results obtained so far suggest that this behaviour can indeed be modelled in the laboratory ferret. Thus, unfamiliar male scent produced a behavioural profile consistent with proxemic avoidance in relation to the scent block. Importantly, this response was consistent and robust over several trials, suggesting the biologically relevant nature of the model. Similarly, studies using female scent indicated that these observations were associated with a specific avoidance of unfamiliar male conspecific odour.

Initial studies suggest that pretreatment with the reference benzodiazepine anxiolytic, diazepam, attenuated territorial avoidance and released the inhibition of scent-marking in the presence of opponent odour, an action associated with dominance and/or increased aggression. Ongoing studies will further validate the pharmacological sensitivity of this response.

SUMMARY

In this chapter we have described two examples which illustrate the utility of ethology in behavioural pharmacology. Human anxiety disorders involve cognitive, affective and behavioural elements. The theoretical paradox in attempting to produce a model of this pathological state in healthy, non-human species is self-evident. Therefore, the only available compromise lies in the development of a model which provides an analogue of human anxiety disorder in animals. Such a model must be considered analogous not only due to obvious species differences, but also due to the adaptive, rather than pathological nature of the behaviour under observation. It is with this goal and with these limitations in mind that the application of ethology is best appreciated.

As a consequence of natural selection, species-specific behaviours have evolved to enable the organism to respond adaptively to 'stressful' environmental stimuli. Clearly, a stimulus which constitutes a stressor to one species may be innocuous to another, and this relationship will be determined by such factors as social organization and the position of the animal in the food chain, i.e. number and nature of predators in the natural habitat. In this context, the feral rat is subject to a high level of predatorial threat and the adaptive aversion to open unprotected spaces, and complementary thigmotaxis and risk assessment behaviour observed in the elevated zero-maze reflect this vulnerability in the laboratory animal. Similarly, maintenance of intrasexual territoriality provides the basis of an important adaptive behavioural repertoire in the feral ferret. The present model has reproduced this phenomenon within the laboratory environment with promising results.

REFERENCES

Barnett, S.A. (1966) *The Rat: A Study in Behavior*. Aldine, Chicago, IL.

Barrett, J.E. and Gleeson, S. (1991) Anxiolytic effects of 5-HT$_{1A}$ agonists, 5-HT$_3$ antagonists and benzodiazepines: conflict and drug discrimination studies. In: *5-HT$_{1A}$ Agonists, 5-HT$_3$ Antagonists and Benzodiazepines: Their Comparative Behavioural Pharmacology* (eds R.J. Rodgers and S.J. Cooper). Wiley, Chichester, pp. 59–105.

Benjamin, D., Lal, H. and Meyerson, L.R. (1990) The effects of 5-HT$_{1B}$ characterizing agents in the mouse elevated plus-maze. *Life Sci.*, **47**, 195–203.

Blanchard, D.C. and Blanchard, R.J. (1988) Ethoexperimental approaches to the biology of emotion. *Annu. Rev. Psychol.*, **39**, 43–68.

Blanchard, D.C., Weatherspoon, A., Shepherd, J.K. and Rodgers, R.J. (1991) 'Paradoxical' effects of morphine on antipredator defense reactions in wild and laboratory (*R. norvegicus*) rats. *Pharmacol. Biochem. Behav.*, **40**, 819–828.

Blanchard, R.J., Blanchard, D.C. and Hori, K. (1989) An ethoexperimental approach to the study of defense. In: *Ethoexperimental Approaches to the Study of Behaviour* (eds R.J. Blanchard, P.F. Brain, D.C. Blanchard and S. Parmigiani). Kluwer, Dordecht, pp. 114–136.

Blanchard, R.J., Blanchard, D.C., Weiss, S.M. and Meyer, S. (1990) The effects of ethanol and diazepam on reactions to predatory odors. *Pharmacol. Biochem. Behav.*, **35**, 775–780.

Brammer, N., Ennis, C. and Minchin, M.C.W. (1993) [^{3}H]-Serotonin binding to 5-HT$_{1D}$ receptors in the ferret cortex. *Neuroscience, Meetings Abstract* 481.14.

Clapperton, B.K. (1989) Scent-marking behaviour of the ferret, *Mustela furo* L. *Anim. Behav.*, **38**, 436–446.

Clapperton, B.K., Minot, E.O, and Crump, D.R. (1988) An olfactory recognition system in the ferret *Mustela furo* L. (Carnivora: Mustelidae). *Anim. Behav.*, **36**, 541–553.

Cole, J.C. and Rodgers, R.J. (1994) An ethological analysis of the effects of chlordiazepoxide and bretazenil (Ro 16–6028) in the murine elevated plus-maze. *Behav. Pharmacol.*, **4**, 573–580.

Costall, B. and Naylor, R.J. (1991) Anxiolytic effects of 5-HT$_3$ antagonists in animals. In: *5-HT$_{1A}$ Agonists, 5-HT$_3$ Antagonists and Benzodiazepines: Their Comparative Behavioural Pharmacology* (eds R.J. Rodgers and S.J. Cooper). Wiley, Chichester, pp. 133–157.

Costall, B., Kelly, M.E., Tomkins, D.M. and Tyers, M.B. (1989) Profile of action of diazepam and 5-HT$_3$ receptor antagonists in the elevated X-maze. *J. Psychopharmacol.*, **3**, 10P.

Critchley, M.A.E. and Handley, S.L. (1987) Effects in the X-maze anxiety model of agents acting at 5-HT$_1$ and 5-HT$_2$ receptors. *Psychopharmacology*, 93, 502–506.

Critchley, M.A.E., Njung'e, K. and Handley, S.L. (1992) Actions and some interactions of 5-HT$_{1A}$ ligands in the elevated X-maze and effects of dorsal raphe lesions. *Psychopharmacology*, 106, 484–490.

Dourish, C.T. (1987) Brain 5-HT$_{1A}$ receptors and anxiety. In: *Brain 5-HT$_{1A}$ Receptors* (eds C.T. Dourish, S. Ahlenius and P.H. Hutson). Ellis Horwood, Chichester, pp. 261–277

Dunn, R.W., Corbett, R. and Fielding, S. (1989) Effects of 5-HT$_{1A}$ receptor agonists and NMDA receptor antagonists in the social interaction test and the elevated plus-maze. *Eur. J. Pharmacol.*, 169, 1–10.

Falter, U., Gower, A.J. and Gobert, J. (1992) Resistance of baseline activity in the elevated plus-maze to exogenous influences. *Behav. Pharmacol.*, 3, 123–128.

File, S.E. and Johnston, A.J. (1989) Lack of effects of 5-HT$_3$ receptor antagonists in the social interaction and elevated plus-maze tests of anxiety in the rat. *Psychopharmacology*, 99, 248–251.

Gosling, L.M. (1982) A reassessment of the function of scent marking in territories. *Z. Tierpsychol.*, 60, 89–118.

Grant, E.C. and Mackintosh, J.H. (1963) A comparison of the social postures of some common laboratory rodents. *Behaviour*, 21, 246–259.

Griebel, G., Misslin, R., Pawlowski, M. and Vogel, E. (1991) *m*-Chlorophenylpiperazine enhances neophobic and anxious behaviour in mice. *Neuroreport*, 2, 627–629.

Grossen, N.E. and Kelley, M.J. (1973) Species-specific behavior and acquisition of avoidance behavior in rats. *J. Comp. Physiol. Psychol.*, 81, 307–310.

Handley, S.L. and Mithani, S. (1984) Effects of alpha-adrenoceptor agonists and antagonists in a maze-exploration model of 'fear'-motivated behaviour. *Naunyn Schmiedebergs Arch. Pharmacol.*, 327, 1–5.

Handley, S.L. and McBlane, J.W. (1993) 5HT drugs in animal models of anxiety. *Psychopharmacology*, 112, 13–20.

Kaesermann, H.P. (1986) Stretched attend posture, a non-social form of ambivalence, is sensitive to a conflict-reducing drug action. *Psychopharmacology*, 89, 31–37.

Kaesermann, H.P. and Dixon, A.K. (1986) Further validation of the stretched attend posture test, a simple behavioral conflict test in mice. *Psychopharmacology*, 89, S19.

Kahn, R.S. and Wetzler, S. (1991) *m*-Chlorophenylpiperazine as a probe of serotonin function. *Biol. Psychiatry*, 30, 1139–1166.

Kennett, G.A. and Curzon, G. (1988) Evidence that mCPP may have behavioural effects mediated by central 5-HT$_{1C}$ receptors. *Br. J. Pharmacol.*, 94, 137–147.

Kennett, G.A. Whitton, P., Shah, K. and Curzon, G. (1989) Anxiogenic-like effects of mCPP and TFMPP in animal models are opposed by 5-HT$_{1C}$ receptor antagonists. *Eur. J. Pharmacol.*, 164, 445–454.

Klint, T. (1991) Effects of 8-OH-DPAT and buspirone in a passive avoidance test and in the elevated plus-maze test in rats. *Behav. Pharmacol.*, 2, 481–489.

Lee, C. and Rodgers, R.J. (1990) Antinociceptive effects of elevated plus-maze exposure: influence of opiate receptor manipulations. *Psychopharmacology*, 102, 507–513.

Lister, R.G. (1987) The use of a plus-maze to measure anxiety in the mouse. *Psychopharmacology*, 92, 180–185.

Lister, R.G. (1990) Ethologically based animal models of anxiety disorders. *Pharmacol. Ther.*, 46, 321–340.

Montgomery, K.C. (1955) The relation between fear induced by novel stimulation and exploratory behaviour. *J. Comp. Physiol. Psychol.*, 48, 254–260.

Moors, P.J. and Lavers, R.B. (1981) Movements and home ranges of ferrets (*Mustela furo*) at Pukepuke Lagoon, New Zealand. *NZ J. Zool.*, 8, 413–423.

Moser, P.C. (1989) An evaluation of the elevated plus-maze test using the novel anxiolytic buspirone. *Psychopharmacology*, 99, 48–53.

Moser, P.C., Tricklebank, M.D., Middlemiss, D.N. *et al.* (1990) Characterization of MDL 7300EF as a 5-HT$_{1A}$ selective ligand and its effects in animal models of anxiety: comparison with buspirone 8-OH-DPAT and diazepam. *Br. J. Pharmacol.*, 99 343–349.

Pellow, S. and File, S.E. (1986) Anxiolytic and anxiogenic drug effects on exploratory activity in an elevated plus-maze: a novel test of anxiety in the rat. *Pharmacol. Biochem. Behav.*, 24, 525–529.

Pellow, S., Chopin, P., File, S.E. and Briley, M. (1985) Validation of open:closed arm entries in an elevated plus-maze as a measure of anxiety in the rat. *J. Neurosci. Methods*, 14, 149–167.

Pellow, S., Johnston, A.L. and File, S.E. (1987) Selective agonists and antagonists for 5-hydroxytryptamine receptor subtypes, and interactions with yohimbine and FG 7142 using the elevated plus-maze test in the rat. *J. Pharm. Pharmacol.*, 39, 917–928.

Pollard, G.T. and Howard, J.L. (1988) Effects of chlordiazepoxide, pentobarbital, buspirone, chlorpromazine, and morphine in the stretched attend posture (SAP) test. *Psychopharmacology*, 94, 433–444.

Poole, T.B. (1967) Aspects of aggressive behaviour in polecats. *Z. Tierpsychol.*, 24, 351–369.

Powell, R.A. (1979) Mustelid spacing patterns: variations on a theme by *Mustela*. *Z. Tierpsychol.*, 50 153–165.

Rodgers, R.J. (1991) A step in the right direction: comment on '5-HT and mechanisms of defence'. *J. Psychopharm.*, 5, 316–319.

Rodgers, R.J., Cole, J.C., Cobain, M.R. *et al.* (1992a) Anxiogenic-like effects of fluprazine and eltoprazine in the mouse elevated plus-maze: profile comparisons with 8-OH-DPAT, CGS12066B, TFMPP and mCPP. *Behav. Pharmacol.*, 3, 621–634.

Rodgers, R.J., Lee, C. and Shepherd, J.K. (1992b) Effects of diazepam on behavioural and antinociceptive responses to the elevated plus-maze in male mice depend upon treatment regimen and prior maze experience. *Psychopharmacology*, 106, 102–110.

Russell, P.A. (1973) Relationships between exploratory behaviour and fear: a review. *Br. J. Psychol.*, 64, 417–433.

Shepherd, J.K. (1992) Preliminary evaluation of an elevated 'zero-maze' as a model of anxiety in laboratory rats. *J. Psychopharm.*, 6, A56, 223.

Shepherd, J.K., Flores, T., Rodgers, R.J. and Blanchard, R.J. (1992) The anxiety/defense test battery: influence of gender and ritanserin treatment on antipredator defensive behavior. *Physiol Behav.*, 51, 277–285.

Shepherd, J.K. Grewal, S.S., Fletcher, A. *et al.* (1993) Pharmacological evaluation of the elevated 'zero-maze' as a model of anxiety in rats. *Br. J. Pharmacol.*, 110, 13P.

Shepherd, J.K., Grewal, S.S., Fletcher, A. *et al.* (1994) Behavioural and pharmacological characterization of the elevated 'zero-maze' as an animal model of anxiety. *Psychopharmacology* (in press).

Soderpalm, S., Hjorth, S. and Engel, J.A. (1989) Effects of 5-HT$_{1A}$ receptor agonists and L-5-HTP in Montgomery's conflict test. *Pharmacol. Biochem. Behav.*, 32, 259–265.

Suzuki, T., Inayama, M. and Misawa, M. (1990) The effect of diazepam on exploratory behavior and its strain differences in inbred rats. *Jpn. J. Psychopharmacol.*, 10, 307–314.

Tomkins, D.M., Costall, B. and Kelly, M.E. (1990) Release of suppressed behaviour of rats on the elevated X-maze by 5-HT$_3$ antagonists injected into the basolateral amygdala. *J. Psychopharmacol.*, 4, 262.

Treit, D. (1991) Anxiolytic effects of benzodiazepines and 5-HT$_{1A}$ agonists: animal models. In: *5-HT$_{1A}$ Agonists, 5-HT$_3$ Antagonists and Benzodiazepines: Their Comparative Behavioural Pharmacology* (eds R.J. Rodgers and S.J. Cooper). Wiley, Chichester, pp. 107–131.

Treit, D. and Fundytus, M. (1988) Thigmotaxis as a test for anxiolytic activity in rats. *Pharmacol. Biochem. Behav.*, **31**, 958–962.

Treit, D., Menard, J. and Royan, C. (1993) Anxiogenic stimuli in the elevated plus-maze. *Pharmacol. Biochem. Behav.*, **44**, 463–469.

Upton, N. and Blackburn, T.P. (1991) Anxiolytic-like activity of the selective 5-HT$_3$ receptor antagonist, BRL 46470A, in the rat elevated X-maze. *Br. J. Pharmacol.*, **102**, 253P.

Van der Poel, A.M. (1979) A note on "stretched attention", a behavioural element indicative of an approach–avoidance conflict in rats. *Anim. Behav.*, **27**, 446–450.

Vasar, E., Peuranen, E., Oopok, T. *et al.* (1993) Ondansetron, an antagonist of 5-HT$_3$ receptors, antagonises the anti-exploratory effect of caerulein, an agonist of CCK receptors, in the elevated plus-maze. *Pychopharmacology*, **110**, 213–218.

Wilkinson, L.O. and Dourish, C.T. (1991) Serotonin and animal behaviour. In: *Serotonin Receptor Subtypes: Basic and Clinical Aspects* (ed. S.J. Peroutka). Liss, New York, pp. 149–212.

Wright, I.K., Heaton, M., Upton, N. and Marsden, C.A. (1992) Comparison of acute and chronic treatment of various serotonergic agents with those of diazepam and idazoxan in the rat elevated X-maze. *Psychopharmacology*, **107**, 405–414.

5 Prediction of Antidepressant Activity from Ethological Analysis of Agonistic Behaviour in Rats

PAUL J. MITCHELL
Department of Neuropharmacology, Wyeth Research (UK) Ltd, Taplow, Maidenhead, UK

INTRODUCTION

Antidepressants and animal models of depressive illness

Following the introduction of the monoamine oxidase inhibitors (MAOIs) and tricyclic antidepressants (TCAs) for the treatment of depressive illness in the 1950s (see Coppen, 1967; Kline and Cooper, 1980) various drug-screening tests have been developed to help identify novel compounds with potential antidepressant activity (Willner, 1985). The majority of the early screening tests (e.g. potentiation of the behavioural effects of L-dopa or amphetamine, or reversal of the behavioural effects of 5-hydroxytryptophan (5-HTP) or reserpine) were based entirely on the acute effects of antidepressants available at the time. Thus, while the predictive validity of these tests is apparently high, both their face validity and construct validity as models of depressive illness are highly questionable (Willner, 1985). Hence, the utility of these tests is strictly limited to the identification of 'me-too' drugs.

More recently, a number of animal models have been developed which better address the theoretical requirements of a good model of depressive illness. Such models (e.g. learned helplessness, behavioural despair, chronic unpredictable stress) possess potential construct validity with regard to depressive illness (Willner, 1985). At the present time, the learned helplessness and behavioural despair models are probably the most common behavioural models used to identify potential antidepressant activity (Danysz *et al.*, 1991; Willner, 1991). While these animal models are arguably superior to the pharmacological screening test, doubts have been expressed regarding certain aspects of their use both in terms of their ability to accurately predict antidepressant drug activity and as animal models of depressive illness.

Ethology and Psychopharmacology. Edited by S.J. Cooper and C.A. Hendrie
© 1994 John Wiley & Sons Ltd

For example, the questionable pharmacological specificity of the learned helplessness model (see Porsolt et al., 1991) raises doubts about the predictive validity of this model (Willner, 1985). Moreover, the relationship between the helpless behaviour exhibited by rodents and depressive illness is unclear, which questions this model's face validity (Willner, 1985). The predictive validity of the behavioural despair test is also limited (Willner, 1985) since this model identifies both false positives and false negatives (Porsolt et al., 1991). Furthermore, both models, and also the screening tests referred to above, respond both to acute and/or subchronic drug treatments and therefore do not correspond to the latency for clinical efficacy experienced with antidepressant drugs (Eisen, 1989; Khan et al., 1989; Oswald et al., 1972). Thus, although there have been clear advances in the animal models used to identify potential antidepressant activity, even models with greater apparent construct validity to depressive illness still fail in terms of their predictive validity (i.e. pharmacological specificity) or face validity (i.e. relationship of observed behaviour to depressive illness, sensitivity to acute drug treatment).

We have taken a fundamentally different approach to the problem of identifying the antidepressant activity of psychotropic compounds. We have based our work on an ethological analysis of rodent social behaviour.

Rationale for models based on rodent social behaviour

The ethological studies of Dixon and co-workers (Dixon et al., 1989) have shown that increased flight and impaired sociability are significant features of the non-verbal behaviour of patients with depressive illness. Clinical studies also indicate that such abnormal behavioural responses/reactions of patients with depressive illness to environmental and social stimulation are progressively modified during remission from the illness (Eisen, 1989; Khan et al., 1989; Oswald et al., 1972). Thus recovery from a depressive episode is associated with progressively reduced self-criticism and feelings of guilt (Priest et al., 1980) which leads to increased physical and/or verbal interaction with the environment or social events (Kaplan et al., 1961). The reversal of impaired sociability may therefore prove to be an important index of the recovery process from depressive illness. The ability of antidepressant treatments to modify the behavioural responses/reactions of patients with depression has generally been ignored in the search for a definitive animal model of depressive illness. The resident–intruder studies described below were designed to determine whether antidepressant treatments modify the social and agonistic behaviour patterns of experimental animals in ways that may be related to their ability to modify human reactive behaviour. The experimental paradigm relies exclusively upon the concepts and techniques of ethological analysis of rodent social and agonistic behaviour since ethology provides a method of precise and quantitative assessment of natural animal behaviour.

Ethology: historical perspectives, techniques and concepts

Ethology (defined as the science or study of the function and evolution of animal behaviour) is typically concerned with the analysis of natural action patterns of animal behaviour in a natural environment, and early studies of wild animals examined how such behaviour contributed to the survival of both the species in general and the individual animal in particular (e.g. Tinbergen, 1960). It was only during the late 1950s and early 1960s that the utility of natural action patterns in the study of both the behaviour of laboratory animals *per se* and the behavioural effects of drugs was first recognized by Michael Chance, Ewen Grant, John Mackintosh and Paul Silverman at the Ethology Laboratory, University of Birmingham. Their publications (e.g. Chance and Silverman, 1964; Grant, 1963; Grant and Chance, 1958; Grant and Mackintosh, 1963: Silverman, 1965) have become landmarks in the development of ethological techniques in behavioural pharmacology. Even so, it is only within the last 10–15 years that behavioural pharmacologists have capitalized on ethological techniques to study the behaviour of laboratory animals, and it is no coincidence that the increasing use of ethological techniques in behavioural pharmacology has occurred with the rapid advances in computer technology to facilitate data recording and analysis.

The ethogram

An ethogram is a behavioural catalogue of identifiable behavioural elements that closely approximates the complete repertoire of behaviours or postures exhibited by a given species under a variety of environmental conditions.

The classic paper by Grant and Mackintosh (1963) described and classified the various elements of non-social, social and agonistic behaviour that comprise the behavioural repertoires of a number of laboratory rodents (i.e. mouse, rat, guinea-pig, golden hamster), and ethograms described in the majority of subsequent ethopharmacological experiments on laboratory rodents have predominantly been derived from this paper. An ethogram listing the behavioural elements exhibited by laboratory rats is shown in Table 1, which has been adapted from Grant (1963), and Grant and Mackintosh (1963). These publications also demonstrated how, firstly, the various behavioural elements for a given species fall into behavioural pathways, indicating an inherent progression from one behaviour or posture to the next, and, secondly, that these behaviours may be grouped according to the motivational category in which they occur (see Figure 1).

The ethogram thus provides the foundation from which the behaviour of laboratory animals may be qualitatively measured. There are four important points to note here: firstly, observation and analysis of all the observable components of behaviour increases the chance of detecting unexpected changes

Table 1 Summary of the various elements of rat behaviour, grouped according to motivational category, expressed during social encounters. Adapted from Grant (1963)

Motivational category	Element	Description/comment
Exploration	Locomotion	Orientation to the physical environment with ambulation
	Rearing	As locomotion but static and upright
Investigation and mating	Approach	Directed locomotion towards the other rat
	Follow	Approach when the conspecific moves away
	Stretched attention	Elongation of the body extending the head towards the conspecific
	To–fro	Rapid ambulation away from (retreat) and toward (approach) the other rat
	Walk round/circle/side	Movement broadside to the conspecific
	Nose and investigate	Orientation to the other rat's head and body
	Attempt mount	Incomplete or disorientated mount
	Mount	Full male sexual activity, as full as possible between males
	Sniff genitalia	Orientation to the conspecific's genitalia
	Tail rattle	Beating movement of the tail
Aggression	Aggressive groom	As aggressive posture with nibbling of the conspecific's fur (the latter in a submit, crouch or elevated crouch posture)
	Aggressive posture	Head over and at 90° to the conspecific which is in the submit, crouch or elevated crouch posture
	Attack	Rapidly to and partly over the conspecific
	Bite	Seizing the skin of the conspecific but rarely penetrating
	Offensive sideways	Broadside approach with head orientated towards the conspecific
	Offensive upright	On hind legs with head orientated towards the conspecific
	Pull	As bite but then moving backwards
	Threat/thrust	Head and body rapidly orientated towards the conspecific
Flight–submit	Defensive sideways	Broadside stance with the ventral surface rotated to the conspecific but with the head orientated away from the other rat
	Defensive upright	On hind legs facing the conspecific (as offensive upright) but the head is orientated away from the conspecific
	Submit	Lies flat on back with ventral surface towards the conspecific

Table 1 Continued

Motivational category	Element	Description/comment
Flight–escape	Attend	Orientation directed towards the other rat, often with crouch
	Crouch	On all four paws with shoulders lowered, sometimes with one forepaw raised. The hind legs may be extended
	Elevated crouch	As crouch but on hind legs with forepaws on the wall of the cage. May be envisaged as crouch with rear
	Flag and evade	Head and forebody turned away from the conspecific, sometimes followed by a rapid movement away (retreat)
	Retreat	Rapid movement away from the conspecific usually to a place of safety
	Under food hopper	Place to retreat to
Maintenance	Digging	Burrow into the sawdust on the floor of the cage
	Drinking	Self-explanatory
	Eating	Self-explanatory
	Licking	Licks own body fur
	Lick penis	Self-explanatory. Invariably follows attempt mount or mount
	Scratching	Scratch own body fur usually with hind limbs
	Shaking	Wriggles body
	Washing	Wipe face with licked forepaws

Reproduced from Mitchell and Redfern (1992a) by kind permission from Elsevier Science Ltd, The Boulevard, Langford Lane, Kidlington OX5 1GB, UK.

in behaviour and may reveal important potentially useful or dangerous behavioural effects of drugs. The sensitivity of ethological analysis enables even subtle effects of drugs on animal behaviour, which may be missed by more traditional experimental paradigms, to be readily identified and quantified.

Secondly, evaluation of the changes in either concomitant behaviours or the association between sequential behaviours (as determined by cluster analysis, Jones and Brain, 1985) may reveal the selectivity of drug effects on behaviour.

Thirdly, the awareness that no single behavioural element can be understood without reference to the complete dynamic structure of behaviour is inherent in the ethological approach (Dixon, 1982). For example, laboratory rats frequently exhibit grooming behaviour when quiescent. However, grooming may also be indicative of displacement behaviour, implying motivational conflict (Bastock et al., 1953), when, for example, the subject is uncertain whether to display aggressive or flight behaviour in response to the aggressive behaviour of a conspecific. The role or function of grooming behaviour may

90

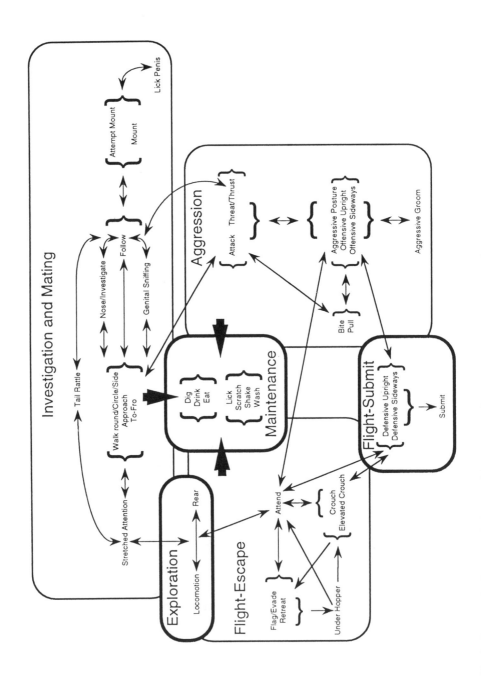

therefore only be understood in the context of the overall behaviour of the subject.

Finally, the limitations of ethologically based studies of animal behaviour are not the various behaviours exhibited by the subject(s), but primarily the behaviours that the observer can identify and record. Thus the accuracy and ultimate value of ethological analysis are dependent on the observer's skill and experience.

Ethologically obtained measures provide a wide profile of meaningful behaviours that are relevant to the survival of the species. Ethological techniques require extensive training of the observer and are very time consuming, but such disadvantages are clearly outweighed by the accuracy, sensitivity and detail of the behavioural profiles obtained.

METHODOLOGICAL CONSIDERATIONS

A major problem in observing animal behaviour, especially when using social behaviour as a pharmacological tool, is to ensure that the subject animals perform at an intensity and at the time required by the experimenter. The environment plays a very important role in determining which behaviours a given species is predisposed to display. Lighting conditions (File and Hyde, 1978), social experience and familiarity of partner(s) (Bolles and Woods, 1964; Einon et al., 1978; File and Pope, 1974; Latane, 1969), familiarity of experimental arena (File and Hyde, 1978), territorial advantage (Barnett, 1975; Latane, 1969) and hierarchical position within a closed social group (Gentsch et al., 1988; Koolhaas et al., 1980) all affect the social behaviour of rats (for discussion see Mitchell, 1993).

General experimental conditions

Rats are nocturnal. The circadian locomotor activity expressed throughout a 12 h:12 h light–dark cycle demonstrates that while rats are generally quiescent during the light phase, activity occurs immediately at the onset of the dark phase and lasts until the onset of the subsequent light phase (Figure 2). To identify and record as many behaviours and postures from a subject's behavioural repertoire as possible observations should be made when the subjects are at their most active. For nocturnal animals observations during the dark phase of the light–dark cycle are clearly warranted. In the studies described here all animals were housed under reverse-daylight conditions from weaning for at

---

Figure 1   Simplified schematic representation of the pathways of non-social, social and agonistic behaviour of the rat. The individual behaviours or postures are grouped according to motivational category (see Table 1 for description of each element). Arrows indicate the normal progression of behavioural elements, while the large arrow-heads indicate displacement activity. (Adapted from Grant, 1963; reproduced from Mitchell, 1993, by permission of the Institute of Animal Technology.)

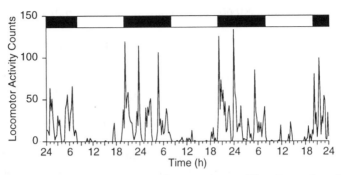

Figure 2 Circadian locomotor activity of grouped rats ($N = 3$) monitored continuously over 72 h. The x-axis indicates time in hours (24 h clock). Rats were housed under a 12 h/12 h light–dark cycle (lights on 0800). Black bands indicate the dark period of the light–dark cycle. The y-axis indicates locomotor activity counts per 15 min epoch. Locomotor activity was recorded continuously by infrared photo cell units, positioned in the wall of the cage, linked to a microcomputer. (Reproduced from Mitchell, 1993, by permission of the Institute of Animal Technology.)

least five weeks before the start of each experiment to allow full entrainment to the reverse-daylight cycle. Furthermore, all experiments were performed during the dark phase when rats are most active.

The structure of social behaviour in a number of different orders of vertebrates is dependent on the agonistic behaviour appropriate to the antagonism between males. When male laboratory rats are housed in closed groups such behaviour arranges the males in order of rank (Chance and Silverman, 1964). The respective rank position of each group member is related to the level of aggressive behaviour exhibited by each rat when they are initially housed together. Thus higher aggressors achieve higher rank positions. Generally, the social hierarchy develops over a period of about two to three weeks, but once established both the hierarchical structure and the level of aggressive behaviour exhibited by each group member remain essentially constant (Grant and Chance, 1958). Furthermore, a rat's rank position appears to be maintained through success in social and agonistic encounters with the cage partners (Koolhaas *et al.*, 1980). In the resident–intruder paradigm, all animals were housed in closed social groups for at least three weeks prior to and throughout each experiment. This not only allowed the development and maintenance of a stable social hierarchy in each group but also provided constancy of social experience from the same time point following weaning (Bolles and Woods, 1964; Einon *et al.*, 1978; Latane, 1969).

Resident–intruder paradigm

Both domesticated and in-bred strains of male rats exhibit agonistic behaviour to defend their territory when confronted with an unfamiliar intruder conspecific (Barnett, 1975). The term 'agonistic behaviour', first used by Scott (1958), refers to the spectrum of conflict-related behaviours, including not only aggressive behaviours, but also the elements indicative of escape, defence and submission. In Table 1, these elements are grouped according to the motivational categories aggression, flight–escape and flight–submit. Even under certain laboratory conditions the agonistic behaviour of in-bred laboratory rats contains all the behavioural elements of the agonistic behaviour of wild rats (Blanchard *et al.*, 1975). If two rats are placed in a neutral environment where neither rat has a territorial advantage, then very few aggressive episodes will be observed, even if the active contact is quite intense (Latane, 1969). In contrast, if an unfamiliar intruder conspecific is introduced into the home cage of an isolated resident rat, then intense social and agonistic behaviour will ensue. Such social and agonistic behaviour is initiated predominantly by the resident rat and is indicative of the degree of territorial advantage enjoyed by the resident rat over the intruder. The territorial advantage is even apparent after the resident rat has been singly housed for only a few days. Figure 3 summarizes the behavioural profiles of both resident and intruder male Wistar rats observed during such encounters. The predominant behaviour of the resident rat is investigation of the intruder which frequently progresses into aggression. In response, the intruder rat displays high levels of flight behaviour (i.e. flight–escape and flight–submit). In these studies, the resident and intruder rats were obtained from different parental groups to ensure that all social encounters were between rats which were unfamiliar to each other. The resident rats were isolated before each experimental day (to provide territorial advantage) and returned to the social group immediately

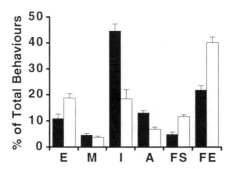

Figure 3   Behavioural profiles of resident rats (black columns) and intruder rats (white columns) exhibited during social encounters performed under low-intensity (2 lux) red light during the dark phase of the light–dark cycle. Both resident and intruder rats were unfamiliar to each other and had been housed in groups of four for at least five weeks since weaning. The resident rats were housed individually for three days before the social encounter, whereupon an intruder rat was placed in the cage and the social behaviour recorded on videotape. Data were grouped according to motivational category as indicated in the text. E, exploration; M, maintenance; I, investigation; A, aggression; FS, flight–submit; FE, flight–escape. $\chi^2 = 1568$, d.f. = 5, $p < 0.0001$.

following each social encounter (to re-establish each group member's rank position within the social hierarchy), while the intruder animals were housed in social groups throughout. Furthermore, social encounters were performed in familiar conditions (i.e. standard laboratory polypropylene cages) so that the experimental environment was not aversive to the subjects, thereby promoting the expression of agonistic behaviour (File and Hyde, 1978; File and Pope, 1974; Latane, 1969).

Initially the effect of acute drug treatment was determined to identify the minimum effective dose of each drug on the social behaviour of the resident rats when confronted with an unknown intruder conspecific. To examine the effects of chronic treatment, each drug was administered at the minimum effective dose when given acutely, but over 24 h via subcutaneously (s.c.) implanted osmotic mini pumps. The use of mini pumps obviates the need for repeated handling of the subjects which itself may modify the subsequent social and agonistic behaviour of rodents. In order to follow any progressive changes in the social behaviour of rats associated with chronic treatment of psychotropic drug, all animals were repeat-tested during the course of each experiment. It is accepted that previous social experience may help determine subsequent social behaviour in an agonistic situation (Baenninger, 1974; Bolhuis et al., 1984). However, the advantages of observing progressive drug-induced changes in the behaviour of the same animal may outweigh the disadvantages of conditioning associated with repeat-testing regimes. For consistency, animals used in the initial acute treatment studies were also repeat-tested (where the subjects received a different dose on each occasion) to ensure that the social experience of these animals was similar to that of the animals used in the chronic drug treatment studies.

The effect of psychotropic drugs on social behaviour may depend on the social position of the treated subject (File and Pope, 1974; Raleigh et al., 1985). If the social position of an animal predetermines that animal's response to psychotropic drugs then a significant contribution to 'biological variation' or 'experimental error' may reflect the differential responses of animals in various social positions. Indeed, Silverman (1965) argued the case for using stable social groups in behavioural experiments. This is especially important in acute drug studies since repeat-testing schedules ensure the various rank positions are spread equally throughout all treatment groups. Previous studies (Mitchell and Redfern, 1992b) have also demonstrated that chronic drug treatments (administered to a single rat in a social group) which modify rodent social and agonistic behaviour also modify the hierarchical structure of the group. In closed social groups of rats, therefore, chronic administration of the various group members with different treatments (i.e. drug vehicle and various doses of drug) which differentially modify the social and agonistic behaviour of rodents would ultimately be reflected by a disruption of the original hier-archical structure of the group. The only way to minimize these effects in chronic treatment studies (and therefore maintain the original hierarchical structure of grouped rats) is to administer the same dose of drug or drug vehicle to each group member.

RESIDENT–INTRUDER STUDIES

Method

In each study, age-matched male Wistar rats were housed in two groups of eight rats per group (designated 'resident' and 'intruder' respectively). Each group was further subdivided into two groups of four animals at least three weeks prior to the experiment.

In all studies only the resident rats received drug or vehicle. Each group of animals was tested on four occasions on a weekly cycle. Resident rats were isolated for three days prior to each test day and housed individually with food and water available *ad libitum*. At the start of each social encounter test the home cage containing the resident rat was positioned inside the recording cabinet (for details see Mitchell and Redfern, 1992a) for 30 min, following which the relevant intruder conspecific was introduced. The resulting social encounter was recorded on videotape for 10 min under low-intensity (2–4 lux at the cage floor) red light illumination by a video camera positioned above the recording cabinet. At the end of the recording session both resident and intruder rats were returned to their respective group cages.

In the acute drug studies resident rats were injected s.c. with drug or vehicle prior to the social encounter and returned to their home cage. Each study ensured that all resident rats within a particular group received the drug vehicle and three doses of drug and encountered each of the corresponding intruder conspecifics over the four test sessions.

In the chronic drug studies resident rats were tested on the first occasion without any drug or vehicle treatment. The subjects were then anaesthetized and osmotic mini pumps containing drug or vehicle were implanted into an s.c. pocket lying along the midline of the back. Social encounter tests were then performed after seven and 14 days of treatment after which the mini pumps were removed. A final social encouter was performed seven days later. The social encounters were arranged to ensure that each resident rat encountered each of the corresponding intruder conspecifics over the four test sessions.

The occurrence of each behaviour or posture exhibited by the resident and intruder rats during each social encounter was identified and recorded during video playback. The scores for each behaviour/posture were grouped according to their motivational category (see Table 1) for each animal and the total score for each category expressed as a percentage of the total number of behaviours observed for that animal. The data from the two groups of four resident rats were grouped (i.e. $N = 8$ per treatment) and the mean and standard error of the mean (s.e.m.) for both the percentage values of each motivational category and the total number of behaviours/postures observed within each treatment group were calculated. Data for the corresponding intruder groups were treated similarly.

Results and discussion

Compared to vehicle-treated controls, acute treatment of resident rats with either the antidepressant drug clomipramine, 10, 30 and 90 μmol/kg (equivalent to 3.14, 9.41 and 28.4 mg/kg base concentration, respectively), or the anxiolytic drug diazepam, 3.3, 10 and 30 μmol/kg (equivalent to 0.94, 2.85 and 8.54 mg/kg base concentration, respectively), induced a dose-related reduction in aggressive behaviour directed at the conspecific intruder, concomitant with a dose-related increase in flight behaviour (Figure 4). None of the doses of clomipramine examined significantly modified either investigatory behaviour or maintenance behaviour of the resident rats, while the highest dose tested increased exploratory behaviour. The diazepam-induced changes in agonistic behaviour were also associated with reduced exploratory and investigatory behaviour and increased maintenance behaviour. In comparison, the drug-free intruder rats in both drug groups exhibited decreased flight behaviour, generally concomitant with increased exploratory behaviour, that appeared to be related to the doses of drug administered to the resident rats.

Although both clomipramine and diazepam induced similar dose-related changes in the agonistic behaviour of resident rats, the behavioural profiles *per se* provide no indication whether such behavioural changes are due to drug-induced sedation or a selective effect on rodent agonistic behaviour. Comparison of the dose–response curves of clomipramine and diazepam on the aggressive behaviour and total number of behaviours exhibited by resident rats, and also on exploratory locomotor activity (ELA) in a separate group of reverse-daylight entrained rats, demonstrates that while clomipramine markedly reduced aggressive behaviour at doses which had no effect on the total behaviour score or on ELA, diazepam only reduced aggressive behaviour at doses which concomitantly reduced the total behaviour score and ELA (Figure 5). These data indicate that acute treatment with clomipramine has a selective effect on the aggressive behaviour of resident rats, while the behavioural changes induced by acute treatment with diazepam are more likely due to sedation.

Figure 4 The effect of acute treatment with clomipramine and diazepam on the behavioural profiles of drug-treated resident rats (black columns) and non-treated intruder rats (white columns) during social encounters. Values on the y-axis indicate mean ($\pm$ s.e.m.) of the percentage values for each motivational category according to each treatment. On the x-axis V represents drug vehicle while values represent dose (μmol/kg, s.c.). Mann–Whitney U-test: $*p < 0.05$, $**p < 0.01$, $***p < 0.001$ compared to respective vehicle-treated controls. $N = 8$ in all groups. (Reproduced from Mitchell and Redfern, 1992a, by permission of Oxford University Press.)

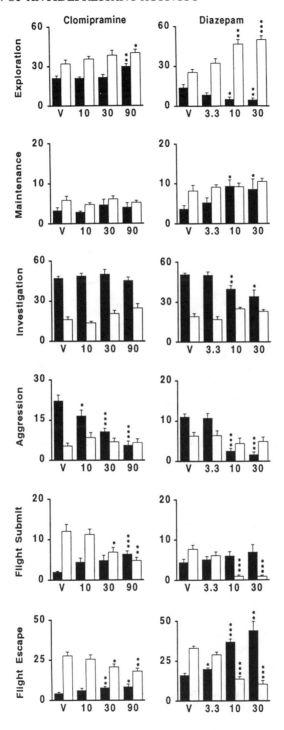

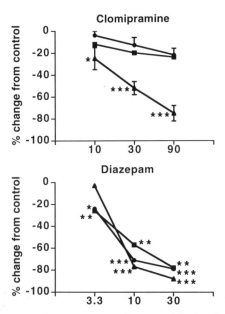

Figure 5   Dose–response curves to acute treatment with clomipramine and diazepam on aggressive behaviour (closed triangles) and total behaviour score (closed circles) exhibited by resident rats during social encounters, and on exploratory locomotor activity (closed squares). Mann–Whitney U-test: $*p < 0.05$, $**p < 0.01$, $***p < 0.001$ compared to respective vehicle-treated controls. For ID_{50} values see Table 2. Where necessary, error bars have been omitted for brevity. (Reproduced from Mitchell and Redfern, 1992a, by permission of the *Journal of Psychopharmacology*.)

Similarly, acute treatment with other antidepressant compounds examined (i.e. fluoxetine, iprindole, mianserin, phenelzine and venlafaxine) also induced a selective reduction in the aggressive behaviour of resident rats (Mitchell and Fletcher, 1993; Mitchell and Redfern, 1992a) (Table 2). In contrast, acute treatment with the antipsychotic drug haloperidol (Table 2) or the 5-HT$_{1A}$ partial agonist, gepirone (Table 2 and Figure 6), only reduced aggression at doses which were either sedative (Mitchell and Redfern, 1992a) or induced components of the 5-HT$_{1A}$ receptor-mediated behavioural syndrome (Mitchell and Forster, 1992), respectively. The close correspondence between the ID_{50} values for haloperidol and diazepam on ELA and the total behaviour score of resident rats (Table 2) suggests that ethological analysis of the behavioural profiles provides an in-built measure of the onset of non-specific behavioural changes, such as the sedation, without recourse to alternative experimental paradigms. Care should be taken, however, when making assumptions about apparent non-specific behavioural changes based on total behaviour scores. The data for gepirone (Figure 6) clearly show that induction of stereotypic behaviours may also markedly reduce the ability of resident rats to exhibit social and agonistic behaviour.

Table 2 Effect of acute treatment with pychotropic drugs on aggressive behaviour and total behaviour score exhibited by resident rats during social encounters, and on exploratory locomotor activity (ELA)

Drug	ID$_{50}$ values (μmol/kg)		
	Aggression	Total behaviours	ELA
Clomipramine[a]	29.5	>90	>90
Fluoxetine[a]	3	>10	>10
Iprindole[a]	3.82	>9	>9
Mianserin[a]	1.19	>3	>3
Phenelzine[a]	5.69	>9	>9
Venlafaxine[b]	24.87	>180	Not tested
Gepirone	4.79	9.45	Not tested
Diazepam[a]	8.73	7.26	8.59
Haloperidol[a]	0.19	0.18	0.18

[a]Data from Mitchell and Redfern (1992a), reproduced by permission of the *Journal of Psychopharmacology*.
[b]Reprinted from Mitchell and Fletcher (1993), with kind permission from Pergamon Press Ltd., Headington Hill Hall, Oxford, OX3 0BW, UK.
Where exact ID$_{50}$ values are not provided the values indicate the highest dose tested.

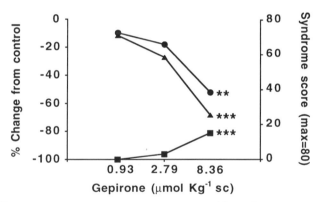

Figure 6 Dose–response curves to acute treatment with gepirone on aggressive behaviour (closed triangles) and total behaviour score (closed circles) exhibited by resident rats during social encounters, and for the induction of the 5-HT$_{1A}$ receptor-mediated behavioural syndrome (closed squares). Mann–Whitney U-test: $^*p < 0.05$, $^{**}p < 0.01$, $^{***}p < 0.001$ compared to respective vehicle-treated controls. For ID$_{50}$ values on aggression and total behaviours see Table 2. Error bars have been omitted for brevity.

Some studies suggest that previous social experience may condition subsequent social behaviour in an agonistic situation (Baenninger, 1974; Bolhuis *et al.*, 1984). However, neither resident rats treated chronically with saline via implanted mini pumps, nor the corresponding non-treated intruder conspecifics, exhibited treatment- or time-dependent changes in their behavioural profile (Figure 7) or total number of behaviours (data not shown) during

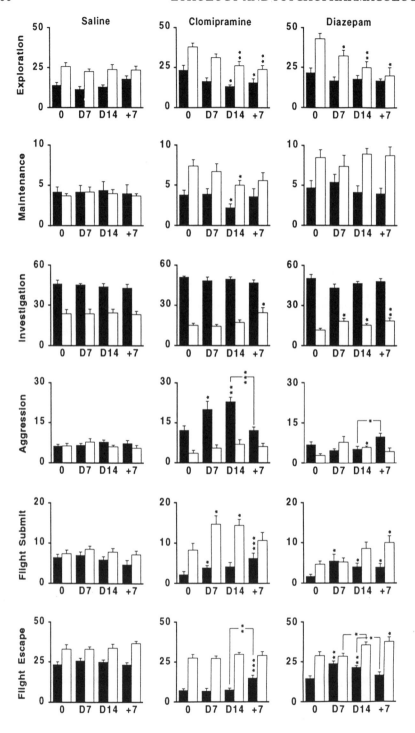

the course of the experiment (Mitchell and Fletcher, 1993). Thus any conditioning effect of social experience appears to have no significant influence on the behavioural profile of either resident or intruder rats subjected to the repeat-testing paradigm.

In contrast, chronic exposure of resident rats to clomipramine, 10 μmol/kg per day s.c. (equivalent to 3.14 mg/kg per day base concentration), increased aggressive behaviour at days 7 and 14 of drug treatment (Figure 7), concomitant with a small increase in flight–submit behaviour (day 7) and reduced exploratory and maintenance behaviour (day 14). By seven days following the removal of the mini pumps the elevated aggressive behaviour had returned to that observed prior to clomipramine treatment, although this was associated with increased flight behaviour. The marked changes in the behavioural profile of clomipramine-treated resident rats was associated with increased flight–submit behaviour and decreased exploratory and maintenance behaviour (day 14) exhibited by the drug-free intruder conspecifics. The other antidepressant drugs examined (i.e. fluoxetine, iprindole, mianserin, phenelzine and venlafaxine) also markedly increased the aggressive behaviour of the resident rats during, but generally not following (phenelzine-treated rats excepted), chronic treatment (Table 3) (Mitchell and Fletcher, 1993; Mitchell and Redfern, 1992a). Interestingly, both electroconvulsive shock (ECS) and the 5-HT_{1A} receptor partial agonist, gepirone, also increased the aggressive behaviour of resident rats (Table 3) during repeated or chronic treatment respectively (Mitchell and Fletcher, 1992; Mitchell and Forster, 1992). Such behavioural changes were generally associated with reduced flight behaviour exhibited by the resident rats, but increased flight behaviour and reduced exploratory behaviour exhibited by the drug-free intruder conspecifics. In comparison, continuous treatment of resident rats with diazepam, 3.3 μmol/kg per day s.c. (equivalent to 0.94 mg/kg per day base concentration), increased flight behaviour but had no significant effect on aggressive behaviour (Figure 7) (Mitchell and Redfern, 1992a). Haloperidol decreased aggressive behaviour and increased exploratory behaviour at day 14 of treatment only (Table 3) (Mitchell and Redfern, 1992a).

The increase in aggressive behaviour induced by chronic treatment of the

---

Figure 7 The effect of chronic treatment with saline (9.72 μl per day), clomipramine (10 μmol/kg per day) and diazepam (3.3 μmol/kg per day), via s.c.-implanted osmotic mini pumps, on the behavioural profiles of drug-treated resident rats (black columns) and non-treated intruder rats (white columns) during social encounters. Values on the y-axis indicate mean ($\pm$ s.e.m.) of the percentage values for each motivational category according to each experimental day. On the x-axis 0 represents day 0 (prior to pump implantation), D7 and D14 indicate days 7 and 14 of treatment, and +7 indicates day 7 following removal of the pumps. Mann–Whitney U-test: $*p < 0.05$, $**p < 0.01$, $***p < 0.001$ compared to day 0 except where indicated. $N = 8$ in all groups. (Saline data reprinted from Mitchell and Fletcher, 1993, with kind permission from Pergamon Press Ltd, Oxford. Clomipramine and diazepam data reproduced from Mitchell and Redfern, 1992a, by permission of the *Journal of Psychopharmacology*.)

Table 3 Effect of chronic treatment with psychotropic drugs and repeated ECS on aggressive behaviour exhibited by resident rats during social encounters

Drug	Dose (μmol/kg per day)	Max. % change in aggression	Recovery to Baseline (days)[c]
Clomipramine[a]	10	$+88.5\ p < 0.01$	7
Fluoxetine[a]	1.1	$+127.0\ p < 0.001$	7
Iprindole[a]	3	$+131.4\ p < 0.001$	7
Mianserin[a]	0.33	$+148.3\ p < 0.001$	7
Phenelzine[a]	1	$+130.7\ p < 0.001$	14
Venlafaxine[b]	20	$+269.6\ p < 0.001$	7
ECS		$+100.0\ p < 0.01$	7
Gepirone	2.79	$+84.8\ p < 0.001$	7
Diazepam[a]	3.3	-31.9 NS	Rebound increase in aggression
Haloperidol[a]	0.11	$-34.1\ p < 0.05$	7

[a]Data from Mitchell and Redfern (1992a), by permission of the *Journal of Psychopharmacology*.
[b]Data from Mitchell and Fletcher (1993), with kind permission from Pergamon Press Ltd., Headington Hill Hall, Oxford, OX3 0BW, UK.
[c]Values indicate the number of elapsed days before the earliest behavioural recording indicated the aggressive behaviour had returned to the predose level.
The p values indicate significant differences from predose baseline aggression scores. NS indicates not significant.

resident rats with the majority of antidepressant drugs tested appears to be dependent on the continued presence of the drug since by seven days after the cessation of drug treatment the level of aggressive behaviour had returned to that observed prior to treatment. The slow return of the elevated aggressive behaviour towards the pretreatment baseline levels exhibited by the resident rats after chronic treatment with the irreversible MAOI, phenelzine (Table 3), probably reflects the time course of MAO regeneration.

GENERAL DISCUSSION AND CONCLUSIONS

The studies described here further demonstrate that ethologically based methodologies provide precise and quantifiable profiles of rodent social behaviour which may be applied to the analysis of the behavioural effects of psychotropic drugs.

The resident–intruder paradigm has shown that acute treatment with a number of antidepressant drugs selectively reduces the aggressive behaviour of resident rats, concomitant with a general increase in flight behaviour (Mitchell and Fletcher, 1993; Mitchell and Redfern, 1992a). In contrast, the antipsychotic drug, haloperidol, and the anxiolytic drug, diazepam, reduced aggression only at sedative doses (Mitchell and Redfern, 1992a), while the 5-HT$_{1A}$ receptor partial agonist, gepirone, reduced aggression only at doses which induced components of the 5-HT$_{1A}$ receptor-mediated behavioural syndrome (Mitchell and Forster, 1992). These data accord well with a limited number of studies which suggest that acute treatment with antidepressant drugs may selectively reduce the aggressive behaviour of rodents in some experimental paradigms designed to model offensive and defensive aggression and predatory behaviour (see Mitchell and Redfern, 1992a). In contrast, neuroleptics and anxiolytics generally reduce aggressive behaviour in rodents only at doses that are sedative (Delini-Stula and Vassout, 1979; Olivier and van Dalen, 1982), although anxiolytic drugs may also increase rodent aggressive behaviour under certain experimental conditions (Olivier et al., 1991). However, such selective antiaggressive effects of acute treatment with antidepressant drugs are generally the exception rather than the rule (Miczek, 1987). A possible explanation for the sensitivity of the resident–intruder paradigm to the selective antiaggressive effects of antidepressant drugs is that this model promotes the expression of the full repertoire of non-social, social and agonistic behaviours rather than aggression alone. The resident–intruder paradigm is not, therefore, a model of rodent aggression per se.

The common ability of a wide range of antidepressant drugs to induce similar changes in rodent agonistic behaviour suggests that the selective decrease in aggressive behaviour, and concomitant increase in flight behaviour, may predict antidepressant activity. However, whether these behavioural changes induced by acute treatment with antidepressant drugs have any relevance regarding the delayed clinical efficacy of this class of drug (Eisen, 1989; Khan et al., 1989; Oswald et al., 1972) is unlikely. It should also be noted that the serenic compounds, fluprazine and eltoprazine (Olivier et al., 1989), have been developed on the basis of their selective antiaggressive properties observed over a wide range of animal models of aggression, including a resident–intruder paradigm in rats. The selective sensitivity of rodent aggressive behaviour to acute treatment with both serenic and antidepressant drugs clearly requires clarification.

In contrast to the effects of acute treatment with antidepressant drugs, chronic treatment with these drugs, and repeated ECS, markedly increased the aggressive behaviour of resident rats, concomitant with reduced flight behaviour (Mitchell and Fletcher, 1992; Mitchell and Redfern, 1992a). In comparison, chronic treatment with neither haloperidol nor diazepam similarly increased aggressive behaviour. Interestingly, while the 5-HT$_{1A}$ receptor partial agonist, gepirone, failed to induce an 'antidepressant-like' change in agonistic behaviour on acute administration, chronic treatment with this compound also enhanced the aggressive behaviour of resident rats. These observations suggest that the elevated aggressive behaviour of resident rats induced by chronic antidepressant drug treatment, and repeated ECS, is a common behavioural effect in the rat of established antidepressant treatments. Indeed, chronic treatment with antidepressant drugs has also been demonstrated to increase both aggressive and submissive/defensive behaviours in a limited number of behavioural studies in rodents (Delini-Stula and Vassout, 1981; Eichelman and Barchas, 1975; Mogilnicka and Przewlocka, 1981; Valdman and Poshivalov, 1986; Willner *et al.*, 1981), which suggests that such treatment augments behavioural expression resulting in exaggerated aggressive or submissive responses appropriate to the social stimulus. Such behavioural changes are also likely to be relevant with respect to the clinical latency of these treatments (Eisen, 1989; Khan *et al.*, 1989; Oswald *et al.*, 1972).

The available data suggest that it is difficult to differentiate between the effects of acute treatment with either antidepressant drugs or serenic compounds on the aggressive behaviour of rodents (see above). Recent studies in rats have shown, however, that the serenic drug, eltoprazine, exhibits a persistent and selective antiaggressive effect even after chronic oral dosing (Mos and Olivier, 1991). It is possible, therefore, that serenic and antidepressant compounds will only be differentiated in terms of their effects on rodent agonistic behaviour following chronic treatment.

In summary, the resident–intruder studies have shown that the antidepressant compounds, clomipramine, fluoxetine, iprindole, mianserin, phenelzine and venlafaxine, induce selective and diametrically opposite effects on the agonistic behaviour of resident rats during social encounters with an unknown intruder conspecific. Similarly, Dixon (1978) showed that acute treatment with imipramine reduced the aggressive behaviour of mice but increased aggressive behaviour when the drug was administered chronically over 14 days via the drinking water.

The enhanced aggressive behaviour associated with chronic antidepressant treatment (including repeated ECS) is particularly important with regard to the ability of this paradigm to predict the antidepressant potential of novel compounds. Thus the resident–intruder data predict the potential antidepressant activity of gepirone (chronic treatment studies only) which has been suggested by other preclinical (Chojnacka-Wojcik *et al.*, 1991; Giral *et al.*, 1988; Wieland and Lucki, 1990) and clinical (Amsterdam *et al.*, 1987; Cassone *et al.*, 1986) studies.

It should be noted, however, that under certain experimental conditions anxiolytic drugs may also increase the aggressive behaviour of rats, but only when the baseline level of aggression has been suppressed (Olivier *et al.*, 1991). It is possible, therefore, that the increased aggressive behaviour exhibited by resident rats exposed to chronic antidepressant treatment in these studies may be due to an anxiolytic effect. Available evidence, however, suggests a crucial difference between animal models which identify anxiolytic and antidepressant activity. The behavioural effects of anxiolytic drugs are consistent with their ability to disinhibit or release previously suppressed behaviours (File and Pellow, 1987; Joly and Sanger, 1991; Treit, 1985). However, in the resident–intruder model there is no evidence indicating suppression of the social and agonistic behaviour of the rats (Mitchell and Redfern, 1992a, 1992b). Furthermore, antidepressant drugs generally fail to disinhibit or release the suppressed behaviour of rats in models of anxiety (Cassella and Davis, 1985; File, 1985;

File and Green, 1984; File and Johnston, 1987; File *et al.*, 1985) although some studies suggest that antidepressants may indeed exhibit anxiolytic activity in some animal models but only after continuous treatment for two to five weeks (Bodnoff *et al.*, 1988; Commissaris and Fontana, 1991). Thus a prerequisite for an animal model to identify anxiolytic activity is suppression of the particular behaviour being observed. In contrast, our studies suggest that antidepressant treatments, administered chronically, appear to enhance the non-suppressed agonistic responses of resident rats resulting in enhanced aggressive behaviour. Furthermore, chronic treatment with the anxiolytic drug, diazepam, failed to increase the aggressive behaviour of resident rats in these studies. The behavioural effects of antidepressant drugs observed in the resident–intruder paradigm are therefore more likely to reflect antidepressant rather than anxiolytic activity.

Thus the increase in aggressive behaviour observed during chronic administration of established antidepressant treatments may represent a disinhibition or release of rodent social and agonistic behaviour (Mitchell and Redfern, 1992a) which, it is argued, may reflect the reversal of intropunitive aggression (Priest *et al.*, 1980) or impaired sociability (Dixon *et al.*, 1989) in depressed patients that leads to the externalization of emotions (Kaplan *et al.*, 1961) associated with the remission from depressive illness.

In conclusion, the resident–intruder paradigm, coupled with an ethological analysis of behaviour, provides a full quantitative analysis of antidepressant drug activity. The model may be used to compare the potency of various treatments on rodent agonistic behaviour and determine the magnitude and direction (*vis-á-vis* acute or chronic treatment) of behavioural changes.

Nevertheless, it should be recognized that the resident–intruder paradigm makes no assumptions about the relationship to depressive illness. By definition, animal models of depressive illness attempt to model the psychological condition. Thus designating the resident–intruder paradigm as a 'model' of depressive illness makes assumptions about the behaviours exhibited by the rats that are clearly not justified. However, the available data suggest that the predictive validity of the paradigm to identify potential antidepressant activity may be high.

ACKNOWLEDGEMENTS

The author wishes to thank Dr P.H. Redfern (School of Pharmacy and Pharmacology, University of Bath), who supported the initial development of the resident–intruder paradigm and whose continued interest and encouragement are much appreciated. Thanks also to colleagues in the Department of Neuropharmacology at Wyeth Research (UK) Ltd, especially Dr C.T. Dourish, Mr A. Fletcher and Dr E.A. Forster, for their encouragement and invaluable technical expertise during recent resident–intruder studies.

REFERENCES

Amsterdam, J.D., Berwish, N., Potter, L. and Rickels, K. (1987) Open trial of gepirone in the treatment of major-depressive disorder. *Curr. Ther. Res.*, **41**, 185–193.

Baenninger, R. (1974) Some consequences of aggressive behaviour: a selective review of the literature on other animals. *Aggress. Behav.*, **1**, 17–37.

Barnett, S.A. (1975) *The Rat: A study in behaviour*, 2nd edn. University of Chicago Press, Chicago.

Bastock, M., Morris, D. and Moynihan, M. (1953) Some comments on conflict and thwarting in animals. *Behaviour*, **6**, 66–84.

Blanchard, R.J., Fukunaga, K., Blanchard, D.C. and Kelly, M.J. (1975) Conspecific aggression in the laboratory rat. *J. Comp. Physiol. Psychol.*, **89**, 1204–1209.

Bodnoff, S.R., Suranyi-Cadotte, B., Aitken, D.H. *et al.* (1988) The effects of chronic antidepressant treatment in an animal model of anxiety. *Psychopharmacology*, **95**, 298–302.

Bolhuis, J.J., Fitzgerald, R.E., Dijk, D.J. and Koolhaas, J.M. (1984) The cortico-medial amygdala and learning in an agonistic situation in the rat. *Physiol. Behav.*, **32**, 575–579.

Bolles, R.C. and Woods, P.J. (1964) The ontogeny of behaviour in the albino rat. *Anim. Behav.*, **12**, 427–441.

Cassella, J.V. and Davis, M. (1985) Fear-enhanced acoustic startle is not attenuated by acute or chronic imipramine treatment in rats. *Psychopharmacology*, **87**, 278–282.

Cassone, V.M., Chesworth, M.J. and Armstrong, S.M. (1986) Entrainment of rat circadian rhythms by daily injection of melatonin depends upon hypothalamic suprachiasmatic nuclei. *Physiol. Behav.*, **36**, 1111–1121.

Chance, M.R.A. and Silverman, A.P. (1964) The structure of social behaviour and drug action. In: *CIBA Symposium: Animal Behaviour and Drug Action* (eds H. Steinberg, A.V.S. De Reuck and J. Knight). Churchill, London, pp. 65–79.

Chojnacka-Wojcik, E., Tatarczynska, E., Golembiowska, K. and Przegalinska, E. (1991) Involvement of 5-HT$_{1A}$ receptors in the antidepressant-like activity of gepirone in the forced swimming test in rats. *Neuropharmacology*, **30**, 711–717.

Commissaris, R.L. and Fontana, D.J. (1991) A potential animal model for the study of anti-panic treatments. In: *Advances in Pharmacological Sciences: Animal Models in Psychopharmacology* (eds B. Olivier, J. Mos and J.L. Slangen). Birkhauser Verlag, Basle, pp. 59–63.

Coppen, A. (1967) The biochemistry of affective disorders. *Br. J. Psychiatry*, **113**, 1237–1264.

Danysz, W., Archer, T. and Fowler, C.H. (1991) Screening for new antidepressant compounds. In: *Behavioural Models in Psychopharmacology: Theoretical, Industrial and Clinical Perspectives* (ed. P. Willner). Cambridge University Press, Cambridge, pp. 126–156.

Delini-Stula, A. and Vasssout, A. (1979) Differential effects of psychoactive drugs on aggressive responses in mice and rats. In: *Psychopharmacology of Aggression* (ed. M. Sandler). Raven Press, New York, pp. 41–60.

Delini-Stula, A. and Vassout, A. (1981) The effects of antidepressants on aggressiveness induced by social deprivation in mice. *Pharmacol. Biochem. Behav.*, **14**, 33–41.

Dixon, A.K. (1978) The effects of antidepressants on the social behaviour of mice after acute and chronic administration. Paper presented to the *2nd World Congress in Biological Psychiatry in Barcelona*, Abstract 111.

Dixon, A.K. (1982) Ethopharmacology: a new way to analyse drug effects on behaviour. *Triangle*, **21**, 95–105.

Dixon, A.K., Fisch, H.U., Huber, C. and Walser, A. (1989) Ethological studies in animals and man: their use in psychiatry. *Pharmacopsychiatry*, 22 (Suppl. 1), 44–50.

Eichelman, B. and Barchas, J. (1975) Facilitated shock-induced aggression following antidepressive medication in the rat. *Pharmacol. Biochem. Behav.*, 3, 601–604.

Einon, D.F., Morgan, M.J. and Kibbler, C.C. (1978) Brief periods of socialization and later behaviour in the rat. *Dev. Psychobiol.*, 11, 213–225.

Eisen, A. (1989) Fluoxetine and desipramine: a strategy for augmenting anti-depressant response. *Pharmacopsychiatry*, 22, 272–273.

File, S.E. (1985) Animal models for predicting clinical efficacy of anxiolytic drugs: social behaviour. *Neuropsychopharmacology*, 13, 55–62.

File, S.E. and Green, A.R. (1984) Repeated electroconvulsive shock has no specific anxiolytic effect but reduces social interaction and exploration in rats. *Neuropharmacology*, 23, 95–99.

File, S.E. and Hyde, J.R.G. (1978) Can social interaction be used to measure anxiety? *Br. J. Pharmacol.*, 62, 19–24.

File, S.E. and Johnston, A.L. (1987) Chronic treatment with imipramine does not reverse the effects of 3 anxiogenic compounds in a test of anxiety in the rat. *Neuropsychobiology*, 17, 187–192.

File, S.E. and Pellow, S. (1987) Behavioral pharmacology of minor tranquilizers. *Pharmacol. Ther.*, 35, 265–290.

File, S.E. and Pope, J.H. (1974) Social interaction between drugged and undrugged rats. *Anim. Learn. Behav.*, 2, 161–164.

File, S.E., Pellow, S. and Chopin, P. (1985) Can animal tests of anxiety detect anti-panic compounds? *Soc. Neurosci. Abstr.*, 11, 273.

Gentsch, C., Lichtsteiner, M. and Feer, H. (1988) Competition for sucrose-pellets in triads of male Wistar rats: the individuals' performances are differing but stable. *Behav. Brain Res.*, 27, 37–44.

Giral, P., Martin, P., Soubrie, P.H. and Simon, P. (1988) Reversal of helpless behavior in rats by putative 5-HT$_{1A}$ agonists. *Biol. Psychiatry*, 23, 237–242.

Grant, E.C. (1963) An analysis of the social behaviour of the male laboratory rat. *Behaviour*, 21, 260–281.

Grant, E.C. and Chance, M.R.A. (1958) Rank order in caged rats. *Anim. Behav.*, 6, 183–194.

Grant, E.C. and Mackintosh, J.H. (1963) A comparison of the social postures of some common laboratory rodents. *Behaviour*, 21, 246–259.

Joly, D. and Sanger, D.J. (1991) Social competition in rats: a test sensitive to acutely administered anxiolytics. *Behav. Pharmacol.*, 2, 205–213.

Jones, S.E. and Brain, P.F. (1985) An illustration of simple sequence analysis with reference to the agonistic behaviour of four strains of laboratory mice. *Behav. Proc.*, 11, 365–388.

Kaplan, S.M., Kravetz, R.S. and Ross, W.D. (1961) The effects of imipramine on the depressive components of medical disorders. *Proc. 3rd World Congress Psychiatry*, 2, 1362–1367.

Khan, A., Cohen, S., Dager, S. *et al.* (1989) Onset of response in relation to outcome in depressed outpatients with placebo and imipramine. *J. Affect. Dis.*, 17, 33–38.

Kline, N.S. and Cooper, T.B. (1980) Monoamine oxidase inhibitors as antidepressants. In: *Psychotropic Agents, Part I: Antipsychotics and Antidepressants* (eds. F. Hoffmeister and G. Stille). Springer-Verlag, Berlin, pp. 369–397, 55/I.

Koolhaas, J.M., Schurmann, T. and Wiepkema, P.R. (1980) The organization of intraspecific agonistic behaviour in the rat. *Prog. Neurobiol.*, 15, 247–268.

Latane, B. (1969) Gregariousness and fear in laboratory rats. *J. Exp. Social Psychol.*, 5, 61–69.

Miczek, K.A. (1987) The psychopharmacology of aggression In: *Handbook of Psychopharmacology, Vol. 19: New Directions in Behavioural Pharmacology* (eds L.L. Iversen, S.D. Iversen and S.H. Snyder). Plenum Press, New York, pp. 183–328.

Mitchell, P.J. (1993) Ethological studies of the social behaviour of the rat. *Anim. Technol.*, **44**, 105–117.

Mitchell, P.J. and Fletcher, A. (1992) Chronic treatment with the new antidepressant, venlafaxine, and repeated electroconvulsive shock increases the aggressive behaviour in resident rats during social interaction. *J. Psychopharmacol.*, **6**, 141.

Mitchell, P.J. and Fletcher, A. (1993) Venlafaxine exhibits pre-clinical antidepressant activity in the resident–intruder social interaction paradigm. *Neuropharmacology*, **32**, 1001–1009.

Mitchell, P.J. and Forster, E.A. (1992) Gepirone exhibits antidepressant-like activity on the social/agonistic behaviour of resident rats. *J. Psychopharmacol.*, Abstracts (BAP/EBPS joint Summer Meeting, Cambridge, 2–7 August), A84 (Abstr. 335).

Mitchell, P.J. and Redfern, P.H. (1992a) Acute and chronic antidepressant drug treatments induce opposite effects in the social behaviour of rats. *J. Psychopharmacol.*, **6**, 241–257.

Mitchell, P.J. and Redfern, P.H. (1992b) Chronic treatment with clomipramine and mianserin increases the hierarchical position of subdominant rats housed in triads. *Behav. Pharmacol.*, **3**, 239–247.

Mogilnicka, E. and Przewlocka, B. (1981) Facilitated shock-induced aggression after chronic treatment with antidepressant drugs in the rat. *Pharmacol. Biochem. Behav.*, **14**, 129–132.

Mos, J and Olivier, B. (1991) Effects of eltoprazine and haloperidol on aggression in male rats after chronic administration. *Biol. Psychiatry*, **29** (11S), 211S.

Olivier, B. and van Dalen, D. (1982) Social behaviour in rats and mice: an ethologically based method for differentiating psychoactive drugs. *Aggress. Behav.*, **8**, 163–168.

Olivier, B., Mos, J., Tulp, M. *et al.* (1989) Modulatory action of serotonin in aggressive behaviour. In: *Behavioural Pharmacology of 5-HT* (eds P. Bevan, A.R. Cools and T. Archer). Erlbaum, Hillsdale, NJ, pp. 89–115.

Olivier, B., Mos, J. and Miczek, K.A. (1991) Ethopharmacological studies of anxiolytics and aggression. *Eur. Neuropsychopharmacol.*, **1**, 97–100.

Oswald, I., Brezinova, V. and Dunleavy, D.L.F. (1972) On the slowness of action of tricyclic antidepressant drugs. *Br. J. Psychiatry*, **120**, 673–677.

Porsolt, R.D., Lenegre, A. and McArthur, R.A. (1991) Pharmacological models of depression. In: *Animal Models in Psychopharmacology* (eds. B. Olivier, J. Mos and J.L. Slangen). Birkhauser, Basle, pp. 137–159.

Priest, R.G., Beaumont, G. and Raptopoulos, P. (1980) Suicide, attempted suicide and antidepressant drugs. *J. Int. Med. Res.*, **8** (Suppl. 3), 8–13.

Raleigh, M.J., Brammer, G.L., McGuire, M.T. and Yuwiler, A. (1985) Dominant social status facilitates the behavioural effects of serotonergic agonists. *Brain Res.*, **348**, 274–282.

Scott, J.P. (1958) *Aggression*. University of Chicago Press, Chicago.

Silverman, A.P. (1965) Ethological and statistical analysis of drug effects on the social behaviour of laboratory rats. *Br. J. Pharmacol.*, **24**, 579–590.

Tinbergen, N. (1960) Comparative studies of the behaviour of gulls (*Laridae*): a progress report. *Behaviour*, **15**, 1–70.

Treit, D. (1985) Animal models for the study of anti-anxiety agents: a review. *Neurosci. Biobehav. Rev.*, **9**, 203–222.

Valdman, A.V. and Poshivalov, V.P. (1986) Pharmaco-ethological analysis of antidepressant drug effects. *Pharmacol. Biochem. Behav.*, **25**, 515–519.

Wieland, S. and Lucki, I. (1990) Antidepressant-like activity of 5-HT$_{1A}$ agonists measured with the forced swim test. *Psychopharmacology*, **101**, 497–504.

Willner, P. (1985) *Depression: A psychobiological synthesis.* Wiley–Interscience, Chichester.

Willner, P. (1991) Animal models of depression. In: *Behavioural Models in Psychopharmacology: Theoretical, Industrial and Clinical Perspectives* (ed. P. Willner), Cambridge University Press, Cambridge, pp. 91–125.

Willner, P., Theodorou, A. and Montomery, A. (1981) Subchronic treatment with the tricyclic antidepressant DMI increases isolation-induced fighting in rats. *Pharmacol. Biochem. Behav.*, **14**, 475–479.

6 The Development of an Animal Model of Panic with Predictive and Face Validity

C.A. HENDRIE AND S.M. WEISS

Department of Psychology, University of Leeds, UK

INTRODUCTION

Although the fossil record may demonstrate the effects of natural selection on morphology, statements about the evolution of behaviour, except in circumstances where morphology dictates activity, must of necessity be somewhat more tentative. However, what can be said is that in circumstances where rapid reaction to environmental events is required, behaviour must invariably be more flexible than genetic change. *A priori*, such behavioural changes eventually feed back into the gene pool through co-variance with already encoded traits, sexual selection or by other mechanisms. The existence of 'phyletic' memory (Marais, 1872–1936, first published in 1969) species-specific defence reactions (Bolles, 1970) and *preparedness* (Seligman, 1970) clearly demonstrates this.

For prey species such as mice, it is likely that selection pressure has also led to the development of strategies that are maximally efficient for the evasion of predation with consequent optimization of reproductive success. In this context, although wild mouse strains have developed coat colours that blend in well with the animal's surroundings, such a strategy must be of limited usefulness to animals that have not also developed appropriate behavioural responses for the detection, recognition and evasion of predators (Bertram, 1978; Endler, 1986).

COSTS OF ANTIPREDATOR DEFENCE

For mice, the evasion of predators may take many forms. In the absence of specific information concerning the location of a predator, an animal may use its camouflage and/or behavioural strategies to reduce the probability of attracting the attention of predators or to avoid locations where predators are likely to be. Each of these strategies has costs, however. The first is untenable for extended periods as animals must meet their energetic needs (that is, they

Ethology and Psychopharmacology. Edited by S.J. Cooper and C.A. Hendrie
© 1994 John Wiley & Sons Ltd

must satisfy the energy requirements of cellular maintenance, thermoregulation and the locomotor costs of obtaining food; Bronson, 1985). The second may limit access to high-quality food resources. This may be a potentially fatal restriction, as for example, small animals may require to eat as much as every 3 s during the winter months simply to maintain body temperature (Gibb, 1960).

It follows, therefore, that each time an animal seeks to satisfy a consummatory need (feeding, fighting, fornication) it is prevented from performing activities which are incompatible with that required behaviour and also, of necessity, places itself at greater risk of predation. This may be expressed as:

cost per unit time = probability of death − probability of successful
               per unit time   completion of consummatory act
                                      per unit time

(after McCleery, 1978).

It follows therefore that, for example, a foraging animal reduces its ability to defend itself from predatory attack and simultaneously increases the risk of such exposure. In this situation animals are required to make 'decisions' concerning the relative cost of performing a particular act and, although not explicitly stated in the above expression, must also determine the relative value of the resource. For example, in winter, where energetic costs are high, a higher risk of predation may be accepted in situations where food availability is low (e.g. Crowcroft and Rowe, 1963).

The risk of predation, and hence probability of death, may be influenced, although not removed, by a prey species' own behaviour. For example, bank voles (*Clethrionomys glareolus*), like many other rodent prey species, maximize their activities during the twilight hours around dusk and dawn (Erkinaro, 1972)—a strategy which serves to reduce the efficiency of a potential predator's exteroceptors (de Ruiter, 1963). Unfortunately, the pigmy owl (*Glaucidium passerinum*), a primary predator of the bank vole, has an activity pattern which exactly matches that of its prey (Mikkola, 1970) and like many owl species has night vision which is around 100 times more sensitive to light than diurnally active birds and which overlaps with the sensitivity of cats (Martin, 1986). Therefore, as is the case with other prey species (Curio, 1976), small rodents have developed strategies which reduce the risk of predation from *a number* of different diurnally active predators (e.g. Mustalides, including stoat (*Mustela erminea*), weasel (*M. nivalis*), mink (*M. vison*), polecat (*M. putorius*); fox (*Vulpes vulpes*), cat (*Felix catus*) and many hunting birds such as the kestrel (*Falco tinnunculus*)). However, this has had little effect on their vulnerability to attack from owls.

PREDATOR-SPECIFIC DEFENCE STRATEGIES

Strategies for antipredator defence fall into at least two categories. There are those that are appropriate for all predator species and those that are species specific, or at least only appropriate for species using a particular hunting technique. That is, whilst the detection of a predator leads to the activation of defence mechanisms, the specific defence strategy employed should relate to the *recognition* of the category to which the predator belongs.

For example, visual camouflage is only an appropriate defence against species that primarily use vision for prey location. Conversely, flight (used in the sense of the prey attempting to remove itself from the predator's immediate vicinity) is only an adaptive strategy when the prey is faster than its pursuer or can adopt flight strategies (protean behaviour) which have an appreciable probability of leading to escape (Driver and Humphries, 1988). Other factors which influence the relative intensity of threat posed by each predator species include the degree of dependence each predator species has on each prey species, the extent to which the predator selects between different classes and species of rodent available to it, and environmental variables such as cover, weather and the availability of alternative prey (King, 1985).

Initial defence depends on the ability of a prey species to recognize its predators (Endler, 1986), while the hunting strategy of the predator determines the defensive strategy of the prey. Weasels are active-searching predators. They use sight, vision and, secondarily, scent to locate their prey and run in irregular patterns examining likely parts of the microenvironment where rodents may hide. The physical size of a weasel limits access to very few burrows or nest sites and they hunt whenever they are hungry (Powell, 1978). In contrast, the prey-capture technique of the tawny owl (*Strix aluco*) is 'perch and pounce'. That is, the owl relies almost exclusively on a technique where it waits on a fixed perch and then drops or swoops on nearby prey. Unlike the barn owl (*Tyto alba*), tawny owls in woodlands rarely, if ever, hunt on the wing (Martin, 1990). Also, environmental variables can play an important role in influencing the tawny owl's hunting efficiency since rainfall can affect hearing and reduce the noise that mice make when moving across foliage. Furthermore, hunting becomes more 'speculative' (Yarnall, 1969) on dark nights as the strike rate becomes less accurate (Clarke, 1985; King, 1985). However, there is apparently a compensation, reflecting a possible increased reliance on sound, as owls will approach the prey at a slower speed and extend the talons more widely than on clear nights (Martin, 1990).

With such different hunting techniques, mice may be expected to exhibit widely different defensive strategies based on predator recognition *per se*. For weasels, killing behaviour is triggered by movement (Powell, 1978). In contrast, under conditions of low illumination, which are common in woodland canopies, to the extent that light levels fall below an owl's absolute visual threshold (Goodman and Glynn, 1988), movement (or at least, the sound of movement) *inhibits* an owl striking, as they use the termination of the last locatable sound source to predict the position of the prey (Knudsen, 1980).

Although exact forms of defence reactions are obviously related to the distance between predator and prey (the distance-dependent defence hierarchy (Gallup, 1974; Ratner, 1977)), it may be expected that mice, having detected a predator in close proximity, should exhibit different strategies. Woodmice freeze or leap when exposed to stoats (Erlinge *et al.*, 1974), while their most common fugitive reaction is to bolt for a hole (King, 1985) or 'scamper away' (Bolles, 1970). Such predator-specific defensive behaviour is exhibited by many other species and serves to either remove the prey animal from the vicinity of the potential predator or to make it difficult for the predator to find the prey after it has stopped moving (Driver and Humphries, 1988).

Other findings also demonstrate powerfully the existence of prey animals' abilities to differentiate predators. These include the ability of several species to emit predator-specific alarm calls. For example, vervet monkeys (*Cercopithecus aethiops*) emit different calls which depend on the presence of a ground-based or an aerial predator, which, in turn, elicits appropriate defensive behaviour in other members of the troop (Seyfarth and Cheney, 1980, 1986). There have also been demonstrations that domestic chickens (*Gallus gallus*) produce quantitatively and qualitatively different alarm calls to the presence of either terrestrial or aerial predators (Collias, 1987; Gyger *et al.*, 1987), a phenomenon which has recently been elegantly investigated using computer-generated visual stimuli (Evans *et al.*, 1993).

ANTIPREDATOR DEFENCE REACTIONS IN LABORATORY STRAINS

Therefore, there is very good evidence that prey species have developed mechanisms for the recognition of predators which utilize various hunting techniques and these include different avoidance manoeuvres. This evidence accords with the suggested principle that antipredator defence reactions have co-evolved with the development of various predator hunting strategies (Gilbert and Raven, 1975). Importantly for the above assertion, the opportunity to acquire appropriate defence reactions for a number of predators is strictly limited since, having once initiated the final attack sequence, the success rate of many predators rarely falls below 90% (Curio, 1976). By contrast, predators may, of course, learn much about the behaviour of their prey. For example, cats (*Felis domesticus*) will stalk a mouse in the open, yet approach one that is close to cover with great speed (Leyhausen, 1973). These behaviours are presumably related to the probability of detection and success of resultant escape responses. Further, the observations of big cats delaying the kill of a prey to allow cubs to 'practise' their chase and preingestion techniques are well known (Driver and Humphries, 1988).

In view of the strictly limited opportunities for learning, it may be concluded that antipredator defence mechanisms are innate and, as selection is based on reproductive success, the population that possesses innate antipredator defence reactions survives longer, reproduces more and eventually replaces the population without this advantage (Haldane, 1953). Thus, it may be predicted that prey species have developed defence mechanisms that are related in intensity to the extent to which each predator relies on them as a prime source of food. Further, if such mechanisms are genetically encoded, they should still be present in laboratory species *unless these have been actively selected out*.

In this context, it is not surprising that wild rats show defensive threat and attack towards a human (e.g. Blanchard *et al.*, 1990) whereas their laboratory counterparts do not (personal observation)—a difference that is presumably due to selection pressure, applied by normal husbandry techniques, over many generations. Similarly, whilst it is interesting to note that *Microtus* shows clear behavioural reactions to the scent of weasel musk (Stoddart, 1976) and that this activates benzodiazepine-sensitive analgesia mechanisms in feral white-footed mice (*Peromyscus leucopus*) (Kavaliers, 1988) it is critically relevant to the above suggestion that the scent of a cat activates endogenous opioid analgesia mechanisms in laboratory rats (Lester and Fanselow, 1985).

In a visible burrow system, laboratory rats also show intense and unequivocal defence reactions to visual contact with a cat. These reactions include withdrawal, movement constraint (including immobility), risk assessment, suppression of other activities (Blanchard and Blanchard, 1989) and the emission of ultrasonic 'alarm cries' which are eventually taken up by the whole colony (Blanchard *et al.*, 1991). The effect of the sight of a cat on behaviour is very profound and animals can take up to 6 h following exposure to the cat to emerge from the burrow to the surface area.

Therefore, there is a body of evidence which clearly demonstrates that, whilst feral and laboratory species show differences in their reactions to humans, the selection process that led to these differences has left the innate defensive reactions to other potential predators largely unaffected. In view of these findings, a series of studies were undertaken to further examine the influence of predator stimuli on behaviour in an in-bred strain (male DBA/2, Bantin and Kingman, Hull, UK) of laboratory mice.

OWL/MOUSE INTERACTIONS

The initial focus was on tawny owls, rather than on other mouse predators, for the following reasons:

1. Under many circumstances mice are highly territorial (Berry, 1970) and are sedentary, rarely moving from their territory unless forced to by extreme circumstances.
2. Tawny owls are also highly territorial, with the possession of a territory essential not only for successful breeding but for the very survival of each individual throughout the year (Martin, 1990). The annual mortality of territory holders is less than 15% per annum, whilst it is approximately 60% in non-territory holders. These mainly die of starvation (Hirons *et al.*, 1979).

3. Tawny owls are primary small-rodent predators, having been shown to crop greater than 30% of a given woodland mouse population in a two-month period (King, 1985), taking up to 8–10 per night.
4. Tawny owls defend their territory vigorously with calls, threatening behaviour or flying skirmishes, not only from other owls but also from terrestrial predators, including cats, dogs and foxes (Mikkola, 1983).

Together, these factors indicate very strong selection pressure exerted by tawny owls on mice (whilst simultaneously removing pressure from a number of other predators). Further, as observation has shown that woodland mouse populations remain viable, the evolution of an effective antipredator defence mechanism that is specific to tawny owls is strongly suggested.

Since tawny owls are nocturnal aerial predators, the stimuli available to the mouse for detection of an owl are restricted, i.e. in the absence of scent or visual cues, the only indication of an owl being active in a given vicinity are the calls it makes prior to flying to its hunting perch. As such, by employing tape-recordings of the tawny owl's territorial calls, it was possible to present laboratory mice with as much information concerning the presence of an owl as would be available to them in the field. This form of stimulus presentation has the added advantage of being completely controllable by the experimenter in terms of volume, content and timing of presentation. In all studies, mice were group housed ($n = 10$), held under reversed light/dark conditions with food and water available *ad libitum*. Stimulus material was presented in a modified activity arena ($30 \times 40 \times 30$ cm) illuminated under dim red light (2×60 W). The sound level was kept to 60–70 dB and calls were broadcast into the arena by means of a small speaker placed on one wall 25 cm above the floor. Stimulus material for all studies consisted of 3 min human voice followed by 2 min of the particular animal/bird call.

BEHAVIOURAL AND ANTINOCICEPTIVE REACTIONS: DESCRIPTION AND SPECIFICITY

As a first step, it was necessary to demonstrate that the tape-recorded calls of murine predators would produce defensive reactions in mice and to demonstrate the specificity of these effects. The first of this series of studies investigated the influence of a variety of calls on the activation of endogenous analgesia mechanisms in view of the proposed role of these systems in the optimization of behavioural defence strategies (e.g. Liebeskind *et al.*, 1976). We examined the hypothesis that opioid-dependent analgesia is selectively produced by calls that signal the presence of a potential predator.

The measure of antinociception employed was the tail-flick latency to a radiant heat source (e.g. Rodgers and Hendrie, 1983). Animals were hand held for this assessment and were used only once. Calls used in this study were selected as belonging to known mouse predators (red fox (*Vulpes vulpes crucigera*), little owl (*Athene noctua*), tawny owl (*Strix aluco*), barn owl (*Tyto alba*), kestrel (*Falco tinnunculus*)) or to non-mouse predators (mallard (*Anas platyrhyncos*), oystercatcher (*Haematopus ostralegus*), common gull (*Lanus canus*), great tit (*Parus major*), red deer (*Cervus elaphus*)).

Data are presented in Figure 1 and these show that, of the predator species, the calls of both the tawny owl and barn owl induced significant analgesia. Somewhat surprisingly the call of the common gull also produced the same effect. Therefore further studies were carried out and showed that the time-course of these call-induced analgesias were very different. Whilst the tawny owl-induced analgesia was of long duration (greater than 40 min following 2 min exposure to the call), the antinociception induced by the gull and the barn owl lasted for, at most, 5 min post exposure. A further study was also conducted designed to extend the range of predators to include the calls of the weasel (*Mustela nivalis*), stoat (*M. erminea*) and cat (*Felis catus*). Whilst the effects of the tawny owl were replicated, none of the others produced any nociceptive changes, suggesting that mice utilize either scent or sight to detect the presence of these predators.

The involvement of opioids in the mediation of call-induced analgesia are

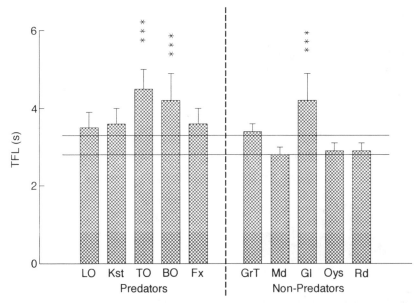

Figure 1 Specificity of call-induced analgesia. All data are presented as mean ($\pm$ s.e.m.). Analysis of the analgesic response to the calls of various animal species revealed that the calls of the tawny owl (TO), barn owl (BO) and common gull (Gl) induced significant analgesia as compared to control (parallel lines, upper line = mean + s.e.m., lower line = mean − sem). Exposure to the calls of the little owl (LO), kestrel (Kst), fox (Fx), great tit (GrT), mallard (Md), oystercatcher (Oys) or red deer (Rd) all failed to influence nociception. ***$p < 0.01$.

summarized in Figure 2, which shows that the response to the tawny owl was largely naloxone reversible. The barn owl effect was only partially antagonized by naloxone and the response to the gull was unaffected by the opioid antagonist (Hendrie, 1991). Together, these data indicate that the gull and tawny owl activate differentially mediated analgesia systems.

Endogenous analgesia may be divided into at least two components. The first is long lasting and opioid mediated which is thought to be released under extreme life-threatening circumstances where it would be maladaptive to express any behaviour other than defence/escape responses (e.g. Liebeskind, 1976; Rodgers and Hendrie, 1983). The second is of much shorter duration (< 10 min) and is mediated by non-opioid mechanisms and can be viewed as being a response to the *anticipation* of threat (Rodgers and Randall, 1987). Therefore, the data (Figure 2) may be taken to indicate that mice interpret the tawny owl call as representing an *actual* threat, whilst the gull's call represents a *potential* threat.

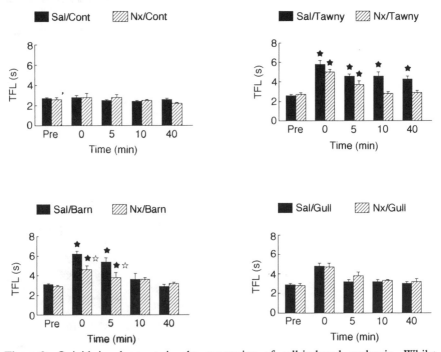

Figure 2 Opioid involvement in the expression of call-induced analgesia. Whilst 5 mg/kg naloxone (Nx) was without effect *per se*, this antagonist fully attenuated tawny owl-induced analgesia from 10 min post exposure. Similarly, naloxone partially antagonized barn owl analgesia but was without effect on the expression of gull-induced analgesia. These data suggest the activation of both opioid and non-opioid analgesia mechanisms by the calls of the tawny and barn owls and the activation of only non-opioid mechanisms by the call of the common gull. ★ = $p < 0.01$ from control (Cont), ☆ = $p < 0.05$ from saline (Sal)-treated animals at the same time point.

This interpretation of the influence of the various calls on murine behaviour was fully supported by the results of the ethological analysis presented in Figure 3. These data show that the increase in defensive behaviour induced by the above-mentioned species could be clearly differentiated. The tawny owl, barn owl (and kestrel) all produced a significant increase in call-orientated behaviour. That is, animals rapidly orientated towards the source of the call, with ears forward with the simultaneous expression of Straub tail and piloerection. In contrast, the gull failed to induce this response. However, there was a significant increase in *attend*—a generalized scanning of the test apparatus (Hendrie and Neill, 1991).

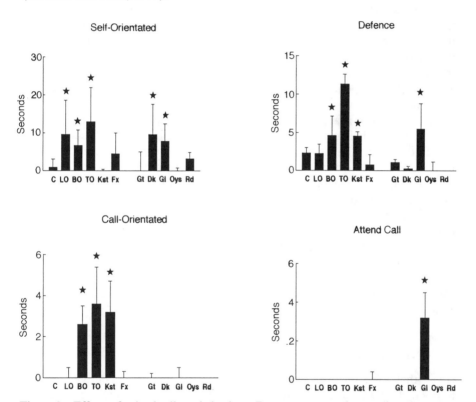

Figure 3 Effects of animal calls on behaviour. Data are expressed as medians (+ upper quartile). Detailed ethological analysis of behaviours expressed by laboratory mice following a 2 min exposure to the calls of various species revealed that the little owl (LO), barn owl (BO), tawny owl (TO), Mallard (Dk) and common gull (Gl) all increased the incidence of self-orientated behaviours (top left panel). The barn owl, tawny owl, kestrel (Kst) and gull increased defence (top right). Only the barn owl, tawny owl and kestrel influenced call-orientated behaviour (bottom left), whilst the effect on defensive behaviour produced by the gull could be attributed to an increase in attend (bottom right). The calls of the fox (Fx), oystercatcher (Oys) and red deer (Rd) were without significant effect as compared to control (C). See text for further details. ★ = $p < 0.05$.

Therefore, it can be concluded that the calls of the tawny owl, and, to a lesser extent of the barn owl, induce endogenous opioid-mediated analgesia and produce an increase in defensive, particularly call-orientated, behaviour. The effects of the gull call—a potential false positive in this paradigm—are qualitatively and quantitatively different in that the observed analgesia is non-opioid mediated and the defensive behaviours seen are indicative of a generalized increase in vigilance rather than a specific investigation of the aerial environment.

There are several explanations for a gull call to elicit a reaction in a mouse. The first and most obvious is that gulls may actually be murine predators. An extensive search of the literature has failed to reveal any evidence to support this assertion. However, personal observation has shown that mice and gulls do interact, particularly when gulls are scavenging. In this situation gulls show non-predatory aggression towards other species which represent competitors for valuable food resources. As such, mice who avoid gulls conserve energy by avoiding this competition—a response which may eventually feed back into the gene pool.

Alternatively, it is apparent that the gull and owl have similarities at the first rising pitch of their calls. Consequently, the reaction to the gull call may be due to transitory similarities between the respective stimuli leading to a very brief period of 'mistaken identity'. As such, these antipredator mechanisms must be viewed as being relatively non-precise. However, it is important to note that errors are of *inclusion* in the set of stimuli representing potential threat rather than *exclusion* errors which may have potentially lethal consequences.

The apparently lower intensity of analgesic and behavioural reaction seen in response to the barn owl as compared to the tawny owl may simply be explained by the former's lesser reliance on small rodents as a food source (Mikkola, 1983). Thus, barn owls may be less of a threat to mice than tawny owls.

SECONDARY SPECIES

Given that mice do react in a relatively specific manner to the calls of the tawny owl, it was of interest to examine whether they could also use another source of information concerning the proximity of an owl, namely the alarm calls of passerine birds. Tawny owls are often mobbed at daytime roost by smaller birds, such as blackbirds (*Turdus merula*), robins (*Erithacus rubecula*) and tits. Owls usually remain at roost when subjected to mobbing, which then dies away. However, if the owl tries to fly, alarm-calling is intensified as the owl is followed by the mobbing birds (Mikkola, 1983). To investigate the effects of passerine alarm-calling on mouse behaviour, the calls of the blackbird, robin and chaffinch (*Fringilla coelebs*) alarming to the presence of three different categories of predator were employed. These were either ground based (cat), diurnal (kestrel) or nocturnal predatory birds (owl). Calls of the chaffinch alarming to a cat and a robin alarming to a kestrel were unfortunately not available.

Studies into the effects of these calls on the activation of endogenous analgesia revealed a significant increase in tail-flick latency in all conditions tested except the human-voice control. While the analysis of the mediation of this analgesic response is not yet complete it is clear that alarm calls of all passerine birds examined activate endogenous analgesia in mice (Hendrie *et al.*, 1992), suggesting that mice interpret any songbird alarm call as indicating potential threat.

These findings were largely paralleled by data derived from ethological analysis of the behaviour of these animals during the 5 min test period, as there was a generalized enhancement of locomotor activity as compared to human-voice control. However, there did appear to be some specificity in other reactions, as a large increase in *rearing* and *stretched attend posture* was seen in the blackbird alarming to the presence of an owl or a cat conditions. Further, increased incidence of *stretched attend posture* induced by the robin alarming to an owl was also seen. These data are presented in Figure 4 and indicate that mice react with appropriate defensive behaviours to the alarm calls of the blackbird and robin—birds which, as stated above, frequently mob tawny owls.

THE CALLBOX AS A MODEL OF PANIC DISORDER

In summarizing these data, it becomes clear that laboratory mice react with remarkable specificity to stimuli indicating the presence of a tawny owl. As such, the phenomena seemed worthy of more intensive pharmacological investigation to determine the relevant neurochemical mechanisms. In order to facilitate these studies, a test arena (callbox) was constructed which was designed to allow the ready measurement of the defensive responses exhibited by mice when exposed to owl calls. This was achieved by inserting a false floor with a small burrow ($8 \times 20 \times 6$ cm) attached underneath into the arena described above. The test time was also extended by 5 min of blank tape to model the hunting pattern of the owl. Once they have displayed a territorial call, owls fly to a hunting perch and then search for prey in *complete silence*. Thus, for all the following studies, animals were introduced into the test arena and exposed to 3 min human voice, 2 min tawny owl call and 5 min of silence. The dependent measure was the time spent within the burrow.

In the absence of specific information concerning the neurochemical mediation of tawny owl call-induced defensive behaviour, a practical first step was to examine the effects of a variety of compounds. A summary of these data are presented in Table 1. It is noteworthy that there are no effects on burrow time of diazepam, chlordiazepoxide or buspirone. These are known to be anxiolytic

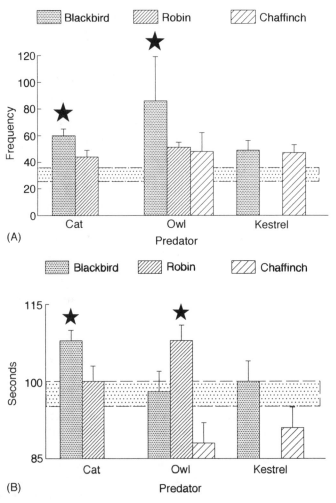

Figure 4 Influence of the alarm calls of passerines on murine behaviour. Following a generalized increase in analgesic responding induced by all alarm calls examined, ethological analysis revealed there to be an increase in rearing behaviour produced by a blackbird alarming to a cat and an owl (A), and a modest but significant increase in the level of stretched attend posture produced by the blackbird alarming to a cat and the robin alarming to an owl (B). Data are expressed as medians (+ upper quartile). ★ = $p < 0.05$ from human voice control (the upper and lower quartiles of which are represented by the shaded areas).

in a variety of animal tests and in the clinic. Therefore, it is unlikely that the current test situation is equivalent to models of anxiety such as the elevated plus-maze (Montgomery, 1958) or the light/dark model of exploration (Crawley and Goodwin, 1980). Consequently, it was necessary to seek an alternative interpretation.

Table 1 Summary of the effects of representative compounds in the callbox model of panic in mice. Data reveal that old- and new-generation anxiolytics appear to be without influence in this model. By contrast, clinically active antipanic agents and CCK_B antagonists do have activity. These findings strongly suggest that the callbox is a model with predictive validity for the detection of novel agents for the treatment of panic disorder in the clinic

Compound	Dose range (mg/kg)	Treatment	MED (mg/kg)
Diazepam	0–2.5	Acute, chronic	No effect
CDP	0–20	Acute, chronic	No effect
Buspirone	0–2.0	Acute, chronic	No effect
d-Amphetamine	0–2.5	Acute	No effect
Haloperidol	0–0.1	Acute	No effect
Devazepide	0–0.5	Acute	No effect
L-365,260	0–0.005	Acute	0.00005
LY 288513	0–0.1	Acute	0.01
Imipramine	0–10	Acute	No effect
Imipramine	0–10	Chronic	10
Alprazolam	0–1.0	Acute	0.5
Alprazolam	0–1.0	Chronic	1.0

MED, minimum effective dose.

Firstly, although the DSM-III-R (American Psychiatric Association, 1987) lists generalized anxiety disorder (GAD), panic, phobia, obsessive-compulsive disorder (OCD) and post-traumatic stress syndrome amongst others, it has been suggested that animal models of 'anxiety' reflect only one aspect of this complex, namely GAD (Green and Hodges, 1989). Further, GAD and panic disorder in particular, are differentially sensitive to pharmacological intervention. Even now, the class of drug most frequently prescribed for the treatment of GAD are benzodiazepines. This has led to the hypothesis that anxiety may be mediated via an, as yet unidentified, benzodiazepine inverse agonist (e.g. Nutt and Lawson, 1992). The situation with panic disorder is much less clear as, although the high-potency benzodiazepine alprazolam (e.g. Ballenger *et al.*, 1988) is effective in this disorder, flumazenil *provokes* panic attacks (Nutt *et al.*, 1990). As such, although panic disorder is currently preferentially treated with the tricyclic antidepressant imipramine or alprazolam (Brandon, 1990), the latter stands out as being atypical amongst its class.

Nonetheless, it was of interest that, in the present model (callbox), both imipramine and alprazolam were effective, especially as the antidepressant was only active when given chronically. Further, although devazepide, a cholecystokinin$_A$ (CCK_A) antagonist was ineffective, both the CCK_B antagonists examined (L-365,260; LY288513) produced effects in the same direction as imipramine and alprazolam.

These findings have led to the conclusion that the callbox may be a model of panic disorder with 'panic' being expressed as increased escape/flight responses

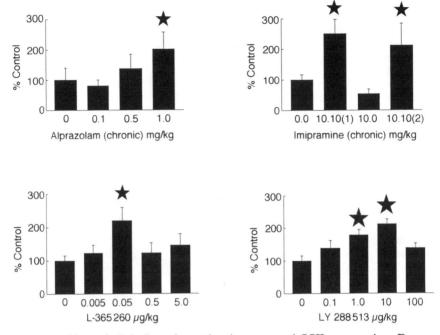

Figure 5   Effects of clinically active antipanic agents and CCK_B antagonists. Data are expressed as per cent control time spent in the strategically defensible burrow location (medians + upper quartiles). The top left panel shows the effects of chronic alprazolam. The top right panel summarizes two studies with chronic imipramine and shows that 10 days administration of 10 mg/kg of this tricyclic antidepressant (10,10) increased burrow time as compared to saline control (0,0), whilst 10 days chronic treatment, with saline given on the last day, did not (10,0). These data indicate that chronic history plus acute treatment are essential for the expression of this response. The two bottom panels show the effects of L-365 260 and LY 288 513 and suggest that these may be potential novel agents for the treatment of panic disorder. ★ = $p < 0.05$ from saline control.

on the surface of the test chamber. Antipanic agents would appear to replace these protean flight attempts with a more organized defensive response; that is, hiding in the burrow, which is reflected as an increase in time spent in this strategically defensible location (Hendrie and Neill, 1992a).

CCK AND PANIC

In this context, an impressive body of evidence has grown to suggest an important role for CCK in the mediation of panic disorder. Firstly, microiontophoretic studies have shown that benzodiazepine agonists *antagonize* the excitatory effects of CCK-8S on rat hippocampal pyramidal neurones (Bradwejn and de Montigny, 1984). Secondly, CCK peptide fragments (CCK-4, pentagastrin) have been shown to induce panic attacks in patients with panic disorder (Abelson and Neese, 1990; Bradwejn *et al.*, 1990) and healthy volunteers (de Montigny, 1989). Patients with panic disorder also show lowered tonic concentrations of CCK-8S (Lydiard *et al.*, 1992)—a finding which has been interpreted as indicating that these patients may have an increased sensitivity to CCK (Bradwejn *et al.*, 1992). Lastly, CCK-4 has been shown to induce 'fear/panic'-like behaviours in primates—an effect which may be attenuated by alprazolam (Ervin *et al.*, 1991). Where panicogenic effects of CCK-4 have shown, they have also been shown to be attenuated by CCK_B antagonists.

In view of these data, a further study was conducted to examine the effects of CCK-4 in the callbox model. Data from this study are presented in Figure 6 and reveal that the effects of this peptide in the callbox are to reduce time spent in the burrow to 50% less than controls. As such, data from the callbox closely parallel studies in the clinic. That is, CCK_B antagonists are indicated as being antipanic agents and CCK-4 is shown to be panicogenic in the callbox, primate studies and the clinic.

With such evidence indicating the importance of the CCK_B receptor subtype in the mediation of *panic* disorder, it may be viewed as unfortunate that the water has been somewhat muddied by evidence indicating CCK_B antagonists to be active in animal models of GAD. Unsurprisingly, there is a degree of controversy surrounding these effects, as several groups show CCK_B antagonists to be active in the elevated plus-maze (e.g. Ravard and Dourish, 1990) and black/white model of exploration (e.g. Hughes *et al.*, 1990; Singh *et al.*, 1991) whilst at least one group has failed to show any involvement of this receptor subtype in anxiety *per se*. Rather, the CCK_A receptor subtype has been indicated (Hendrie *et al.*, 1993). Further, where CCK_B antagonist activity has

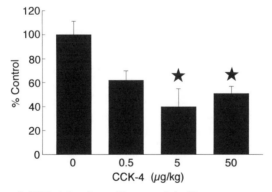

Figure 6 Effects of CCK-4 in the callbox model. Data are expressed as medians (+ upper quartiles) of control time spent in the burrow and indicate that CCK-4 produces a marked increase in time spent on the surface of the test apparatus, with consequent effects on burrow time. These data accord remarkably well with studies showing this tetrapeptide to have panicogenic effects in humans. ★ = $p < 0.05$ from saline control.

been shown, there are wild fluctuations in dose–response data (e.g. Hughes *et al.*, 1990; Singh *et al.*, 1991).

These data have been viewed as indicating that environmental factors may have an important influence on the expression of CCK antagonist effects. A detailed analysis of studies showing CCK_B antagonists to be active has revealed that the light cycle (and hence the part of the light cycle where studies were conducted) is of prime importance. Where animals are kept under 'normal' light/dark cycle and tested during the light phase, CCK_B antagonists have activity (e.g. Hughes *et al.*, 1990; Ravard and Dourish, 1990; Singh *et al.*, 1991). Conversely, where animals are housed under reversed light/dark conditions and tested during the dark phase, CCK_B antagonists are inactive, whereas CCK_A antagonists are active (e.g. Hendrie *et al.*, 1993). Recent studies in this laboratory have demonstrated this point experimentally (Hendrie and Weiss, 1994).

In view of these findings we have formulated a heuristic model of the actions of CCK-8S (CCK) in the mediation of a number of activities essential for an animal's survival. In brief, when CCK levels are high animals are disposed to sleep and rest. When they are low, they are motivated to forage and feed. For example, CSF and plasma levels of CCK peak at around 30 min post onset of feeding (Sodersten and Linden, 1992), which parallels the onset of rest in the satiety sequence (e.g. Dourish, 1992). Further, peripheral or central injections of CCK have been shown to influence sleep (Zetler, 1980) and induce hypolocomotion (Crawley *et al.*, 1981; Van Ree *et al.*, 1983). This latter effect is antagonized by devazepide but not L-365,260 (O'Neill and Dourish, 1992) suggesting that CCK_A receptors are involved in the mediation of satiety-induced hypolocomotion. These effects, of CCK on activity *per se*, have obvious and important consequences for the interpretation of CCK antagonist activity in exploration models, such as those commonly used as measures of 'anxiety'.

It has been suggested that the effects of CCK agonists in animal models of anxiety may be mediated by their influence on *motivation to explore* (Harro and Vasar, 1991). Consequently, the apparent anxiogenic effects of CCK in exploration models such as the plus-maze, black/white exploration model, hole board test etc. (e.g. Harro and Vasar, 1991; Vasar *et al.*, 1992; Guimaraes *et al.*, 1992) may depend on the initial starting point in the apparatus. Animals showing movement arrest in a closed arm of the plus-maze indicate CCK to be anxiogenic, whilst those moving less from the starting white section of the black/white box suggest the opposite case (Neill and Hendrie, 1992). Consequently, the effect of CCK antagonists may be nothing more than the attenuation of the effects of endogenous CCK on movement, especially when animals are tested during the light phase of the light/dark cycle.

With regard to the second aspect of the above heuristic model of the effects of CCK-8S, the period of activity, vigilance/defence mechanisms should be activated as risk of predation is at its greatest—responses which should be correlated with low levels of CCK. As such, it is predictable that panic patients have lower levels of CCK than normal controls, which they do (Lydiard *et al.*, 1992). Consequently, the unequivocal observations that CCK$_B$ agonists *induce* panic in mice, primates and man (see above) must be viewed as paradoxical.

However, animals are motivated to forage when energy resources are low. Extreme physical exertion should obviously be avoided under such circumstances except where the probability of predation is so great as to make this impossible. Therefore, it is entirely feasible that the mechanisms governing protean behaviour and the cognitive symptomatology associated with imminent attack are indistinguishable since they should always be expressed together. As such, it is not surprising that the physical manifestations of panic disorder in many ways resemble the effects of extreme, possibly anaerobic, physical activity (e.g. rapid heart rate, sweating, faintness, shaking/trembling, nausea, choking, paraesthesia, hot flushes/chills) and that the cognitive components are appropriate for the motivation of intense flight (anxiety/fear/apprehension, *fear* of dying, *fear* of losing control, *fear* of going insane).

In this context, it is interesting that many agents used to provoke panic attacks (e.g. sodium lactate/bicarbonate, hypercapnia, hyperventilation, hypoglycaemia (for review see Nutt and Lawson, 1992) either reduce blood sugar availability or mimic the physiological effects of intense physical activity. As such, it is particularly noteworthy that intravenous CCK-4 markedly *increases* serum levels of insulin (Rehfeld, 1971) with consequent effects on blood glucose availability. Similarly, the ability of flumazenil to induce panic attacks is attenuated when it is administered in conjunction with glucose (Nutt, 1993). The above analysis may also serve as an explanation for the phenomenon of exercise-induced endorphin release and analgesia (e.g. Shyu *et al.*, 1982), as a system that induces intense flight, analgesia and fear of death has obvious adaptive significance, *when activated under appropriate circumstances*.

The above model therefore suggests that panic may be viewed as being a cognitive consequence of physiological indications of physical stress. As such, it may be predicted that either high levels of carbon dioxide, lactate and/or low levels of blood sugar should be correlated with the expression of panic in animals and man. It also suggests that manipulations designed to increase availability of blood sugar or normalize blood carbon dioxide levels may be the most effective antipanic agents.

SUMMARY AND CONCLUSIONS

In view of evidence indicating a strong selection pressure by tawny owls on mice, a model was constructed to readily measure the defensive behaviour indicated by ethological analysis following exposure to such calls. From a series to studies with a broad range of compounds it is evident that the callbox model is selectively sensitive to antipanic agents rather than anxiolytics. Further, examination of the effect of CCK-4 and CCK antagonists revealed that the current model produced data that closely parallel the findings from studies utilizing human and primate subjects. The callbox may, therefore, represent an ethologically valid animal model of panic.

However, in conclusion, findings suggest that the effects of CCK-4 on panic may be secondary to its stimulatory effects on the release of insulin, whilst the apparent anxiolytic activity of CCK antagonists in forced exploration models may merely reflect the inhibitory effects of CCK on activity *per se*. Consequently, further research is indicated to examine in more detail the role of these more fundamental mechanisms in the mediation of human anxiety disorders.

ACKNOWLEDGEMENTS

CAH is grateful to his dog Glenn, the border collie, for not being able to tell the difference between broadcast presentation of horses trotting and the real thing. He barks at both and thereby provided the basis for the initial idea. The authors would like to thank Wyeth Research (UK), Huntercombe Lane South, Taplow, UK, for their generous support in funding this project.

REFERENCES

Abelson, J.L. and Neese, R.M., (1990) Cholecystokinin-4 and panic. *Arch. Gen. Psychiatry*, **47**, 395.

American Psychiatric Association (1987) *Diagnostic Criteria from DSM-IIIR*. APA, Washington, DC.

Ballenger, J.C., Burrows, G.D., Dupont, R.L. *et al.* (1988) Alprazolam in panic disorder and agoraphobia: results from a multicenter trial I: efficacy in short term treatment. *Arch. Gen. Psychiatry*, **45**, 413–422.

Berry, R.J. (1970) The natural history of the house mouse. *Field Stud.*, **3**, 219–262.

Bertram, B.C.R. (1978) Living in groups: predators and prey In: *Behavioural Ecology: An Evolutionary Approach* (eds J.R. Krebs and N.B. Davies). Blackwell, Oxford, pp. 64–96.

Blanchard, R.J. and Blanchard, D.C. (1989) Antipredator defensive behaviours in a visible burrow system. *J. Comp. Psychol.*, **103**, 70–82.

Blanchard, D.C., Blanchard, R.J. and Rodgers, R.J. (1990) Pharmacological and neural control of anti-predator defense in the rat. *Aggressive Behav.*, **16**, 165–175.

Blanchard, R.J., Blanchard, D.C., Agullana, R. and Weiss, S.M. (1991) Twenty-two kHz alarm cries to presentation of a predator, by laboratory rats living in visible burrow systems. *Physiol. Behav.*, **50**, 967–972.

Bolles, R.C. (1970) Species-specific defense reactions and avoidance learning. *Psychol. Rev.*, **77**, 32–48.

Bradwejn, J. and de Montigny, C. (1984) Benzodiazepines antagonise cholecystokinin-induced activation of rat hippocampal neurons. *Nature*, **312**, 363–364.

Bradwejn, J., Koszycki, D. and Meterissian, G. (1990) Cholecytsokinin-tetrapeptide induced panic attacks in patients with panic disorder. *Can. J. Psychiatry*, **35**, 83–85.

Bradwejn, J., Koszycki, D., Couetoux du Terte, A. *et al.* (1992) The cholecystokinin hypothesis of panic and anxiety disorders: a review. *J. Psychopharmacol.*, **6**, 345–351.

Brandon, S. (1990) Clinical use of benzodiazepines in anxiety and panic disorders. In: *Benzodiazepines: Current Concepts* (eds I. Hindmarch, G. Beaumont, S. Brandon and B.E. Leonard). Wiley, Chichester, pp. 111–141.

Bronson, F.H. (1985) Mammalian reproduction: an ecological perspective. *Biol. Reprod.*, **32**, 1–26.

Clarke, J.A. (1985) Moonlight's influence on predator/prey interactions between short-eared owls (*Asio flammeus*) and deermice (*Peromyscus maniculatis*). *Behav. Ecol. Sociobiol.*, **13**, 205–209.

Collias, N.E. (1987) The vocal repertoire of the red junglefowl: a spectrographic classification and the code of communication. *Condor*, **89**, 510–524.

Crawley, J.N. and Goodwin, F.K. (1980) Preliminary report of a simple animal behaviour model for the anxiolytic effects of benzodiazepines. *Pharmacol. Biochem. Behav.*, **13**, 167–170.

Crawley, J.N., Hays, S.E., Paul, S.M. and Goodwin, F.K. (1981) Cholecystokinin reduces exploratory behaviour in mice. *Physiol. Behav.*, **27**, 407–411.

Crowcroft, P. and Rowe, F.P. (1963) Social organisation and territorial behaviour in the wild house mouse. *Proc. Zool. Soc. (Lond.)*, **140**, 517–531.

Curio, E. (1976) *The Ethology of Predation.* Springer-Verlag, Berlin.

Dourish, C.T. (1992) Behavioural analysis of the role of CCK_A and CCK_B receptors in the control of feeding. In: *Multiple Cholecystokinin Receptors in the CNS* (eds C.T. Dourish, S.J. Cooper, L.L. Iversen and S.D. Iversen). Oxford University Press, Oxford, pp. 235–253.

Driver, P.M. and Humphries, D.A. (1988) *Protean Behaviour: The Biology of Unpredictability.* Oxford University Press, Oxford.

Endler, J.A. (1986) Defense against predators. In: *Predator–Prey Relationships* (eds M.E. Feder and G.V. Lauder). University of Chicago Press, Chicago, pp. 109–134.

Erkinaro, E. (1972) Seasonal changes in the phase position of circadian activity rhythms in some voles and their endogenous component. *Aquilo Ser. Zool.*, **13**, 87–91.

Erlinge, S., Bergsten, B. and Kristiansson, H. (1974) The stoat and its prey: hunting behaviour and fugitive reactions. *Fauna Flora Stockholm*, **69**, 203–211.

Ervin, F., Palmour, R. and Bradwejn, J. (1991) A new primate model for panic disorder. *144th Meeting of the American Psychiatric Association*, New Orleans, NR216: 100.

Evans, C.S., Macedonia, J.M. and Marler, P. (1993) Effects of apparent size and speed on the response of chickens, *Gallus gallus*, to computer generated simulations of aerial predators. *Anim. Behav.*, **46**, 1–11.

Gallup, G.G. (1974) Animal hypnosis: factual status of a fictional concept. *Psychol. Bull.*, **81**, 836–853.

Gibb, J.A. (1960) Populations of tits and goldcrests and their food supply in pine plantations. *Ibis*, **102**, 163–208.

Gilbert, L.E. and Raven, P.E. (1975) *Coevolution of Animals and Plants.* University of Texas Press, Austin.

Goodman, S.M. and Glynn, C. (1988) Comparative rates of nocturnal osteological disorders in a collection of Paraguayan birds. *J. Zool. (Lond.)*, **214**, 167–177.

Green, S. and Hodges, H. (1989) Animal models of anxiety. In: *Behavioural Models in Psychopharmacology* (ed. P. Willner). Cambridge University Press, Cambridge pp. 21–49.

Guimaraes, F.S., Russo, A.S., De Aguiar, J.C. *et al.* (1992) Anxiogenic-like effect of CCK-8 microinjected into the dorsal periaqueductal grey of rats in the elevated plus-maze. In: *Multiple Cholecystokinin Receptors in the CNS* (eds C.T. Dourish, S.J. Cooper, L.L. Iversen and S.D. Iversen). Oxford University Press, Oxford, pp. 149–154.

Gyger, M., Marler, P. and Pickert, R. (1987) Semantics of an avian alarm call system: the male domestic fowl, *Gallus domesticus. Behaviour*, **102**, 15–40.

Haldane, J.B.S. (1953) Animal populations and their regulation. *Modern Biol.*, **15**, 9–24.

Harro, J. and Vasar, E. (1991) Cholecystokinin-induced anxiety: how is it reflected in studies of exploratory behaviour? *Neurosci. Biobehav. Rev.*, **15**, 473–477.

Hendrie, C.A. (1991) The calls of murine predators activate endogenous analgesia mechanisms in laboratory mice. *Physiol. Behav.*, **49**, 569–573.

Hendrie, C.A. and Neill, J.C. (1991) Exposure to the calls of predators of mice activates defensive mechanisms and inhibits consummatory behaviour in an inbred mouse strain. *Neurosci. Biobehav. Rev.*, **15**, 479–482.

Hendrie, C.A. and Neill, J.C. (1992a) An animal model of panic. *J. Psychopharmacol.*, **6**, 125.

Hendrie, C.A. and Neill, J.C. (1992b) CCK and anxiety. In: *Multiple Cholecystokinin Receptors in the CNS* (eds C.T. Dourish, S.J. Cooper, L.L. Iversen and S.D. Iversen). Oxford University Press, Oxford, pp. 132–142.

Hendrie, C.A. and Rodgers, R.J. (1990) Microcomputer based data logging and analysis in pharmacoethology. In: *Microcomputers, Psychology and Medicine* (eds R. West, M.J. Christie and J. Weinman). Wiley, New York, pp. 187–201.

Hendrie, C.A. and Weiss, S.M. (1994) The effects of light cycle on anxiolytic versus antipanic activity of CCK antagonists. *Br. J. Pharmacol.* (submitted).

Hendrie, C.A., Noyce, G. and Turner, T. (1992) Alarm calls of passerine birds activate defense mechanisms in laboratory mice. *J. Psychopharmacol.* (meetings suppl.), 334.

Hendrie, C.A., Neill, J.C., Shepherd, J.K. and Dourish, C.T. (1993) The effects of CCK-A and CCK-B antagonists on activity in the black/white exploration model of activity in mice. *Physiol. Behav.*, **54**, 689–693.

Hirons, G.J.M., Hardy, A.R. and Stanley, P. (1979) Starvation in young tawny owls. *Bird Study*, **26**, 59–63.

Hughes, J., Boden, P., Costall, B. *et al.* (1990) Development of a class of selective cholecystokinin type B receptor antagonists having potent anxiolytic activity. *Proc. Natl. Acad. Sci. USA*, **87**, 6728–6732.

Kavaliers, M. (1988) Brief exposure to a natural predator, the short-tailed weasel, induces benzodiazepine-sensitive analgesia in white footed mice. *Physiol. Behav.*, **43**, 187–193.

King, C.M. (1985) Interactions between woodland rodents and their predators. *Symp. Zool. Soc. Lond.*, **55**, 219–247.

Knudsen, E.I. (1980) Sound localisation in birds. In: *Comparative Studies of Hearing in Vertebrates* (eds A.N. Popper and R.R. Fay). Springer-Verlag, Berlin, pp. 289–322.

Lester, L.S. and Fanselow, M.S. (1985) Exposure to a cat produces opioid analgesia in rats. *Behav. Neurosci.*, **99**, 756–759.

Leyhausen, P. (1973) *Verhaltsstudien an Katzen*, 3rd edn. Parey, Berlin.

Liebeskind, J.C., Giesler, G.J. and Urca, G. (1976) Evidence pertaining to an endogenous mechanism of pain inhibition in the central nervous system. In: *Sensory Functions of the Skin in Primates* (ed Y. Zotterman). pp. 561–573.

Lydiard, R.B., Ballenger, J.C., Laraia, M.T. *et al.* (1992) CSF cholecystokinin concentrations in patients with panic disorder and in normal comparison subjects. *Am. J. Psychiatry*, **149**, 691–693.

Marais, E. (1969) *The Soul of the Ape*. Anthony Blond, London.

Martin, G.R. (1990) *Birds by Night*. Poyser, Carlton.

Martin, G.R. (1986) Sensory capacities and the nocturnal habit in owls. *Ibis*, **128**, 266–277.

McCleery, R.H. (1978) Optimal behaviour sequences and decision making. In: *Behavioural Ecology: An Evolutionary Approach* (eds J.R. Krebs and N.B. Davies). Blackwell, Oxford, pp. 377–410.

Mikkola, H. (1970) On the activity and food of the pygmy owl *Glaucidium passerinum* during breeding. *Ornis Fenn.*, **47**, 10–14.

Mikkola, H. (1983) *Owls of Europe*. Poyser, Carlton.

Montgomery, K.C. (1958) The relation between fear induced by novelty stimulation and exploratory behaviour. *J. Comp. Physiol. Psychol.*, **48**, 254–260.

Montigny, C., de (1989) Cholecystokinin-tetrapeptide induces panic-like attacks in healthy volunteers. *Arch. Gen. Psychiatry*, **46**, 511–517.

Neill, J.C. and Hendrie, C.A. (1992) Effects of CCK agonists in the black/white exploration model in mice. *J. Psychopharmacol.*, **6**, 123.

Nutt, D.J. (1993) Benzodiazepine receptors and panic. *J. Psychopharmacol.* (meetings suppl.), 167.

Nutt, D.J. and Lawson, C.W. (1992) Panic attacks: a neurochemical overview of models and mechanisms. *Br. J. Psychiatry*, **160**, 165–178.

Nutt, D.J., Glue, P., Lawson, C.W. *et al.* (1990) Flumazenil provocation of panic attacks: evidence for altered benzodiazepine sensitivity in panic disorder. *Arch. Gen. Psychiatry*, **47**, 917–925.

O'Neill, M.F. and Dourish, C.T. (1992) Evidence that hypolocomotion induced by peripheral or central injection of CCK in the mouse is mediated by peripherally located CCK_A receptors. In: *Multiple Cholecystokinin Receptors in the CNS* (eds C.T. Dourish, S.J. Cooper, L.L. Iversen and S.D. Iversen). Oxford University Press, Oxford, pp. 254–259.

Powell, R.A. (1978) A comparison of fisher and weasel hunting behaviour. *Carnivore*, **1**, 28–34.

Ratner, S.C. (1977) Immobility in invertebrates: what can we learn? *Psychol. Rev.*, **1**, 1–14.

Ravard, S. and Dourish, C.T. (1990) Cholecystokinin and anxiety. *Trends Pharmacol. Sci.*, **11**, 271–273.

Rehfeld, J.F. (1971) Effect of gastrin and its C-terminal tetrapeptide on insulin secretion in man. *Acta Endocrinol.*, **66**, 169–176.

Rodgers, R.J. and Hendrie, C.A. (1983) Social conflict activates status-dependent analgesic and hyperalgesic mechanisms in male mice: effects of naloxone on nociception and behaviour. *Physiol. Behav.*, **30**, 775–780.

Rodgers, R.J. and Randall, J.I. (1987) On the mechanisms and adaptive significance of intrinsic analgesia systems. *Rev. Neurosci.*, **1**, 185–200.

Ruiter, L. de (1963) The physiology of vertebrate feeding behaviour: towards a synthesis of the ethological and physiological approaches to problems of behaviour. *Z. Tierpsychol.*, **20**, 498–516.

Seligman, M.E.P. (1970) On the generality of the laws of learning. *Psychol. Rev.*, **77**, 406–418.

Seyfarth, R.M. and Cheney, D.M. (1980) The ontogeny of vervet alarm calling behaviour: a preliminary report. *Z. Tierpsychol.*, **54**, 37–56.

Seyfarth, R.M. and Cheney, D.M. (1986) Vocal development in vervet monkeys. *Anim. Behav.*, **34**, 1640–1658.

Shyu, B.C., Andersson, S.A. and Thoren, P. (1982) Endorphin mediated increase in pain threshold induced by long lasting exercise in rats. *Life Sci.*, **30**, 833–840.

Singh, L., Lewis, A.S., Field, M.J. *et al.* (1991) Evidence for an involvement of the brain cholecystokinin B receptor in anxiety. *Proc. Natl. Acad. Sci. USA*, **88**, 1130–1133.

Sodersten, P. and Linden, A. (1992) Plasma and cerebrospinal fluid concentrations of CCK and satiety. In: *Multiple Cholecystokinin Receptors in the CNS* (eds C.T. Dourish, S.J. Cooper, L.L. Iversen and S.D. Iversen). Oxford University Press, Oxford, pp. 222–233.

Stoddart, D.M. (1976) Effect of the odour of weasels (*Mustela nivalis* L.) on trapped samples of their prey. *Oecologia*, **22**, 439–441.

Van Ree, J.M., Gaffori, O. and De Wied, D. (1983) In rats, the behavioural profile of CCK-8 related peptides resembles that of antipsychotic agents. *Eur. J. Pharmacol.*, **93**, 63–78.

Vasar, E., Harro, J., Pold, A. and Lang, A. (1992) CCK receptors and anxiety in rats. In: *Multiple Cholecystokinin Receptors in the CNS* (eds C.T. Dourish, S.J. Cooper, L.L. Iversen and S.D. Iversen). Oxford University Press, Oxford, pp. 144–148.

Yarnall, J.L. (1969) Aspects of the behaviour of *Octopus cyanea* Gray. *Anim. Behav.*, **17**, 747–754.

Zetler, G. (1980) Effects of cholecystokinin-like peptides on rearing activity and hexobarbital-induced sleep. *Eur. J. Pharmacol.*, **66**, 137–139.

7 Opponent Environmental Targets and Sensorimotor Systems in Aggression and Defence

ROBERT J. BLANCHARD[a] **AND D. CAROLINE BLANCHARD**[b]

[a]*Department of Psychology and Bekesy Laboratory of Neurobiology, and* [b]*Pacific Biomedical Research Center and Department of Anatomy, John A. Burns School of Medicine, University of Hawaii, Honolulu, Hawaii, USA*

INTRODUCTION

A basic premise of ethopharmacology is that behaviour should be analysed and understood to the same degree as the pharmacological mechanisms involved. In the description and analysis of conspecific attack and defensive behaviours of rats, the pioneering studies of Grant, Chance and MacKintosh some 30 years ago (Grant and Chance, 1958; Grant, 1963; Grant and MacKintosh, 1963) constituted an enormous step forward. Although new schemes for categorizing or conceptualizing aggressive and defensive behaviours have since been proposed, it is significant that for most investigators the basic understanding of which behaviours constitute conspecific attack or defence in the rat follows the results of their studies. In fact, many of the changes proposed (e.g. at a workshop on a standardized nomenclature for rodent agonistic behaviour at the meetings of the International Society for Research on Aggression, in 1980) simply involved applying different names to the same actions, to reduce the use of affect- or intent-implying terminology in favour of terms that are more physically descriptive.

In the studies of Grant and his colleagues, while the individual labels given to behavioural components might have had some theoretical overtones, the attack/defence distinction was empirical and atheoretical. The distinction was based on the finding that, particularly in well-practised animals with a history of agonistic encounters, attack behaviours tended to cluster in the action pattern of one combatant, with rather consistent sequential relationships among these, while the behaviours of the other animal tended not to include these, but included a different set, again with relatively consistent sequential dependencies among them. The detailed descriptions of attack and defence

Ethology and Psychopharmacology. Edited by S.J. Cooper and C.A. Hendrie
© 1994 John Wiley & Sons Ltd

behaviours, and the distinction between them, were particularly timely since much of the contemporary work on rat aggression involved 'reflexive fighting' or 'pain–aggression' paradigms and behaviours that were labelled aggressive on the basis of dubious analogies to actions sometimes seen in human combat (e.g. boxing, striking and kicking). In addition to their superior descriptive and empirical bases, the analyses of Grant *et al.*, together with the well-described cat attack/defence distinction of Leyhausen (1979) and the pioneering mouse work of John Paul Scott (1966), also stressed that agonistic behaviours in non-human animals must be analysed species by species. This is because the precise form of these behaviours may differ between species even if the organizational principles are similar.

Although subsequent behavioural work on aggression and defence has taken many different directions, one trend has retained an emphasis on detailed behavioural description and analysis, while expanding attention to the ecological relevance of the test situation and the functions (as expressed by typical outcomes) of individual behaviours and behaviour patterns in these enriched environments. The combination of this behavioural approach with manipulation of biological variables has been labelled 'ethoexperimental analysis'. Much of the work to be described here falls under this rubric.

Such analyses have resulted in the discovery of several additional features of aggressive, defensive (and some other) behaviours. First, both aggression and defence are strongly targeted towards specific sites on the body of the opponent, and this targeting is a major determinant of the specific actions involved in conspecific aggression and defence. Second, the importance of such directed behavioural strategies can be seen also in situations in which threat is anticipated rather than present, resulting in a high-intensity, long-term 'risk assessment' pattern that is a major component of defensive behaviour. An understanding of the defence pattern and its normal progression over time indicates that both the magnitude and also the type of defensive actions seen are functions of the characteristics and intensity of the threat stimulus. These behavioural analyses have a number of implications for investigation of the effects of drugs on aggressive and defensive behaviour, and they also suggest the importance of analysing the neural correlates of aggression and defence as sensorimotor response systems.

TARGET SITES FOR OFFENSIVE AND DEFENSIVE BITES

If rats are grouped in mixed-sex colonies, then fighting among males may be quite severe, commonly with wounding. The wounds are sustained much more often by intruders than residents (Blanchard, R.J. and Blanchard, 1977), or by subordinates compared to dominants (Blanchard, R.J. *et al.*, 1992), indicating an important characteristic of offensive attack compared to defence, that it more often wounds the opponent. Moreover, when attackers wound the opponent the wounds cluster on the opponent's back, whereas the comparatively few wounds found on the opponents of defensive animals were virtually restricted to the snout (Blanchard, R.J. and Blanchard, 1977; Pellis and Pellis, 1987).

Was the biter or the bitten responsible for this clustering of wounds on the back? Were the bites consistently aimed, or, were they located so consistently because the defender was somehow making this site the easiest to reach and bite? A study involving terminally anaesthetized intruders, presented such that only their dorsal or ventral aspect was offered, answered these questions. Attacking rats seldom bit the ventrum of their opponent even when it was freely available and unprotected, but quickly bit the dorsum (Blanchard, R.J. et al., 1978). However, anaesthetized intruders were bitten on the head as well, indicating that a conscious and intact defender does something that is useful in protecting this head site. Thus there are a variety of mechanisms that determine the sites of wounds produced by attacking conspecific rats.

1. Some areas of the body (in rats, the ventrum) are protected by a sort of inhibition that operates even when the defender is unconscious.
2. Some body sites are actively protected by the defender. In rats, the head is protected by the defender's manipulation of a physical structure, the mystacial vibrissae. These are fanned, out and forward, by defensive rats and apparently provide a tactile barrier when they are touched by the attacker's vibrissae, preventing further movement toward the defender's head. When the defender's vibrissae are trimmed away, many more bites result (Blanchard, R.J. et al., 1977b).
3. Some body sites (in rats, the back) are frequent targets for conspecific biting attack, while predatory attack is often aimed at the neck.

TARGET SITES AS DETERMINANTS OF CONSPECIFIC ATTACK AND DEFENSIVE BEHAVIOURS

How might these protected as well as targeted areas contribute to the form of attack and defensive behaviours? Analysis of fighting in pairs of male rats (Blanchard, R.J. and Blanchard, 1977) suggested that, if the opponent's back is readily available to an attacker, it is bitten. However, if it is initially unavailable because of the defender's behaviour, then the attacker's behaviour changes so as to reach this area, regardless. For example, if the back is not available because the defender is running away, then the attacker will chase the defender and bite its back if and when this area can be reached. However, in the small cages typically used for such studies, the defender will stand on its hind limbs, orientated towards the attacker in a defensive upright posture. This orientation places the defender's raised ventrum in the path of the attacker, and also interposes the fanned-forward vibrissae, providing a barrier to head bites. Attackers faced with such a defence tend to show the lateral attack, with the attacker aligning the long axis of its body perpendicularly to that of the upright defender, then crowding sideways into the defender (sometimes pushing it off balance) and/or lunging around the defender to reach its back. An experienced defender may further counter this attack by pivoting on its hind feet to follow the attacker's trajectory. Another common defence for a laboratory rat is lying on its back, which often occurs as a gradual but continuous movement from the upright defensive stance. The upright defender leans further and further back, until it is supine. The attacker counters by standing 'on top' and, often, digging at the side of the supine defender. If the back is exposed in this fashion, a bite is the likely result.

These analyses suggest that specific attacker behaviours occur in response to particular defender behaviours. The specific defence–attack dyads that show the closest relationships are those outlined in Table 1. Because each of these defensive behaviours conceals the defender's back target from the attacker, and each of the corresponding attack behaviours tends to thwart that specific defence and enable access to the back, we have suggested that the organization of these specific defence–attack dyads reflects a defender 'back-defence' strategy, while offensive behaviour constitutes a 'back-attack' strategy (Blanchard, R.J. and Blanchard, 1977). Each such 'strategy' involves a group of movement patterns, each coordinated with other patterns in the group and, often, to movements or features of the opponent.

TARGET SITES FOR DEFENSIVE BITING

To be useful as a criterion for distinguishing attack from defence, it is important that the target for offensive attack is different from the target for defensive attack. In addition to the snout target for attack by defensive rats (e.g. intruders, colony subordinates) in free encounters, bites in situations where an extraneous pain is applied also involve a snout target. This is true even when the subjects have had previous experience as a colony resident, making offensive, back-targeted, biting attacks. Thus when resident–intruder pairs were run in the resident's home cage, the resident bit its opponent on the back. However, when the same pairs were run in a 'reflexive fighting' situation with foot shock, bites by both members of the pair were on the snout of the opponent (Blanchard R.J. et al., 1978). In addition, bites to an anaesthetized conspecific by rats receiving tail shock while confined in a tube were directed at the opponent's snout/head. They almost never bit the back, leg or tail of the anaesthetized conspecific when this was offered as a target during shock.

Table 1 Defence–attack dyads

Defender behaviour	Attacker behaviour
Flight	Chase
Defensive upright	Lateral attack
On the back	Standing on top

Bites by rats directed at a predator are defensive. Although there are some early (e.g. Yerkes, 1913; Stone, 1932) as well as recent (e.g. Blanchard, R.J. *et al.*, 1986; Nanumenko *et al.*, 1989) studies of the defensive behaviours of wild rats to human approach and contact, prey–predator size differential and the natural reluctance of the experimenter to make body parts available for this purpose act against analysis of bite targets on the body of the threatening stimulus in such studies. There is also need to minimize trauma to a non-human predator. However, the adventitious event of a laboratory cat with an untreatable illness, therefore to be euthanized, enabled us to compare the target sites for antipredator defence with those of defensive bites to a conspecific (Blanchard, R.J. *et al.*, 1980). Laboratory rat subjects were confined in a tube with an electrode fixed to the tail. When the snout, forepaw or tail of the terminally anaesthetized cat was presented, a sex difference in defensive attack appeared: no site on the cat was bitten by male rats prior to tail shock, but high levels of snout-biting appeared after shock had been given, even on subsequent non-shock trials. The forepaw was bitten on shock trials only, while the tail was virtually never bitten, even when shock was given. Female rats bit the cat's snout (but not other sites) even before any shock. These findings indicate a clear hierarchy of defensive attack sites, with the snout the major target, although the paw may also be a target during shock (Blanchard, R.J. *et al.*, 1980).

Interpretations of the function of the snout/head target, common to both defensive (conspecific) and antipredator attack, tend to focus on the deterrent effect of potential damage to these sites, particularly the eyes. This interpretation is consonant with the finding (Herzog and Bern, 1992) that animals as different from rats as garter snakes also strike differentially, and more frequently, at the eyes of a threatening target.

TARGET SITES IN WILD RATS AND OTHER MUROID RODENTS

For a behaviour pattern to be of some value in pharmacological research at least some aspects of the behaviour should have considerable degree of generality across species, i.e. the behaviour pattern should *not* be species specific. Thus target sites for biting, even if different for offensive and defensive attack, would be less interesting if they occur only in domesticated rats.

To determine if these phenomena appear in much the same form in wild as in laboratory rats, *Rattus norvegicus* were wild trapped in both stable and recently harvested sugar-cane fields, and carefully examined for the number and sites of wounds (Blanchard, R.J. *et al.*, 1985). The harvesting of cane was clearly stressful and very few immature and subadult animals were trapped on the edges of fields that had recently been harvested and burned. These animals also had more wounds, doubtless reflecting enhanced agonistic behaviour when refugees from the burned areas invaded adjacent fields. However, the sites of wounds were only slightly different in the disturbed and undisturbed areas, with about 70% of wounds on the back in the former, and just over 95% in the latter. Some head, limb and particularly tail wounds were found on animals from disturbed areas, consistent with an invasion by animals that, when attacked, immediately attempted to flee. However, ventrum wounds were extremely rare in both the undisturbed and the harvested-cane situations.

The dyadic interactions of attacking and defending wild-trapped wild *R. norvegicus* and also *R. rattus* were examined by Takahashi and Blanchard (1982). First, the target sites for attack in these laboratory settings were very similar for laboratory rats (87.1% back bites), wild *R. norvegicus* (79.6% back bites) and *R. rattus* (80.9% back bites). Also, total durations of the attack behaviours of a specific defence–attack dyad were very similar to the durations of the corresponding defence component of that dyad, as would be predicted by a view that these attack and defensive behaviours 'go together' because the attack behaviour counters the defence tactic offered. The wild versus laboratory rat differences that were seen appeared to reflect alterations of defensive behaviour. Wild rats tended to show more flight, on-the-back, and defensive attack behaviours, and less freezing and boxing or defensive upright, and these changes were precisely mirrored in the durations of the corresponding attack component of the relevant dyad. Later studies of antipredator defence (Blanchard, R.J. *et al.*, 1986) suggested a substantial difference in the incidence of specific defences between wild and laboratory rats even when both were bred and raised in a laboratory. The essential point, however, is that the basic form of defensive behaviours was similar for wild and laboratory rats, just as their bite targets had been found to be similar. The durations of these defences were precisely matched by the durations of the appropriate attack behaviours in intrastrain encounters. It is also of interest to note that the same attack–defence dyads were obtained in wild-trapped *R. rattus*. These dyadic attack–defence relationships and the behaviours they include are thus not 'species specific', although they are species typical.

The phenomenon extends to other muroid rodents as well. In resident–intruder tests, resident Swiss–Webster mice made nearly 80% of their bites on the back of the opponent, while the most common target of intruder bites was the opponent's head. Mouse bites do not, however, appear to be quite so rigidly targeted as those of rats: residents made over 10% of their bites at the opponent's ventrum. Consonant with the view that defensive behaviours depend upon target sites for attack, one defensive behaviour, lying on the back, that appears to be effective because ventral bites are inhibited, is much less common in these mice than in rats (Blanchard R.J. *et al.*, 1979; Pellis *et al.*, 1992a). Bites to the back of a territorial intruder, particularly to the lower dorsum or rump, are seen also in hamsters (Pellis and Pellis, 1989) and voles (Pierce *et al.*, 1991; Pellis *et al.*, 1992b). As with mice, however, the targets for offensive attack may be somewhat flexible in some species. In prairie voles, if the defender turns to face the attacker, the attacker may switch its attack from the initial target site, the rump, to the defender's head. Consequently, few such facing defences were seen, with defenders fleeing instead. In montane voles, however, the resident continued to attack its opponent's rump, even when a facing defence was offered (Pellis et al., 1992b).

TARGET SITES FOR OTHER AIMED BEHAVIOURS

Offensive and defensive attack are only two of a number of dyadic behaviours that involve relatively specific target sites on the body of an opponent. In fact, such targets appear to be so common that they may constitute an important organizing principle in the analysis of dyadic behaviour patterns (and some others, such as grooming: Sachs, 1988; Fentress, 1988), with particular behaviours adaptive in facilitating or denying access to these targets. In particular, recognition and localization of targets may be important in analysis of the adaptive significance of more complex and extended behaviour patterns in which both the target of behaviour, and the behaviour made to the target, can change over time.

Predation

The nape target appears to be common in predatory attack, particularly against prey for which a swift and certain kill is particularly desirable. Ben-David et al. (1991) reported that wild-trapped marbled polecats (Vormela peregusna syriaca) used nape bites against larger and potentially dangerous prey, suggesting that it may combine effectiveness (damage to spinal cord) with an angle of approach that reduces the danger of retaliatory attack. However, the polecats also used other prey-killing methods, including thorax bites for small prey and ventral bites for prey presenting the ventrum. Tigers also alter the form of attack in response to variation in prey size (Seidensticker and McDougal, 1993). Deer-sized prey are often killed by nape bites, while buffalo-sized prey are killed by throat bites that typically result in suffocation. This difference is apparently based on the greater protection of the vertebra afforded by the thick neck of buffalo or sambar, such that even an adult tiger's teeth cannot penetrate to achieve spinal cord damage. Notably, young tigers use throat bite against smaller prey than do adults, again emphasizing the adaptive function of this variation in bite target.

Juvenile play 'fighting'

Play 'fighting' of juvenile rodents has been described in detail (Pellis and Pellis, 1987, 1991). In play, one rat attempts to contact the other's nape, and the other defends by actions making this target unavailable for contact—a general schema similar to that of adult fighting. However, the targets of attack in play and adult fighting are often different and the play-fighting targets may be related to those for amicable social behaviours (Pellis, 1988), including sexual activity. The view that play fighting involves targets that will later be important in precopulatory behaviour is supported by data for a variety of other animals: golden hamsters (Pellis and Pellis, 1988), prairie and montane voles (Pellis et al., 1992b) and djungarian hamsters (Pellis and Pellis, 1989). A further link between play and male sexual activity is suggested by the finding that juvenile play is virtually absent among house mice—a species with only rudimentary precopulatory behaviour (Pellis et al., 1991).

'Targets' in antipredator defensive behaviour

In conspecific defence, the defender attempts to conceal or protect target sites on its own body. However, some conspecific defences, and much more of antipredator defensive behaviour, consists of actions taken at a distance from the threat stimulus, but aimed or directed with reference to that threat source. In that sense, the threat stimulus and other especially relevant environmental features serve as 'targets' for a wide variety of antipredator defensive behaviours.

Flight, for example, is clearly orientated with reference to the threat, and its parameters change with decreasing distance between the threat source and the subject (Ydenberg and Dill, 1986). Flight also involves targets for approach and not merely an orientation away from threat. In a series of elegant studies Ellard and his colleagues have shown that gerbils respond to a threat stimulus by running towards and entering a place of refuge, if available (Ellard and Goodale, 1988). In a large circular enclosure containing no refuge, gerbils established a place preference during a 15 min exploratory period. Later presentation of an overhead threat stimulus produced flight responses that, rather than responding only to the threat stimulus, maximized the value of the function (distance to the threat stimulus minus the distance to the preferred area in the open field). When two small refuge boxes were available in the same test situation, the subjects showed a significant preference for the refuge they had preferred prior to the threat. However, this preference was not absolute, and the non-preferred refuge was often chosen when it was closer than the other (Ellard, 1993). Even when no refuge is present, being out of visual contact with a threat source is favoured. Rats in an oval runway divided by a partition wall run forward and away from the threat until it is out of sight because of the wall. They stop and assume an immobile posture until the (chasing) threat stimulus reappears and again elicits forward running (Blanchard, R.J. et al., 1986). Thus flight represents a defensive strategy that may be targeted away from an approaching predator or conspecific, towards a place of safety, or both.

Risk assessment: a target-seeking strategy

A situation in which there is no other animal or specific stimulus to serve as either a danger or an attractant might be regarded as constituting the limiting case for targeting of behaviour. However, when a predator or attacking conspecific is not actually present, but is suggested by a partial stimulus (e.g. odour) or by a conditioned (e.g. situational) stimulus, a pattern of response is typically shown in which the major activity is risk assessment. Risk assessment involves investigatory (e.g. visual scanning, sniffing, approach and contact) activities orientated towards the potentially dangerous area or partial stimulus (Blanchard, D.C. et al., 1991). In high threat situations risk assessment may consist only of orientation, while the subject avoids the potential danger and freezes. As the situation becomes less threatening (e.g. following a period in which no further evidence of danger appears), more active risk assessment, including approach, is seen. This approach involves stereotyped movements, with a 'stretch attend' or 'stretch approach' involving lowering of the back, and an intermittent movement pattern. These behaviours, seen also in the 'vigilance' responses of animals in their natural habitat, have been interpreted as representing the attempt to localize and identify a specific target (threat stimulus)—an action that is adaptive in permitting more precise and orientated defences such as flight or defensive threat and attack to occur (Blanchard, D.C. et al., 1991).

We believe that risk assessment reflects the activity of a distinct neurobehavioural system, the function of which is to gather information. Since this information, if negative (i.e. indicating that the threat is not present) serves to reduce defensiveness, risk assessment can be regarded as the defensive behaviour that limits defence. However, this view would not be accurate if risk assessment results in localization and/or identification of the threat, since risk assessment in that situation would give way to more specific defensive behaviours and, likely, a heightening of defensiveness. Finally, for most animals in the real world, failure to localize/identify a particular threat stimulus simply results in continuation of the risk assessment pattern, with any reduction in defensiveness being extremely gradual and incremental. Thus risk assessment is a pivotal activity in the defence pattern, capable of changing both the magnitude and the pattern of defence. However, it is also highly conservative and quite resistant to the effects of negative feedback, although positive feedback can result in a very rapid change in behaviour.

PATTERNING OF OFFENSIVE AND DEFENSIVE BEHAVIOURS

These analyses of offensive and defensive behaviours suggest an important feature in addition to target site involvement. In ecologically valid situations, both, but particularly defence, have a consistent but complex pattern over time. The offence pattern, consisting of approach, sniffing at the anogenital area, and piloerection, followed by the various components of the back-attack strategy (chase, lateral attack, on-top-of and bite), tends to be shorter (typically ending in defeat or disappearance of one combatant) and less complex. In contrast, some type of defence continues as long as a threat or potential threat is present and the subject capable of response.

In the real world and in laboratory situations designed to provide an analogue of these real-world conditions, defence may be a very long-duration response. Thus a single, 15 min presentation of a non-attacking cat to rats living in a visible burrow system produces withdrawal to the burrows, followed by active risk assessment peaking at about 7–10 h after cat exposure, with residual effects lasting 24 h or more (Blanchard, R.J. and Blanchard, 1989). The defensive behaviours change with feedback from risk assessment even if there is no change in the environment itself. This persistence of defensiveness and the different behaviours by which it is expressed over time independent of situational change have important implications for analysis of the biological systems controlling defence and its psychological or motivational designations 'fear' and 'anxiety'.

SENSORIMOTOR INTERACTIONS IN AGGRESSION AND DEFENCE

The notion that both aggressive and defensive behaviours involve particular targets towards (or away from) which behaviour is orientated, and by which individual behaviours are selected and guided, places further emphasis on an understanding of the sensorimotor interactions underlying these behaviours. The analyses described above suggest that while most individual aggressive and defensive behaviours have some targeting component, the individual actions that make up each pattern may differ considerably in the degree to which they reflect a relatively low-level 'reflex-type' sensorimotor behaviour as opposed to a more complex neural (as well as behavioural) system. As an example of the former, the potentiated auditory startle response, as outlined by Michael Davis and his colleagues (e.g. Davis, 1992), involves a known (hindbrain) reflex pathway for auditory startle, which is potentiated by input from limbic forebrain structures following relevant aversive conditioning.

In terms of the latter, more complex, system identification (and localization) of the opponent may involve motivated response chains of considerable complexity and duration. Thus offence tends to occur after a straightforward process of 'identification' that includes (particularly olfactory) investigation of the potential attackee. Defence may occur to minimal stimulation (e.g. sudden sounds or movement) but, in order for specific defences to be effective, more information about the threat stimulus is necessary. Thus in highly social species, such as vervet monkeys, there are not only 'alarm calls' but different calls that are elicited by aerial, terrestrial or subterranean predators (Cheney and Seyfarth, 1990), and that produce appropriately different defensive behaviours in the listener. The need for information on a threat source may also be seen in the incidence and duration of risk assessment behaviour, which have no parallel in the identification process leading to offensive aggression. In this context it is notable that the major response to potential threat stimuli, such as odours from predators (Blanchard, R.J. *et al.*, 1990; Zangrossi and File, 1992a, 1992b; Weldon, 1990) or novel stimuli (Garbe *et al.*, 1993), involves some type of risk assessment rather than the specific defences, e.g. flight, or defensive threat and attack.

A second source of influence on the selection of an offence versus a defence mode, and of particular defensive behaviours as well, is environmental. Thus, even though a stimulus may be identified as one to which offensive attack is often given, the location of the encounter (within subject's home range or territory versus outside this area) can reduce offence and enhance defence. For the defensive animal, such features as location, presence of burrows or other hiding places, and space available for flight can all importantly determine the form of the defensive behaviour given. Such environmental stimuli function both to select particular behaviours and to guide them as they occur.

Target-site analyses also emphasize the importance of sensory guidance of offensive and defensive behaviours, particularly by visual and tactile stimuli. However, in addition to specific target sites on the body of an opponent, sensory guidance may be seen as a component of general orientation towards relevant stimuli such as an opponent, a place of safety or a potential threat stimulus; or, away from an approaching or chasing threat source. These tend to occur over greater threat-to-subject distances than does conspecific defence.

Sensory biasing may represent the remaining limb of a bidirectional relationship between sensation and aggressive/defensive behaviour. Enhanced 'defensiveness', for example, appears to involve enhanced reactivity to threatening stimuli. Thus a handclap or sudden motion produces a systematically higher-magnitude startle response when it is made at successively shorter prey–predator distances. Reduced defensive distance appears to enhance reactivity to dorsal but not ventral contact, and reactivity to vibrissal stimulation (Blanchard R.J. *et al.*, 1986). As will be seen later, stimulation of brain areas associated with defence systems may reduce the threshold for a variety of defensive responses to relevant stimuli.

BRAIN SYSTEMS UNDERLYING SENSORY AND MOTOR INTERACTIONS IN DEFENCE AND AGGRESSION

Much less is known of the brain systems in offensive aggression than of brain systems in defence (Blanchard, D.C. and Blanchard, 1988), and this is as true of the sensory and motor systems involved as of any others. Pellis *et al.* (1992c) report that decortication in infancy does not massively disrupt motor patterning of adult offensive aggression, suggesting that the cortex is either not importantly involved, or is replaceable at this developmental stage. However, it is not known if the circumstances in which aggression normally occurs are altered by decortication, nor if decorticates improve their agonistic skills with fighting experience, as do normal rats. Potegal (1992) has recently reported c-fos expression in corticomedial amygdala (COA), for female hamsters during attack; selective reductions in agression following COA lesions; and reduced latency to attack with stimulation of the same area. Since both aggression and the medial amygdala are strongly associated with olfactory functions, these findings may (or, indeed may not) directly reflect olfactory processes.

For defensive behaviours, in contrast, there has recently been a veritable explosion of information on brain systems mediating these behaviours and the sensory and motor interactions that they represent (see Depaulis and Bandler, 1991, for reviews). Notably, the focus is not merely on specific sensory modalities, but on topographic or other qualities within the modality that correspond to environmentally important threat features. Most of these phenomena involve specific defences such as are made to an approaching and contacting threat stimulus, and they demonstrate a close relationship to sensorimotor relationships that have been demonstrated at a behavioural level.

First, in terms of visual control of defensive behaviours, Redgrave and Dean (1991) discuss a model in which retinal input to the superior colliculus (SC) is organized into zones subserving visual stimuli either in the upper visual field, or, in the lower visual field: electrical stimulation of the SC in the former area produces upward head movements while stimulation of the latter produces downward head movements. In addition, stimulation of only the most superficial layers of SC in the 'upper field stimulus' zone elicited avoidance and other defensive responses. Similar stimulation of the 'lower field stimulus' zone elicited orienting and approach responses—a finding that fits well with the behavioural observation that unexpected overhead movement is more likely to produce flight than is movement at floor level. They also report that some cells in the SC respond specifically to suddenly expanding stimuli such as might be produced by a rapidly oncoming object (Redgrave and Dean, 1991).

The SC is both directly and indirectly connected to the periaqueductal grey (PAG), particularly to the dorsal half of the caudal PAG (Redgrave et al., 1987, 1988). Stimulation of this caudal and dorsolateral PAG site in rats tends to produce forward avoidance (flight), alternating with periods of immobility (Bandler and Depaulis, 1991). A major indirect connection between SC and PAG is through the cuneiform area—a site in which microinjections of excitatory amino acids (EAA) also produce freezing and running (Mitchell et al., 1988). Both of these reactions are prominent in the defensive response of rats to approaching threat stimuli, and occur at defensive (stimulus–subject) distances that strongly suggest a primary role for visual input in the initiation of these behaviours (Blanchard, R.J. et al., 1986). In view of the highly conservative nature of mammalian defences, it is also notable that avoidance movements of the head to visual looming stimuli can also be obtained in human babies and adults. The latter, however, display such movements only when strongly distracted (in this case by a computer tracking game; King *et al.*, 1992). The latency for avoidance was lower than that for orientation under distraction conditions, perhaps suggesting a more direct anatomical route for the former.

A variety of tactile stimuli are also clearly involved in the elicitation and modulation of brain stimulation-elicited defensive behaviours. In rats, stimulation of the (anterior–posterior; A–P) intermediate third of the lateral PAG produces 'backward defences' including backing away and an upright posture, while stimulation of the caudal PAG in the same lateral column (a site apparently similar to the target for the SC projections described by Redgrave and Dean, 1991) produces 'forward avoidance' that can clearly be seen as flight when the animal is tested in a large area (Depaulis, 1993). Contralateral tactile stimulation of the head, but not the flank or hindlimb, increased 'backward defences' of rats with kainic acid (KA) injections in the (A–P) intermediate lateral PAG. However, 'forward avoidance' reactions following KA administration in more caudal portions of the lateral and dorsolateral PAG were facilitated by tactile stimulation of sites throughout the entire A–P extent of the body, with a greater effect of contralateral contact. These findings fit well with the results of behavioural studies, in that a major eliciting stimulus for upright (thus 'backwards') defences in conspecific attack is stimulation of the mystacial vibrissae.

In the cat, EAA stimulation of the same area that in the rat produces 'backwards defences' elicits a threat display of hissing or howling, piloerection, ear retraction and backing. These are a prominent feature of cat conspecific defensive behaviours to close approach (Leyhausen, 1979), although they may also appear in an antipredator context. Following KA injection into these more anterior and lateral PAG areas, both visual approach and tactile (muzzle or upper body) stimulation to the contralateral side increased the intensity of the threat display, or, elicited striking or biting (Bandler and Depaulis, 1991). In both rats and cats, defensive biting tends to occur at even shorter defensive distances than does defensive threat, and contact with the defender's head or upper back (a common target for offensive bites in cats) should be a particularly effective stimulus for such retaliatory action.

Bandler and his co-workers have also recently outlined two pain modalities and their differential connections to regions of the PAG in which stimulation elicits distinct behaviour patterns (Bandler, 1993). Tactile stimuli, such as radiant heat of the skin of the neck, led to *c-fos* expression in the lateral columns of the PAG, while deep pain (injection of formalin into the neck muscles) produced *c-fos* expression in the ventrolateral columns (Keay and Bandler, 1993). EAA stimulation of the ventrolateral column produced 'hyporeactive immobility' in which the animal is unresponsive to external stimulation, and hypotension (Bandler and Depaulis, 1991), while stimulation of the lateral columns tended to produce active responses and hypertension. Although immobility was sometimes seen during periods of active defence following stimulation of the lateral column, this was associated with heightened reactivity to body contact rather than hyporeactivity, and lateral column stimulation produced hypertension rather than the hypotension associated with the ventrolateral column (Carrive, 1991).

The differentiation between the lateral and ventrolateral columns extends to the major somatosensory input pathways to the two PAG regions (Bandler, 1993), and to autonomic effects of stimulation in addition to blood pressure changes. Stimulation of the lateral (and particularly caudal) PAG increased heart rate, and rate and depth of respiration, vasodilation in hindlimb muscle, and pupillary dilation. However, EAA stimulation of the ventral PAG produced a very different pattern, with decreased blood pressure and heart rate, but increased hindlimb muscle blood flow (with a much longer latency, however) and greatly enhanced depth of respiration (Lovick, 1991).

These studies suggest that the PAG serves as a crucial integration area for a number of sensorimotor systems involved in defence. The mechanisms being described in this area make it very clear that the concept of sensorimotor interactions in the control of specific defensive behaviour systems is very meaningful. It should be noted, however, that the dorsal and lateral column behaviours—flight, freezing, defensive threat/attack—correspond very well to those seen in situations involving predator or conspecific attack, not those involving potential threat. Risk assessment appears to represent a very different defence system and one for which the neural correlates are, at present, totally unknown.

IMPLICATIONS OF TARGET-SITE AND BEHAVIOUR-PATTERNING ASPECTS OF AGGRESSION AND DEFENCE

The relationship between a target-site analysis and 'display' concepts

One remarkable aspect of the history of scientific attention to agonistic behaviour is the persistence of the interpretation that conspecific aggression and defence in animals consists of threat and submission displays, respectively, by which disputes are painlessly and bloodlessly settled. One reason for such persistence may be that the actions leading up to the bite or blow, or by which the bite or blow is deflected or avoided, appear unnecessarily stereotyped or ritualized in terms of the basic functions of aggression and defence, to deliver, or thwart, pain or damage. Thus, the defensive upright and lying on the back might appear to have no strategic value in defence if it is believed that the attacker might well bite the defender's easily accessible ventral surface and limbs. Similarly, the lateral attack pattern would make little sense as an attack strategy if attack bites were delivered indiscriminately on the body of the opponent.

Since the lateral attack, and defensive upright and on-the-back occur with great regularity, however, they need some other explanation. Interpretation of the lateral attack as a 'threat display' indicates that the effectiveness of the action in promoting victory, success or enhanced access to resources is mediated solely by the response of the opponent. However, although a previously defeated rat is quite likely to become defensive in the presence of the rat that has previously defeated him (and, indeed, can do so to the odour alone of a dominant rat; Williams, 1989), there is presently no evidence that this effect is mediated through the actions designated as a 'threat display'. Laboratory rats without experience of defeat appear not to respond defensively to resident attack, including repeated 'threat displays' until they are bitten (unpublished observations), suggesting that response to the 'threat display' must be learned, at least in laboratory rats. The 'threat display' may indeed serve as a conditioned stimulus eliciting fear or defensiveness in previously defeated animals, but this would not suggest that it has evolved as a preprogrammed communication mechanism.

In experienced animals, defensive upright and lying on the back are successful defences; comparatively few completed bites occur when the defender is engaged in these activities. This had led to the interpretation that they are 'submission' displays terminating the agonistic encounter without further (or any) damage, because they communicate to the attacker that the defender has 'submitted' and offers no further defence. In terms of a target-site analysis, lying on the back *constitutes* a defence, since it conceals the area, the back, that is the target for conspecific offensive biting. Thus a target-site analysis, providing a clear rationale for the success of activities such as the lateral attack in promoting the goals of the attacker, and upright and on-the-back defences in promoting the goals of the defender, provides an alternative to 'display' interpretations of the same behaviours. This view suggests that interpretation of a given behaviour as an agonistic 'display' should be disallowed unless it can be demonstrated that the success of the action is not related to its effectiveness in achieving or denying access to a bite target.

Implications of aggression/defence analyses for pharmacological research

The preceding findings and analyses suggest that both aggression and defence involve multiple levels of stimulus and motor control. First, animals must identify relevant stimuli such as potential competitors, or predators, using criteria that are in part based on previous experience but may also reflect preprogramming. Subsequently, a behavioural strategy must be selected, and this is determined by the characteristics of the threatening stimulus and the environment in which it occurs. Again, both individual experience and genetic/neural systems variation can modify the relationship between environmental/threat stimuli and the response given, but in the absence of specific training or strong manipulation of biological factors these relationships tend to be quite consistent within a species. The specific strategy chosen then involves the activation of particular sensorimotor systems involving aimed motor patterns with intermittent or continuous feedback from target stimuli. Both the target stimuli and the motor patterns are, again, heavily preprogrammed.

These analyses suggest an organization of attack and defence that needs to be considered in pharmacological analyses of these systems. As one rather simple example, viewing attack or defence patterns from the perspective of a strong target orientation suggests that specific changes in responsivity to contact with particular body sites may serve as a valid index of changes in the 'motivational' aspects of aggression or defence. Thus increased defensiveness can be seen in heightened responsivity to dorsal as opposed to ventral stimulation, a feature of wild as opposed to laboratory rats or rats with lesions producing the so-called 'septal syndrome' (Blanchard, D.C. et al., 1979). These features suggest a range of new measures for pharmacological research that may be particularly specific and sensitive.

Another relatively straightforward implication of these analyses for pharmacological research is that, in conspecific interactions, although attack elicits defence, the form of attack tends to depend very precisely on the form of defence. The phenomenon of drugged intruders eliciting altered attack from aggressive residents may, in some cases, represent a direct example of the latter phenomenon alone, rather than requiring the more elaborate interpretation of drugged intruder eliciting different attack, which in turn alters the intruder's defence. The choice of which interpretation to make probably depends on the specificity of what is measured. When only composite attack and defence scores are given, it would not be possible to determine the major direction of influence. However, if an alteration of a specific defender behaviour is accompanied by a corresponding alteration of the attack component of that specific defence–attack dyad, it would be unparsimonious to interpret the change in the defender's behaviour as the result of alterations in attack.

The patterning aspect of aggression and defence also has implications for pharmacological research. First, it draws attention to variability (from external manipulations, or from individual or genetic differences) in the progression from one behaviour to another within each of these patterns. In terms of individual differences, a recent study of dominance–subordination relationships in rat groups suggests that it is not the latency to attack but the consistency of progression through the attack pattern, and the number of terminal elements (e.g. bites) that determines if a rat will be dominant in its group (Blanchard, R.J. et al., 1992). Since bites have hardly any duration compared to other attack pattern elements, these findings also suggest that composite aggression scores based on duration may be insensitive or even misleading in the context of response to pharmacological or other independent variable manipulation.

A particularly important (and possibly related) example of patterning differences in both aggression and defence may be found in comparison of short-attack-latency (SAL) versus long-attack-latency (LAL) rats and mice (Koolhaas, 1993). The two groups of animals share the majority of actual attack or defence elements, but their timing of these elements, and their responsivity to outside influences and stimuli, are so divergent as to represent different 'strategies' for aggression, defence, sexual, parental, and other important behaviours. The strong and consistent difference of the two groups in responsivity to external stimuli (Benus *et al.*, 1987, 1990) suggests a possible link to the risk assessment activities that have been most specifically characterized in an antipredator defence context. If so, and given that risk assessment is the major behaviour involved in an 'anxiolytic profile' of effects of a variety of anxiolytic drugs, the SAL and LAL rats may provide an excellent model system for investigation of the interaction of risk assessment (RA) and other important behaviours.

Aside from the effects of variations in RA on the patterning of other behaviours, RA itself represents an important example of behaviour whose normal patterning must be understood in order to interpret the effects of drugs on that behaviour. First, a variety of anxiolytic drugs differentially affect RA, as opposed to more specific defences to present threat stimuli (Blanchard, R.J. *et al.*, 1993a). These anxiolytics (e.g. diazepam) consistently *increased* RA behaviour when behaviour was tested against a baseline of freezing and avoidance, but *decreased* RA in a situation in which RA was initially an important (though not predominant) response. This consistent but puzzling finding for anxiolytic drugs may be explained by the particular patterning of RA in the context of long-term responsivity to potential threat (Blanchard, D.C. *et al.*, 1991). Freezing and proximic avoidance of the threatening situation are initial reactions to very high level potential threat, followed by RA over time and as the intensity of threat declines. A further decline in threat intensity, as RA reveals no actual threat source, results eventually in decreased RA and a return to normal, non-defensive behaviour. Thus when the intensity of the potential threat source is very high (i.e. freezing/avoidance baseline) a drug-induced decrease in such defensiveness acts to increase RA. When defensiveness is moderate, and RA is already an important baseline defensive behaviour, drug-induced decreases in defensiveness reduce RA, and return the animal to normal.

Strain- or line-linked differences in defence are even more striking when defensive behaviour has been part of the criterion for selection of animals for these strains or lines. Comparison of wild and laboratory rats suggests that the behavioural components as well as the patterns of defensive behaviour are greatly altered by domestication (Blanchard, R.J. *et al.*, 1986). Defence and defence patterns are also much altered in wild rats selected specifically for the presence or absence of defensive threat/attack to human handling (Naumenko *et al.*, 1989; Blanchard, D.C. *et al.*, in press). These behavioural differences are also associated with particular alterations of neurotransmitter systems

(Naumenko *et al.*, 1989; Blanchard, R.J., 1990), a potential factor in interpretation of the effects of pharmacological agents on defence in the polarized lines.

Finally, attention to the intensity-based patterning of conspecific defensive behaviour may suggest an alternative interpretation of findings such as those of Piret *et al.* (1991). They report that chronically administered diazepam (5 mg/kg over 24 h) increases defence (freezing and defensive upright) while decreasing 'submission' (lying on the back) in rats under attack by a conspecific. A benzodiazepine partial agonist, ZK 91296, tended also to increase defensive upright, while an inverse agonist, FG 7142, decreased defensive upright and increased freezing—results that were interpreted as supporting differential benzodiazepine effects on 'defence' versus 'submission'.

A more parsimonious explanation is that these effects simply reflect benzodiazepine receptor-mediated alterations in the intensity of defensiveness. Defensive upright is seen relatively early in conspecific defence and to fewer assaults, while lying on-the-back tends to occur as a later component, with an animal that has been repeatedly assaulted and may be more defensive. Thus these findings may represent an intensity effect, rather than specific alteration of different neural systems underlying particular defensive behaviours. No doubt this question will also be clarified in the context of detail on the neural systems involved (in this case, caudal portions of the lateral column of the PAG?), but an awareness of the patterning of natural defensive behaviours is also important in directing the behavioural aspects of research on the neural systems involved. In this context, changes in the intensity of defensiveness may be reflected not only in the intensity (frequency, duration, magnitude) of a specific behaviour, but also in the transitions from one behaviour to another.

The role of psychopharmacology in analysis of aggression and defence systems

Most research on the psychopharmacology of aggression- and defence-related behaviour is driven straightforwardly by the continuing and legitimate need to predict the effects of drugs on emotion-related psychopathologies, including anxiety, depression, panic disorder, post-traumatic stress disorder and the like. As precise and comprehensive analyses of aggression and defence become available, we suggest that preclinical research in these areas should increasingly focus on the pharmacology of specific aggressive and defensive behaviours, and of their patterning. Ideally, parallel research on the relationship between specific alterations of aggressive/defensive behaviours and the target symptoms of particular human psychopathologies would provide an improved basis for using drug effects on specific agonistic behaviours to predict their effects on these clinical conditions.

The latter type of information may be more difficult to obtain than the former. In the case of aggression, for example, there is close agreement about what constitutes a good offensive aggression model, for example, that a conspecific opponent should be involved, and that some or all of the behaviours classified as part of the attack pattern by Grant and his colleagues should be seen. This long-term agreement has led to a body of research on the pharmacology of offensive behaviour that has produced very consistent results (for reviews see Olivier and Mos, 1990; Olivier et al., 1984). Exceptions to the consistency have primarily involved situations or subjects in which there were alterations of defensiveness, along with aggression, e.g. when timid versus aggressive resident mice were used as subjects (Krsiak, 1989). This is because defence is so much more powerful a neurobehavioural system than is aggression, and alterations of defence have profound effects on aggressive response.

In contrast to this good body of data on drug effects on offensive aggression in animals, there has been very little attention to the question of the relationship between (offensive) aggression in animal models and aggressive or violent behaviours as components of human psychopathology. While it appears clear that offensive aggression is involved in some human violence, it is also increasingly suggested (Albert, 1993; Blanchard and Blanchard, 1985) that defensive attack may also be important, particularly in pathological violence.

However, even in the absence of any specific understanding of the relationship between aggression/defence and emotional psychopathology, the consequences of administration of a variety of drugs, with known efficacy against particular disorders, on a systematic array of agonistic behaviours should provide some indication that the altered behaviours may be particularly involved in that disorder. This variant of a well-used strategem in psychopharmacological research was used in the identification of the 'anxiolytic profile' mentioned earlier, of four particular effects seen selectively after administration of a variety of classic and novel anxiolytics, plus alcohol, and imiprimine, as well as some as yet clinically untested but potentially anxiolytic compounds (Blanchard, R.J., et al., 1993). In that case, one value of the project was that it strongly suggested a particular role for risk assessment, and other defensive reactions to anticipated or potential (as opposed to actual and present) threat, in anxiety.

More recently, Blanchard et al. (1993b) reported that the panicogenic agent yohimbine potentiated flight-related reactions of mice in an antipredator situation in which a variety of defensive behaviours were measured. Chronic administration of the panicolytic agent alprazolam reduced the number of avoidances at low as well as high (0.5–2.0 mg/kg) doses in a similar test situation, while, consonant with its clinical effect, chlordiazepoxide altered the same measure only when given at a very high dose (25 mg/kg) (Griebel et al., submitted). These findings fit well with the suggestion of Deakin and Graeff (1991) that flight (which is very poorly responsive to anxiolytic drugs generally) is particularly involved in panic disorder.

While much of the interest in the results of such studies simply reflects their value in predicting clinical effects of particular drugs, this work also contributes to the understanding of two additional sets of relationships. First, by providing detailed descriptions of those defensive behaviours that are consistently altered by drugs with acknowledged effectiveness against specific clinical disorders, these studies suggest that these particular behaviours may represent the neurobehavioural systems that are most strongly involved in that specific psychopathology. Thus, to a degree, the results of these psychopharmacological studies can detail specific relationships between animal and human emotion-linked behaviour patterns.

Second, these same studies also contribute to a body of data on differential drug effects on various defensive behaviours. At a minimum, these data should suggest hypotheses about the neurotransmitter/neuromodulator control of particular behaviours that might then be tested through research at the systems level. The same body of data may also provide indications of the basic neurobiological organization of aggression and defence systems. For example, the differentiation of 'anxiety' (primarily risk assessment) components of defence from other defence components by patterns of drug response suggests that the underlying systems for these anxiety and non-anxiety defence components are more different from each other than are the systems that underlie, for example, specific risk assessment activities.

'More different from' has implications at both a neurobiological level, and in terms of conceptualization. In terms of the latter, does the differentiation of 'anxiety' and 'fear' aspects of defence suggest that the 'motivation' associated with anxiety is different from that of fear? Based on recent work (e.g. Williams, 1989; Zangrossi and File, 1992a, 1992b) indicating considerable potentiation of defensiveness in a variety of unrelated situations and tests following threat exposure, it seems very likely that there is substantial generality of the enhancement of defensiveness across situations and behaviours. The drug studies, however, make it clear that this generality is not absolute. While there is not yet any satisfactory theoretical analysis of the relationship of these systems, it seems clear that data on the effects of drugs on these behaviours will be an integral component of such analysis when it is attempted.

In summary, pharmacological analysis of these aggression and defence systems should provide information relevant to both applied and basic research concerns. Moreover, the results of both applied and basic research studies should be valuable in providing a more rational basis for the development of psychoactive drugs.

SUMMARY

The views of aggression and defence that are beginning to emerge from ethoexperimental analyses are complex but relatively conservative, agreeing closely, at the crucial observational and descriptive level, with the early analyses of Grant and his colleagues. Methodologically, ethoexperimental studies over the past 30 years have emphasized the provision of relatively natural living and/or test situations. These afford environmental features that make the functional outcomes of both attack and defence more salient to both the experimenter and to the subjects themselves. They also enable a more realistic and detailed view of the time-course and normal outcomes of attack and defence. These analyses have added to traditional ethological views of attack and defence in several ways:

1. through explanatory principles afforded by the target site concept;
2. by the differentiation of defensive behaviours elicited by specific and present threat stimuli, as opposed to those seen in the context of anticipated threat;
3. by conceptualizations of both attack and defence as progressions involving time, an intensity dimension, and the feedback afforded by successful accomplishment of functional goals (e.g. a back bite or escape down a burrow) associated with particular behaviour patterns.

There is consistent evidence that the three systems—aggression; specific defences to present threat stimuli (fear?); and defensiveness to anticipated threat (anxiety?)—are pharmacologically separable. There is less, but increasing, evidence for differential pharmacological control of behaviours within each system, some of which may be mediated by drug manipulation of an intensity dimension or by sedation. Finally, there is an emerging body of literature indicating that the specific defence systems are differentiated and importantly modulated by particular sensorimotor interactions at the level of the PAG. Neither aggression nor defensiveness to potential threat appears to be organized in the PAG, and the neural correlates of these behaviours are, at present, very poorly understood. It is hoped that the delineation of some of the important behavioural and functional differences among these three patterns will serve as a spur to further research on the neurobiology of the systems involved.

ACKNOWLEDGEMENT

This work was supported by USPHS Awards NIH MH42803, AA06220 and RR03061.

REFERENCES

Albert, D. (1993) Presentation at Guggenheim Conference *Neural Systems in Aggression*, Antwerp, Belgium.

Bandler, R. (1993) Presentation at Guggenheim Conference *Neural Systems in Aggression*, Antwerp, Belgium.

Bandler, R. and Depaulis, A. (1991) Midbrain periaqueductal gray control of defensive behavior in the cat and the rat. In: *The Midbrain Periaqueductal Gray Matter:*

Functional, Anatomical, and Neurochemical Organization (eds A. Depaulis and R. Bandler). Plenum, New York, pp. 175–198.

Ben-David, M., Pellis, S.M. and Pellis, V.C. (1991) Feeding habits and predatory behaviour in the marbled polecat (*Vormela peregusna syriaca*): I. Killing methods in relation to prey size and prey behaviour. *Behaviour*, 118, 127–143.

Benus, R.F., Koolhaas, J.M. and Van Oortmerssen, G.A. (1987) Individual differences in behavioural reaction to a changing environment in mice and rats. *Behaviour*, 100, 105–122.

Benus, R.F., Den Daas, S., Koolhaas, J.M. and Van Oortmerssen, G.A. (1990) Routine formation and flexibility in social and non-social behaviour of aggressive and non-aggressive male mice. *Behaviour*, 112, 176–193.

Blanchard, D.C. and Blanchard, R.J. (1988) Ethoexperimental approaches to the biology of emotion. *Annu. Rev. Psychol.*, 39 (Palo Alto: Annual Reviews).

Blanchard, D.C., Blanchard, R.J., Lee, E.M.C. and Nakamura, S. (1979) Defensive behaviors in rats following septal and septal–amygdala lesions. *J. Comp. Physiol. Psychol.*, 93, 378–390.

Blanchard, D.C., Blanchard, R.J. and Rodgers, R.J. (1991) Risk assessment and animal models of anxiety. In: *Animal Models in Psychopharmacology* (eds B. Olivier, J. Mos and J.L. Slangen). Birkhauser Verlag, Basle, pp. 117–134.

Blanchard, D.C., Popova N.K., Plyusnina, I.Z. *et al.* Defensive behaviors of 'wild-type' and 'domesticated' wild rats in a fear/defense test battery. *Aggressive Behav.* (in press).

Blanchard, R.J. and Blanchard, D.C. (1977) Aggressive behavior in the rat. *Behav. Biol.*, 21, 197–224.

Blanchard, R.J. and Blanchard, D.C. (1985) *Animal Aggression and the Dyscontrol Syndrome* (eds M. Girgis and L.E. Kilom). Elsevier, Amsterdam.

Blanchard, R.J. and Blanchard, D.C. (1989) Anti-predator defensive behaviors in a visible burrow system. *J. Comp. Psychol.*, 103, 70–82.

Blanchard, R.J., Blanchard, D.C., Takahashi, T. and Kelley, M. (1977a) Attack and defensive behavior in the albino rat. *Anim. Behav.*, 25, 622–634.

Blanchard, R.J., Takahashi, L.K., Fukunaga, K.K. and Blanchard, D.C. (1977b) Functions of the vibrissae in the defensive and aggressive behavior of the rat. *Aggressive Behav.*, 3, 231–240.

Blanchard, R.J., Blanchard, D.C. and Takahashi, L.K. (1978) Pain and aggression in the rat. *Behav. Biol.*, 23, 291–305.

Blanchard, R.J., O'Donnell, V. and Blanchard, D.C. (1979) Attack and defensive behaviors in the albino mouse (*Mus musculus*). *Aggressive Behav.*, 5, 341–352.

Blanchard, R. J., Kleinschmidt, C.F., Fukunaga-Stinson, C. and Blanchard, D.C. (1980) Defensive attack behavior in male and female rats. *Anim. Learning Behav.*, 8, 177–183.

Blanchard, R.J., Blanchard, D.C., Pank, L. and Fellows, D. (1985) Conspecific wounding in free ranging *Rattus norvegicus*. *Psychol. Rec.*, 35, 329–335.

Blanchard, R.J., Flannelly, K.J. and Blanchard, D.C. (1986) Defensive behaviors of laboratory and wild *Rattus norvegicus*. *J. Comp. Psychol.*, 100, 101–107.

Blanchard, R.J., Blanchard, D.C., Weiss, S.M. and Mayer, S. (1990) Effects of ethanol and diazepam on reactivity to predatory odors. *Pharmacol. Biochem. Behav.*, 35, 775–780.

Blanchard, R.J., Flores, T., Magee, L. *et al.* (1992) Pregrouping aggression and defense scores influence alcohol consumption for dominant and subordinate rats in visible burrow systems. *Aggressive Behav.*, 18, 459–467.

Blanchard, R.J., Yudko, E.B., Rodgers R.J. and Blanchard, D.C. (1993a) Defense system psychopharmacology: an ethological approach to the pharmacology of fear and anxiety. *Behav. Brain Res.*, 58, 155–165.

Blanchard, R.J., Taukulis, H.K., Rodgers, R.J., Magee, L.K. and Blanchard, D.C. (1993) Yohimbine potentiates active defensive responses to threatening stimuli in Swiss-Webster mice. *Pharmacol., Biochem., Behav.*, **44**, 673–681 (b).

Carrive, P. (1991) Functional organization of PAG neurons controlling regional vascular beds. In: *The Midbrain Periaqueductal Gray Matter: Functional, Anatomical, and Neurochemical Organization* (eds A. Depaulis and R. Bandler). Plenum, New York, pp. 67–100.

Cheney, D.L. and Seyfarth, R.M. (1990) *How Monkeys See the World*. University of Chicago Press, Chicago.

Davis, M. (1992) The role of the amygdala in fear-potentiated startle: implications for animal models of anxiety. *Trends Pharmacol. Sci.*, **13**, 35–41.

Deakin, W. and Graeff, F.G. (1991) 5-HT and mechanisms of defence. *Psychopharmacol.*, **5**, 305–315.

Depaulis, A. (1993) Presentation of Guggenheim Conference *Neural Systems in Aggression*, Antwerp, Belgium.

Depaulis, A. and Bandler, R. (eds) (1991) *The Midbrain Periaqueductal Gray Matter: Functional, Anatomical, and Neurochemical Organization*. Plenum, New York.

Ellard, C.G. (1993) Organization of escape movements from overhead threats in the mongolian gerbil (*Meriones unguiculatus*). *J. Comp. Psychol.*, **107**, 242–249.

Ellard, C.G. and Goodale, M.A. (1988) A functional analysis of collicular output pathways: a dissociation of deficits following lesions of the dorsal tegmental decussation and the ipsilateral efferent bundle in the Mongolian gerbil. *Exp. Brain Res.*, **71**, 307–319.

Fentress, J.C. (1988) Expressive contexts, fine structure, and central mediation of rodent grooming. In: *Neural Mechanisms and Biological Significance of Grooming Behavior* (eds D.L. Colbern and W.H. Gispen). NY Academy of Sciences, New York, pp. 18–26.

Garbe, C.M., Kemble, E.D. and Rawleigh, J.M. (1993) Novel odors evoke risk assessment and suppress appetitive behaviors in mice. *Aggressive Behav.*, **19** 447–454.

Grant, E.C. (1963) An analysis of the social behaviour of the male laboratory rat. *Behaviour*, **21**, 260–281.

Grant, E.C. and Chance, M.R.A. (1958) Rank order in caged rats. *Anim. Behav.*, **6**, 183–194.

Grant, E.C. and MacKintosh, J.H. (1963) A comparison of the social postures of some common laboratory rodents. *Behaviour*, **21**, 246–259.

Griebel, G., Blanchard, D.C., Lee, J., Masuda, C.K. and Blanchard, R.J. Differential modulation of antipredator defensive behavior in Swiss-Webster mice by chlordiazepoxide, and, with acute or chronic treatment with alprazolam. (Submitted for publication).

Herzog, H.A. and Bern, C. (1992) Do garter snakes strike at the eyes of predators? *Anim. Behav.*, **44**, 771–773.

Keay, K.A. and Bandler, R. (1993) *Neurosci. Lett.*, **139**, 143–148.

King, S.M., Dykeman, C., Redgrave, P. and Dean, P. (1992) Use of a distracting task to obtain defensive head movements to looming visual stimuli by human adults in a laboratory setting. *Perception*, **21**, 245–259.

Koolhaas, J.M. (1993) Presentation at Guggenheim Conference *Neural Systems in Aggression*, Antwerp, Belgium.

Krsiak, M. (1989) Behavioural effects of fluprazine in aggressive and timid mice during intraspecies conflict. *Activitas Nervous Superior*, **31**, 63–64.

Leyhausen, P. (1979) *Cat Behavior*. Garland Press, New York.

Lovick, T.A. (1991) Interactions between descending pathways from the dorsal and ventrolateral periaqueductal gray matter in the rat. In: *The Midbrain Periaqueductal*

Gray Matter: Functional, Anatomical, and Neurochemical Organization (eds A. Depaulis and R. Bandler). Plenum, New York, pp. 101–120.

Mitchell, I.J., and Dean, P. and Redgrave, P. (1988) The projection from the superior colliculus to the cuneiform area in the rat. II. Defense-like responses to stimulation with glutamate in cuneiform nucleus and surrounding structures. *Exp. Brain Res.*, **72**, 626–639.

Naumenko, E.V., Popova, N.K., Nikulina, E.M. *et al.* (1989) Behavior, adrenocortical activity, and brain monoamines in Norway rats selected for reduced aggressiveness towards man. *Pharmacol. Biochem. Behav.*, **33**, 85–91.

Olivier, B. and Mos, J. (1990) Serenics, serotonin and aggression. *Prog. Clin. Biol. Res.*, **361**, 203–230.

Olivier, B., van Aken, H., Jaarsma, I. *et al.* (1984) Behavioural effects of psychoactive drugs on agonistic behaviour of male territorial rats (resident–intruder model). In: *Ethopharmacology of Agonistic Behavior in Animals and Humans* (eds B. Olivier, J. Mos and P.F. Brain). Martinus Nijhoff, Dordrecht, pp. 137–156.

Pellis, S.M. (1988) Agonistic versus amicable targets of attack and defense: consequences for the origin, function, and descriptive classification of play-fighting. *Aggressive Behav.*, **14**, 85–104.

Pellis, S.M. and Pellis, V.C. (1987) Play-fighting differs from serious fighting in both target of attack and tactics of fighting in the laboratory rat, *Rattus norvegicus*. *Aggressive Behav.*, **13**, 227–242.

Pellis, S.M. and Pellis, V.C. (1988) Identification of the possible origin of the body target that differentiates play fighting from serious fighting in Syrian Golden hamsters (*Mesocricetus auratus*). *Aggressive Behav.*, **14**, 437–449.

Pellis, S.M. and Pellis, V.C. (1989) Targets of attack and defence in play-fighting of the Djungarian hamster *Phodopus campbelli*: links to fighting and sex. *Aggressive Behav.*, **15**, 217–234.

Pellis, S.M. and Pellis, V.C. (1991) Role reversal changes during the ontogeny of play fighting in male rats: attack vs. defense. *Aggressive Behav.*, **17**, 179–189.

Pellis, S.M., Pellis, V.C., Manning, C.J. and Dewsbury, D.A. (1991) The paucity of social play in juvenile *Mus domesticus*: what is missing from the behavioural repertoire? *Anim. Behav.*, **42**, 686–687.

Pellis, S.M., Pellis, V.C., Manning, C.J. and Dewsbury, D.A. (1992a) Supine defense in the intraspecific fighting of male house mice *Mus domesticus*. *Aggressive Behav.*, **18**, 373–379.

Pellis, S.M., Pellis, V.C., Pierce, J.D. and Dewsbury, D.A. (1992b) Disentangling the contribution of the attacker from that of defender in the differences in the intraspecific fighting in two species of voles. *Aggressive Behav.*, **18**, 425–435.

Pellis, S.M., Pellis, V.C. and Whishaw, I.Q. (1992c) The role of the cortex in play fighting by rats: developmental and evolutionary implications. *Brain Behav. Evol.*, **39**, 270–284.

Pierce, J.D., Pellis, V.C., Dewsbury, D.A. and Pellis, S.M. (1991) Targets and tactics of agonistic and precopulatory behavior in montane and prairie voles: their relationship to juvenile play-fighting. *Aggressive Behav.*, **17**, 337–349.

Piret, B., Depaulis, A. and Vergnes, M. (1991) Opposite effects of agonist and inverse agonist ligands of benzodiazepine receptor on self-defensive and submissive postures in the rat. *Psychopharmacology*, **103**, 56–61.

Potegal, M. (1992) Does mediation of aggressive arousal by the hamster corticomedial amygdala involve an LTP-like effect? *Soc. Neurosci. Abstracts*, 364.12.

Redgrave, P. and Dean, P. (1991) Does the PAG learn about emergencies from the superior colliculus? In: *The Midbrain Periaqueductal Gray Matter: Functional, Anatomical, and Neurochemical Organization* (eds A. Depaulis and R. Bandler). Plenum, New York, pp. 199–209.

Redgrave, P., Mitchell, I.J. and Dean, P. (1987) Descending projections from the superior colliculus in rat: a study using orthograde transport of wheatgerm-agglutinin conjugated horseradish peroxidase. *Exp. Brain Res.*, **68**, 147–167.

Redgrave, P., Dean, P., Mitchell, I.J. *et al.* (1988) The projection from superior colliculus to cuneiform area in the rat. I. Anatomical studies. *Exp. Brain Res.*, **72**, 611–625.

Sachs, B.D. (1988) The development of grooming and its expression in adult animals. In: *Neural Mechanisms and Biological Significance of Grooming Behavior* (eds D.L. Colbern and W.H. Gispen). NY Academy of Sciences, New York, pp. 1–18.

Scott, J.P. (1966) Agonistic behavior of rats and mice. *Am. Zool.*, **6**, 683–701.

Seidensticker, J. and McDougal, C. (1993) Tiger predatory behaviour, ecology and conservation. In: *Mammals as Prey* (eds N. Dunstone and M.L. Gorman). Clarendon Press, Oxford, pp. 105–123.

Stone, C.P. (1932) Wildness and savageness in rats of different strains. In: *Studies in the Dynamics of Behavior* (ed. K.S. Lashley). University of Chicago Press, Chicago, pp. 3–55.

Takahashi, L.K. and Blanchard, R.J. (1982) Attack and defense in laboratory and wild Norway and black rats. *Behav. Proc.*, **7**, 49–62.

Weldon, P. (1990) Responses by vertebrates to chemicals from predators. In: *Chemical Signals in Vertebrates 5* (eds D.W. Macdonald, D. Muller-Schwarze and S.E. Natynczuk). Oxford University Press, New York, pp. 500–521.

Williams, J.L. (1989) Ethoexperimental analysis of stress, contextual odors, and defensive behaviors. In: *Ethoexperimental Approaches to the Study of Behavior* (eds R.J. Blanchard, P.F. Brain, D.C. Blanchard and S. Parmigiani). Kluwer, Dordrecht, pp. 214–228.

Ydenberg, R.C. and Dill, L.M. (1986) The economics of fleeing from predators. *Adv. Study Behav.*, **16**, 229–249.

Yerkes, R.M. (1913) The heredity of savageness and wildness in rats. *J. Anim. Behav.*, **3**, 286–296.

Zangrossi, H. and File, S.E. (1992a) Behavioral consequences in animal tests of anxiety and exploration of exposure to cat odor. *Brain Res. Bull.*, **29**, 381–388.

Zangrossi, H. and File, S.E. (1992b) Chlordiazepoxide reduces the generalized anxiety, but not the direct responses, of rats exposed to cat odor. *Pharmacol. Biochem. Behav.*, **43**, 1195–1200.

8 The Application of Ethopharmacology in an Industrial Setting: The Example of Serenics

J. MOS,[a] **R. VAN OORSCHOT,**[a] **B. OLIVIER,**[a,b] **AND J. TOLBOOM**[c]

[a]CNS Pharmacology, Solvay-Duphar, Weesp, The Netherlands,
[b]Psychopharmacology Department, Faculty of Pharmacy, University of Utrecht, The Netherlands, [c]Department of Statistics, Solvay-Duphar, Weesp, The Netherlands

INTRODUCTION

Aggression is one of several categories of behaviour which have been studied intensively using ethological and psychopharmacological techniques. In fact, aggression research provides one of the best examples of the application of these techniques and may be used to illustrate many of the underlying principles of this type of research. Apart from the usual interest people take in aggression (as can be seen during visits to a zoo where the display of aggression evokes many reactions in the visitors), there is a serious clinical need to treat pathological aggression. Many psychiatric patients exhibit some sort of aggressive behaviour that is disturbing to them and to others. Although aggression is not a separate diagnostic entity in the DSM-III-R or the ICD-9, it is often a symptom accompanying a wide variety of different disorders (de Koning and Mak, 1991). Pharmacological treatment of pathological aggression often involves the use of neuroleptics and other drugs that heavily sedate. It would be beneficial if new drugs could be developed that reduce aggression without adversely affecting normal social behaviour. In our studies on animal aggression and drug effects, we have searched for such compounds, the so-called serenics. In this research process we have relied on ethopharmacological methods because pathological aggression is difficult to define and the validity of animal models is an important issue. Our line of thought on how to use ethopharmacology will be put forward and exemplified by data on the serenic drug eltoprazine and on some selected reference compounds. Subsequently, we will present preliminary data on statistical techniques that we applied to our databank on drugs and aggression in the male rat.

Ethology and Psychopharmacology. Edited by S.J. Cooper and C.A. Hendrie
© 1994 John Wiley & Sons Ltd

PRECLINICAL STRATEGY ON SERENICS

For the development of psychoactive drugs aimed at specifically suppressing aggression, some kind of definition of pathological aggression is needed. What are the essential features of pathological aggression in man? Despite many studies on aggression, both preclinical and clinical, this area of pathological aggression is in desperate need of clear definitions and an overall theory that can be tested and verified. Pathological aggression is not a DSM-III-R disorder for which criteria have been set to determine what is normal and what is abnormal. Neither is a satisfactory knowledge of underlying biological factors the starting point for rational research, either preclinical or clinical. Thus a discussion about the nature and characteristics of pathological aggression is needed before successful attempts can be made to develop animal models and new treatment strategies. It will be clear from the foregoing that the lack of clear definitions of pathological aggression puts considerable limitations on the use of animal models.

The multitude of definitions of 'normal' aggression (Moyer, 1968) underlines the complexity of this set of behaviours. Aggression serves many purposes which, at least in the animal kingdom, do not necessarily have a negative connotation. The variety of situations in which aggression occurs, as well as differences between species, make it unlikely that purely biological definitions will account fully for *pathological* aggression. However, the study of the biology of aggression has revealed some basic characteristics that are shared in many situations. These characteristics may be a useful starting point in considering the factors which determine aggression in humans.

Aggression in animals often occurs in situations of competition. The competition may centre around many different items. Huntingford and Turner (1987) mention the immediate biological needs for food, shelter, nesting place, mate, etc. These are usually so obvious that the area of conflict, i.e. the object which evokes aggression because it cannot be shared, is generally well defined. In human situations it is important to have a clear understanding of the area of conflict. Conflict in itself may be unavoidable, but the ways to handle the conflict may vary. Conflict and aggression also include risks like being hurt and losing, so a careful judgement about when and how to fight is needed. The functionality of aggression is largely determined by this balance and the subsequent investment in fighting or in retreat.

The context in which aggression takes place is an important variable. The perception of threat, of the area of conflict, and of the ways to resolve the conflict determines the eventual occurrence of aggressive behaviour. Moreover, the intensity of aggression, both in terms of the frequency of aggressive acts and the character of the behaviour, is of importance. Although this does not immediately lead to a well-established definition of pathological aggression, these variables should be studied carefully.

An erroneous perception of the area of conflict may result in non-functional aggression. If there is no genuine area of conflict, there is no need for aggression. In many psychiatric patients the perception of reality may be affected and lead to aggression in situations which would not escalate for those who do not experience 'inappropriate' threat. The ways to resolve potential areas of conflict may also determine the functionality of aggression. For example, an impulsive reaction could interfere with more effective, non-aggressive interventions in which both parties run less risk of being damaged. However, perception is quite difficult to measure, in contrast to the intensity of aggression which is easier to record and is therefore more objective. The complete scoring of aggressive behaviour is often possible in laboratory studies of attacks, but in humans too, rating scales have been developed which can be used to quantify the intensity of aggressive responses, for example the Overt Aggression Scale (OAS) (Yudofsky and Silver, 1986).

Without suggesting that the foregoing is an exhaustive attempt to define pathological aggression, we conclude that it is not an easy task to define the limits of adaptive and maladaptive aggression by simply looking at the characteristics of aggression in humans and animals. The problems are in reality even greater since in patients comorbidity often distorts the evaluation of adaptive behaviours in humans. When we admit these limitations in the definition of pathological aggression, what can we do with animal models for the study of aggression? How can they be used to test new drugs and how do they relate to the problem of (pathological) human aggression?

ANIMAL MODELS

Since human pathological aggression is so ill defined, it is impossible *a priori* to 'construct' animal models which have a convincing and adequate face validity with respect to the behavioural problems encountered in humans. One has to rely on animal models which have sufficient biologically or pharmacologically relevant characteristics. In the past, models of aggression were quite artificial. Gradually, however, emphasis was placed on more naturalistic models, as excellently summarized by Miczek (1987), who reviewed the history of animal models used in the psychopharmacology of aggression. Especially in the field of aggression research, ethopharmacological approaches have been of great benefit in understanding the neuropharmacology of aggression. Although the ethopharmacological approach has many attractive and convincing advantages, it should be noted that animal models in which aggression is induced by less naturalistic conditions also have their uses. In a sense, their lack of appropriate contextual relevance could turn into an advantage, because pathological aggression could well appear outside the normal context of human behaviour.

During the development of more naturalistic aggression models, an important distinction arose: the differentiation between offensive and defensive aggressive behaviour (Adams, 1979). While offensive agonistic behaviour is characterized by the initiative of the attacker and damage to the opponent

(Blanchard *et al.*, 1977a, 1977b; Mos *et al.*, 1984), defence behaviour, in contrast, lacks active approach (initiative) and wounds (or incidental ones only) are not inflicted by the defensive animal. Several models focus (although not exclusively) upon the 'offensive' components of agonistic interactions. Other models reflect the more defensive aspects of agonistic behaviour. We have used both type of models and the main characteristics have been described earlier (Olivier *et al.*, 1990).

Thus we have chosen to study drug effects in what can be considered to be normal, functional aggression models. There is no compelling evidence that what we measure in these models is pathological aggression, even though our experimental set-up contains artificial elements. An evaluation of the adaptive value of the behaviour in these models is also impossible. However, the models can be considered to provide situations which permit the study of animal behaviour in ethologically understood settings. In these paradigms the effects of drugs are not only studied on aggressive acts, but on non-aggressive behaviours as well. In this way the specificity of antiaggressive effects can be evaluated by comparing the effects on different behaviours occurring under the same conditions.

A final remark on the use of these models is that they often contain many elements of territoriality. Malmberg (1980) is one of the few authors who has studied territoriality in humans and has convincingly shown the importance of the concept of territoriality for our own species. The aspect of territoriality and pathological aggression deserves more careful study in humans than it has received so far.

ETHOPHARMACOLOGICAL STUDIES

The studies that we will describe are some examples of experiments in rats and mice in which we have employed the methods of ethopharmacology. The building blocks of the studies are adequate ethograms which enable us to study the behaviour of animals in a certain context. The studies by Grant and Mackintosh (1963) formed the basis on which we developed our own ethogram for the different types of test situation. The examples we present are necessarily limited, but indicate the potential of ethopharmacology to discriminate between drug effects.

Studies in mice

In an industrial setting it is impossible to test all the potentially interesting compounds using ethopharmacological tests. Therefore we have made extensive use of a simple screening test for aggression in mice (Yen *et al.*, 1959). In this procedure the ED_{50} values to suppress aggression were determined in isolated male mice. Such mice will readily attack intruder mice after several weeks of isolation, although strain differences are important determinants of the level of aggression (Jones and Brain, 1987).

Table 1 lists the ED_{50} values for several serotonergic compounds and the reference drugs. It is clear that 5-HT$_1$ agonists are among the most powerful compounds to suppress aggression in this model. The most effective ones are the mixed 5-HT$_1$ agonists. Selective 5-HT$_{1A}$ agonists marginally suppressed isolation-induced aggression, but it should be realized that in this model the mice are very experienced fighters, with high levels of aggression. When aggression levels are lower, 5-HT$_{1A}$ agonists do reduce aggression. Sanchez *et al.* (1993) reported similar data for 5-HT$_1$ agonists, although 5-HT$_{1A}$ agonists were more potent in reducing aggression in their experiments. The 5-HT$_{2A/2C}$ agonist DOI did not suppress aggression, whereas the 5-HT$_{2A}$ and 5-HT$_{2C}$ antagonists ritanserin and ketanserin did suppress aggression, albeit at higher doses. The 5-HT$_3$ antagonist ondansetron had no effect on isolation-induced aggression over a wide dose range.

It was already clear from the beginning that aggression-suppressing effects may be caused by different behavioural mechanisms, varying from a specific suppression of the motivation to attack, to sedation, muscle relaxation or disturbing inferences of stereotypy.

A subsequent step in testing putative antiaggressive compounds was to study whether the antiaggressive effects are specific or not. Specificity in our sense means that a compound reduces aggression in the test situation, but does not lead to sedation, interfering stereotypes or other trivial behaviours that result

Table 1 Effect of various serotonergic and reference compounds on aggression in isolated male mice expressed as ED_{50} values to suppress attacks. The predominant effect on serotonergic receptor subtypes is indicated in the second column

Compound	Effect on 5-HT receptor	ED_{50} mg/kg (p.o.)
Eltoprazine	1A/1B agon. (part)	0.3
TFMPP	1B/2C agon. (part)	1.0
RU24969	1A/1B agon.	0.7
8-OH-DPAT	1A agon.	>21
Flesinoxan	1A agon.	1.1
Buspirone	1A agon. (part)	>20
Ipsapirone	1A agon. (part)	>20
DOI	2/2C agon.	>10
Ketanserin	2 antagon.	3.2
Ritanserin	2/2C antagon.	4.4
Ondansetron	3 antagon.	>4.6
Chlorpromazine	–	4.7
Haloperidol	–	0.8
Chlordiazepoxide	–	73.0
Diazepam	–	2.5
Oxazepam	–	5.0

Part: partial agonist.

in a blockade of aggression. Therefore, in more ethologically based models of aggression in mice, we scored aggression as well as other behaviours displayed by mice in an aggression test (Olivier and van Dalen, 1982; Olivier *et al.*, 1989). Figure 1 shows an example of drug effects in the social interaction model in mice. Here, in contrast to isolation-induced aggression, buspirone did reduce aggression. The effects were slightly less specific that those obtained by eltoprazine but certainly better than chlorpromazine. Chlorpromazine reduced aggression, but at the same time social interest and exploration

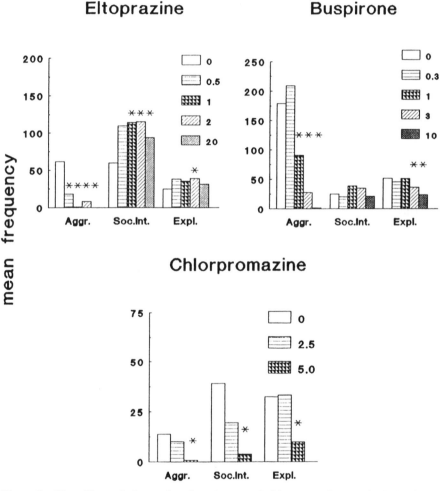

Figure 1 The effects of eltoprazine, buspirone and chlorpromazine on the behaviour of isolated mice confronted with a male intruder in a neutral test arena. Various individual behavioural elements are grouped together into categories. Three important categories are presented here to give an impression of the different behavioural profiles. *$p < 0.05$ against vehicle.

were decreased. Although this drug may be useful as medication to suppress aggression clinically, it also eliminates other important behaviours. Eltoprazine and buspirone, being equally effective in reducing aggression, did not have these profound side-effects.

In this animal model of normal adaptive aggression it can be demonstrated that not all antiaggressive drugs are non-specific reducers of all active behaviours. However, species differences often play an important role in pharmacological studies. Therefore we also tested putative antiaggressive compounds in male and female rats and in guinea-pigs.

Studies in rats

We employed two models of aggression in rats: one for males and one for females, i.e. resident–intruder aggression and maternal aggression during the lactating period.

Figure 2 provides examples of the effects of different drugs on male aggression. Eltoprazine clearly suppressed aggression dose dependently, but did not negatively affect social interest or exploration. In fact it even increased exploration. Only at the highest dose did some increase in inactivity occur, but this was not paralleled by decreased exploration and social interest. It is thus unlikely that this indicates sedation. Buspirone, on the contrary, did reduce aggression, but at the expense of social interest and exploration. Since inactivity increased concomitantly, this profile of antiaggressive actions is clearly non-specific and strongly resembles that of haloperidol (Figure 2). Here a species difference occurs as buspirone was antiaggressive but non-sedative in mice, but is rather sedative at antiaggressive doses in rats. Aggression is not always reduced by drugs. Oxazepam, a benzodiazepine, increased aggression over a wide dose range, but did not lead to sedation. Probably higher doses would reduce aggression as is seen with other benzodiazepines (Mos et al., 1990). Interestingly this observation fits with human studies in which sometimes 'paradoxical' increases in aggression are observed after benzodiazepines are administered. Clearly high doses are needed to suppress aggression in humans and animals. These high doses again result in non-specific suppression of aggression.

Female rats show intense aggression towards intruders during the postpartum period. This period during which aggression occurs is limited, but is long enough to enable pharmacological studies. In Figure 3 the results of some experiments are summarized. The same compounds that were tested in male rats (Figure 2) resulted by and large in similar results, although we sometimes used different doses, based on the experience with male rats. In female rats eltoprazine specifically reduced aggression but did not stimulate exploration as was seen in male rats. Oxazepam induced almost completely similar results in male and female rats. The lower doses of buspirone did not affect aggression significantly, but already started to induce sedation as inactivity increased.

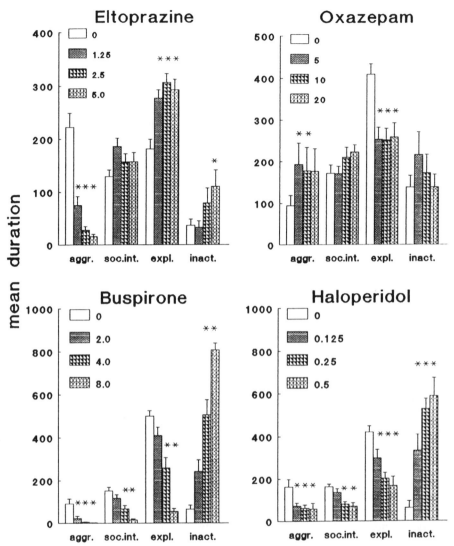

Figure 2 The effects of eltoprazine, oxazepam, buspirone and haloperidol on resident–intruder aggression in male rats are represented by the four major behavioural categories, each comprising different elements. $*p < 0.05$ against vehicle.

Haloperidol, also tested at lower doses than in the male rats, resulted in an almost identical picture. Aggression was not yet significantly reduced, but inactivity was enhanced.

Despite these small differences, drug effects were quite alike in two models with clearly differing neurobiological bases. More extensive studies with other serotonergic compounds confirm these results (Mos *et al.*, 1992a). Again, and like the results obtained in mice, it proved possible to suppress aggression far

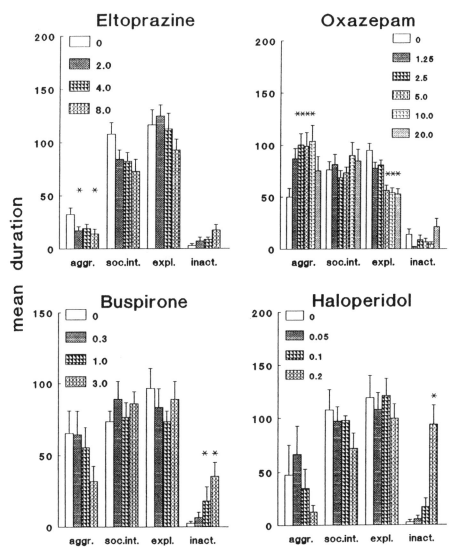

Figure 3 The effects of eltoprazine, oxazepam, buspirone and haloperidol on maternal aggression in female rats are represented by the four major behavioural categories, each comprising different elements. $^{*}p < 0.05$ against vehicle.

more specifically with a mixed serotonergic agonist than with currently used drugs like benzodiazepines and neuroleptics.

MECHANISM OF ACTION

This approach—looking at the specificity of antiaggressive effects in normal aggression—was used by us to search for more effective compounds to treat pathological aggression and finally resulted in the development of eltoprazine, one of the most specific compounds to reduce aggression. However, during the course of the studies it appeared that rats and mice have 5-HT_{1B} receptors, in contrast to most species which have the homologue $5\text{-HT}_{1D\beta}$ receptor. Eltoprazine is a mixed $5\text{-HT}_{1A/1B}$ agonist and has only weak affinity for the 5-HT_{1D} receptor. This made the questions about the mechanism of action even more urgent since extrapolation from rats and mice to man became more critical. Again we applied the ethopharmacological techniques to study these questions. In a preliminary study in pigs, antiaggressive effects in a species without 5-HT_{1B} receptors were observed. Also in green vervet monkeys (McGuire, unpublished data) eltoprazine appeared to reduce aggression far more specifically than haloperidol, albeit at higher doses than in rats and mice.

This raised questions about which receptor subtype was responsible for the observed behavioural effects—the 5-HT_{1A} or the $5\text{-HT}_{1D/1B}$? A first experiment was performed with male guinea-pigs which were allowed to establish a territory. In a design similar to the resident–intruder paradigm in rats we scored various behavioural elements which we grouped into categories on the basis of sequence and cluster analysis. Figure 4 is a summary of the experiments with eltoprazine and the specific 5-HT_{1A} agonist 8-OH-DPAT. Eltoprazine had some limited antiaggressive effects which were neither impressive nor dose related. 8-OH-DPAT had no significant effect on aggression and induces a reduction of social interest at one dose only. Although we did not perform many ethopharmacological studies with the guinea-pig, the impression we had was consistent, i.e. mixed $5\text{-HT}_{1A/1B}$ agonists were less effective in reducing aggression than in rats. Since the data on the 5-HT_{1A} agonist 8-OH-DPAT were somewhat surprising—they suggested no role for 5-HT_{1A} receptors—and the model was difficult to manage experimentally, we switched back to rats in order to study the relative role of pre- and postsynaptic 5-HT_{1A} and 5-HT_{1B} receptors in the control of aggression.

First, some introductory remarks on the localization of relevant serotonergic receptors and earlier studies. 5-HT_{1A} receptors are localized on postsynaptic neurones in the projection areas of the serotonin system emanating from the raphe nuclei. 5-HT_{1A} receptors are also present at the cell bodies and dendrites of the serotonergic neurones in the raphe. Here it acts to reduce serotonin cell-firing, i.e. it reduces the serotonergic neurotransmission. 5-HT_{1B} receptors occur postsynaptically as well as presynaptically, where they act as autoreceptors and reduce serotonin release from the nerve terminal. Lesions of the serotonin cell bodies in the dorsal raphe of male rats by the neurotoxic 5,7-DHT reduce the serotonergic innervation to many different brain areas. These lesions not only abolish almost all somatodendritic 5-HT_{1A} autoreceptors, but also most 5-HT_{1B} presynaptic autoreceptors (Sijbesma *et al.*, 1991). After such lesions, spontaneous resident–intruder aggression was only marginally affected, but eltoprazine still strongly and dose-dependently reduced aggression, even with a tendency of increased efficacy. These studies suggested

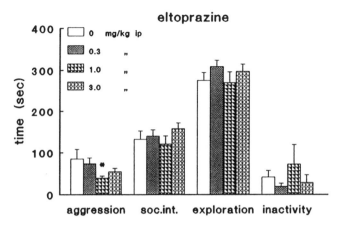

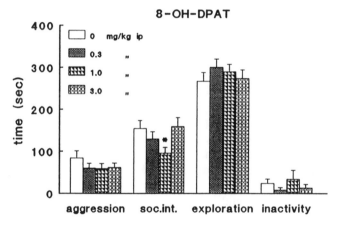

Figure 4 Effect of eltoprazine and 8-OH-DPAT on behaviour displayed by residential male guinea-pigs against intruders. The four major behavioural categories are presented. On the y-axis the mean time spent on the behaviours is given in seconds. $\star p < 0.05$ against vehicle.

important roles for postsynaptic 5-HT_{1A} and/or 5-HT_{1B} receptors in the modulation of aggression. Therefore a further set of experiments was performed.

Mos *et al.* (1992b) injected eltoprazine or 8-OH-DPAT (a prototypical potent and specific 5-HT_{1A} agonist) into the lateral ventricle of male rats which were tested in a resident–intruder paradigm. Eltoprazine reduced aggression, but 8-OH-DPAT did not, strongly suggesting that postsynaptic 5-HT_{1A} receptors do not play a crucial role in the action of eltoprazine, perhaps not at all in the regulation of aggression. One of the mechanisms by which eltoprazine exerts its antiaggressive action is thus by activation of postsynaptic 5-HT_{1B}

receptors. However, systemic administration of 8-OH-DPAT reduces aggression, albeit non-specifically. Thus activation of 5-HT$_{1A}$ receptors directly or indirectly does affect aggression. A second series of experiments was performed in which 8-OH-DPAT was administered directly into the dorsal raphe (Mos *et al.*, 1993). This resulted in a non-specific reduction of aggression, very much the same as after systemic administration. Similarly, administration of eltoprazine into the dorsal raphe led to a non-specific reduction of aggression. Taken together these data suggest that somatodendritic 5-HT$_{1A}$ autoreceptors on the one hand and postsynaptic 5-HT$_{1B}$ receptors on the other hand are involved in the control of aggression. This mechanism of action may explain why eltoprazine is also an effective antiaggressive compound in species without a 5-HT$_{1B}$ receptor, such as the pig. In these species the most likely mechanism of action is via 5-HT$_{1A}$ receptors although the (weaker) agonistic effect of eltoprazine on the 5-HT$_{1D}$ receptor may contribute to the effect. Moreover this may explain why in pigs the behavioural profile of eltoprozine and buspirone is more alike than in the rat. In the rat the 5-HT$_{1B}$ activity of eltoprazine adds considerably to the antiaggressive efficacy, whereas buspirone presumably only acts by its (partial) agonistic activity at the 5-HT$_{1A}$ receptor. Whether the dopamine D$_2$ antagonistic effects of buspirone interfere with buspirone's antiaggressive effects is not clear.

In summary, the animal studies revealed that 5-HT$_1$ agonists are potent antiaggressive compounds, most notably mixed 5-HT$_{1A/1B}$ agonists, at least in rodents. Mechanistic studies support the role of both the 5-HT$_{1A}$ and the 5-HT$_{1B}$ receptor in reducing aggression in rodents. Studies on aggression in higher species also suggest antiaggressive effects of eltoprazine, but these studies have thus far been less detailed and extensive. Moreover, no studies have yet demonstrated that extrapolation from animal studies to human pathological aggression is valid.

CORRESPONDENCE ANALYSIS

Although ethopharmacological studies are very suitable to differentiate the behavioural effects of a drug, they are dependent upon the quality of the drugs used. If a drug is very specific, for example a pure β_1 agonist, it is most likely to assume that the observed effects are related to changes in that receptor-mediated system. However, many drugs are not so clean and specific, thus a number of different molecular mechanisms may play a role in the causation of behavioural changes. If one has a substantial dataset, statistical tools can be used to relate the results of receptor-binding data to the clusters of behavioural changes. In the many years we have studied aggression in the resident–intruder paradigm in male rats we gathered sufficient data on our own and reference compounds to allow such an analysis. Two similar forms of statistical techniques to perform these studies are correspondence analysis and the biplot of a principal component analysis. We applied these techniques to the data on

resident–intruder aggression. The details are given in Gabriel (1971, 1981) and
Greenacre and Hastie (1987). The behavioural data of the resident–intruder
tests were combined into categories. These categories comprise several behavioural elements. A description of these categories has been given previously
(Olivier, 1981). Briefly, the following categories were differentiated: aggression, social interest, exploration, inactivity, self-care and avoidance. As a
measure of drug-induced changes, we calculated the difference between the
square root-transformed duration of behaviour in the separate categories of the
highest dose and the vehicle condition. This difference was normalized in
order to avoid baseline differences and to compensate for unequal duration of
experiments, which were present in these data gathered over a long period.

In Figure 5 the preliminary results of an analysis on 34 compounds is given,
focusing on the behavioural categories only. After the correlation matrix had
been computed, a principal component analysis was performed. The first two
components accounted for 62% and 17% of the total variance respectively.
These are plotted in a so-called biplot, in which these two components of the
correlation matrix are plotted two-dimensionally, ignoring the information in
the remaining components. This results first of all in a projection of the
behavioural categories as illustrated in Figure 5A. Behavioural categories that
are at an angle of 90° are independent, i.e. they are not correlated. An example
in the figure is self-care and avoidance, which are independent in this
experiment. If behavioural categories are projected in the same direction, i.e.
the angle is smaller than 90°, the behavioural categories are not independent.
An example is avoidance and exploration. Social interest and inactivity, are
negatively correlated and are projected under an angle between 90° and 180°.
In this way some behavioural categories can be grouped together, or can be
discriminated. One problem with this method, however, is that if one factor
has much influence, for example the division between inactivity and the other
categories, this factor dominates the graphical representation. A more detailed
look can be obtained if factors 2 and 3 from the analysis are used to create a
biplot (Figure 5B). Aggression and self-care are now much more independent,
while they were grouped more together in the first plot. Aggression is now
opposite, i.e. negatively correlated with exploration. Thus the picture may
change quite profoundly, depending upon the angle at which the plot is looked
at. If only strong factors are studied and plotted, this may override more subtle
relations, which may nevertheless be important for our understanding.

However, the techniques also allow the possibility of locating the compounds in such a biplot (Figure 5B). The projection of a compound on the line
through the origin and the behavioural category gives an estimate of the
original score of the compound on that category. For example, eltoprazine and
RU24969 both have a high and almost equal estimated score on exploration.
For buspirone and oxazepam this score is low (below average). The accuracy of
these estimates depends on the explained total variance and on the distance
from the behavioural categories to the origin. For aggression it is relatively

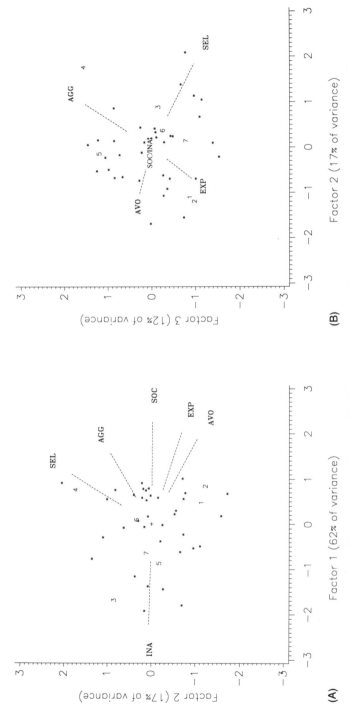

Figure 5 (A) A biplot of the first two factors from a principal component analysis on the behavioural categories and the different drugs. Drugs are marked by an asterisk, or a number. 1: eltoprazine; 2: RU24969; 3: buspirone; 4: oxazepam; 5: haloperidol; 6: DOI; 7: 8-OH-DPAT. (B) A biplot of the second and third factor from the principal component analysis on the behavioural categories and the different drugs. Drugs are marked with an asterisk or a number as in (A). AGG = aggression; AVO = avoidance; EXP = exploration; INA = inactivity; SEL = selfcare; SOC = social interest.

high, for avoidance relatively low. For categories plotted almost at the origin the accuracy would be very poor; it means that such categories are largely ignored in the summary given by the biplot. For compounds, however, a larger distance to the origin indicates more characteristic scores on the behavioural scores. A compound near the origin has average scores in all categories.

The situation for mixed 5-HT$_1$ agonists like eltoprazine and RU24969 is easier to interpret from Figure 5(B) than from Figure 5(A). They reduce aggression and are therefore plotted opposite of the aggression category. Eltoprazine and RU24969 score positively on exploration and are plotted near this category. The opposite holds true for oxazepam (see also Figure 2), which is correctly plotted.

The possibilities can be further extended when the receptor binding data are included. Figure 6(A) shows how the biplot looks for the analysis of receptor binding data. This plot discriminates and clusters 5-HT$_1$ receptors on the one hand and 5-HT$_2$, D$_2$ and α_1-receptors on the other. Again this plot is heavily dominated by factor 1 (affinity) and those drugs that have low affinity for these receptors are all plotted on the left side. Plotting factors 2 and 3 (Figure 6B), which account for 40% of the variance, refines this picture. First of all the 5-HT$_{1B}$ and 5-HT$_{1D}$ receptors are now closely related and discriminated from the 5-HT$_{1A}$ and 5-HT$_{2C}$ receptor. The 5-HT$_2$, D$_2$ and α_1 cluster is now more unravelled. A strange observation which merits further analysis is that the 5-HT$_{2C}$ and the 5-HT$_2$ receptor are not more closely linked. Based on molecular pharmacology these receptors have recently been classified as 5-HT$_{2C}$ and 5-HT$_{2A}$ respectively. Whether this dissociation is related to differences in receptor binding assay or represents a genuine difference remains open for further study.

Finally in Figure 7(A) a combination of receptor binding data and behavioural categories is plotted. This analysis is clearly not very informative as inactivity, being a main contributing factor, is opposed to the other behavioural categories and appears independent from all receptor binding data. We have therefore adopted a different strategy shown in Figure 7(B). In order to relate the receptor binding data to the behavioural categories we have done a canonical correlation analysis. The first two pairs of canonical variables have a 0.69 and 0.57 correlation. The plot has been created in much the same way as before and the compound scores now indicate the behavioural and receptor average. This technique and graphical representation is less dominated by first factors from the principal component analysis. By and large, however, the figure can be read in a similar way as the preceding ones. Inactivity and D$_2$ affinity are now closely linked, in accordance with our knowledge of the effects of neuroleptics. Aggression is negatively coupled to 5-HT$_1$ receptors, while exploration and social interest are more independent from the 5-HT$_1$ cluster.

Clearly these pictures are preliminary as the results are based on relatively few compounds. Athough these figures have to be looked at carefully, they

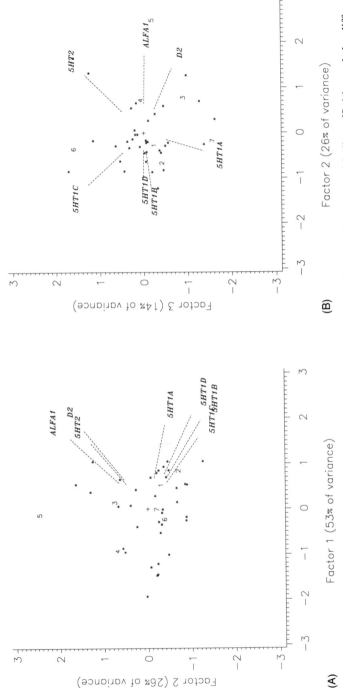

Figure 6 (A) A biplot of the first two factors from a principal component analysis on the receptor binding affinities and the different drugs. Drugs are marked by an asterisk, or a number. 1: eltoprazine; 2: RU24969; 3: buspirone; 4: oxazepam; 5: haloperidol; 6: DOI; 7: 8-OH-DPAT. (B) A biplot of the second and third factor from the principal component analysis on the receptor binding affinities and the different drugs. Drugs are marked with an asterisk or a number as in (A).

175

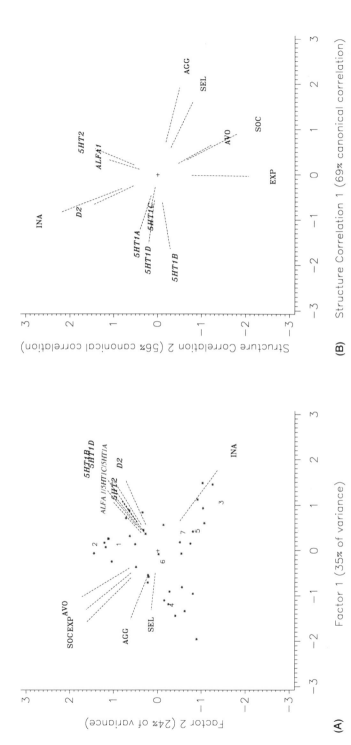

Figure 7 (A) A biplot for the first two components of the principal component analysis of the receptor binding data and the behavioural categories of 34 compounds. See text for details. (B) A biplot representation of the scaled correlations of the first two pairs of canonical variables and the average scores from the canonical correlation analysis of the receptor binding data with the behavioural categories of 34 compounds.

may give rise to new ideas on mechanism of action of antiaggressive compounds. Clearly, this approach is limited by our current selection of drugs, but it is the start of a more statistically-based type of research into new varieties of antiaggressive compounds. It is an interesting possibility to combine receptor binding data with an ethopharmacological profile of compounds in aggression tests. Thus the careful collection of ethopharmacological data in an industrial setting can be used to evaluate our concepts about behavioural clusters and categories.

REFERENCES

Adams, D.B. (1979) Brain mechanisms for offense, defense and submission. *Behav. Brain Sci.*, **2**, 201–241.

Blanchard, R.J., Blanchard, D.C., Takahashi, T. and Kelley, M.J. (1977a) Attack and defensive behaviour in the albino rat. *Anim. Behav.*, **25**, 622–634.

Blanchard, R.J., Takahashi, L.K. and Blanchard, D.C. (1977b) The development of intruder attack in colonies of laboratory rats. *Anim. Learning Behav.*, **5**, 365–369.

Gabriel, K.R. (1971) The biplot-graphic display of matrices with application to principal component analysis. *Biometrika*, **58**, 453–467.

Gabriel, K.R. (1981) Biplot display of multivariate matrices for inspection of data and diagnosis. In: *Interpreting Multivariate Data* (ed. V. Barnett). Wiley, Chichester, pp. 147–174.

Grant, E.C. and Mackintosh, J.H. (1963) A comparison of the social postures of some common laboratory rodents. *Behaviour*, **21**, 246–259.

Greenacre, M. and Hastie, T. (1987) The geometric interpretation of correspondence analysis. *J. Am. Statist. Assoc.*, **82**, 437–447.

Huntingford, F.A. and Turner, A.K. (1987) *Animal Conflict*. Chapman & Hall, London.

Jones, S.E. and Brain, P.F. (1987) Performance of inbred and outbred mice in putative tests of aggression. *Behav. Genet.*, **17**, 87–96.

Koning De, P. and Mak, M. (1991) Problems in human aggression research. *J. Neuropsychiatry*, **3** (Suppl. 1), s61–65.

Malmberg, T. (1980) *Human Territoriality: Survey of Behavioural Territories in Man with Preliminary Analysis of Meaning*. Mouton, The Hague.

Miczek, K.A. (1987) The psychopharmacology of aggression. In: *Handbook of Psychopharmacology*, Vol. 19 (eds L.L. Iversen, S.D. Iversen and S.H. Snyder). Plenum Press, New York, pp. 183–328.

Mos, J., Olivier, B., Van Oorschot, R. and Dijkstra, H. (1984) Different test situations for measuring offensive aggression in male rats do not result in the same wound patterns. *Physiol. Behav.*, **32**, 453–456.

Mos, J., Olivier, B. and van Oorschot, R. (1990) Behavioural and neuropharmacological aspects of maternal aggression in rodents. *Aggressive Behav.*, **16**, 145–163.

Mos, J., Olivier, B. and Tulp, M.Th.M. (1992a) Ethopharmacological studies differentiate the effects of various serotonergic compounds on aggression in rats. *Drug Dev. Res.*, **26**, 343–360.

Mos, J., Olivier, B., Poth, M. and van Aken, H. (1992b) The effects of intraventricular administration of eltoprazine, 1-(3-trifluoromethylphenyl)piperazine hydrochloride and 8-hydroxy-2-(di-n-propylamino)tetralin on resident intruder aggression in the rat. *Eur. J. Pharmacol.*, **212**, 295–298.

Mos, J., Olivier, B., Poth, M. *et al.* (1993) The effects of dorsal raphe administration of eltoprazine, 1-(3-trifluoromethylphenyl)piperazine hydrochloride and 8-hydroxy-2-(di-n-propylamino)tetralin on resident intruder aggression in the rat. *Eur. J. Pharmacol.*, **238**, 411–415.

Moyer, K.E. (1968) Kinds of aggression and their physiological basis. *Commun. Behav. Biol.*, **2**, 65–87.

Olivier, B. (1981) Selective antiaggressive properties of DU 27725: ethological analysis of intermale and territorial aggression in the male rat. *Pharmacol. Biochem. Behav.*, **14**, 61–77.

Olivier, B. and van Dalen, D. (1982) Social behaviours in rats and mice: an ethological base for differentiating psychoactive drugs. *Aggressive Behav.*, **8**, 163–168.

Olivier, B., Mos, J., Van der Heyden, J. and Hartog, J. (1989) Serotonergic modulation of social interactions in isolated male mice. *Psychopharmacology*, **97**, 154–156.

Olivier, B., Mos, J. and Rasmussen, D.L. (1990) Behavioural pharmacology of the serenic, eltoprazine. *Drug Metab. Drug Interact.*, **8**, 31–85.

Sánchez C., Arnt, J., Hyttel, J. and Moltzen, E.K. (1993) The role of serotonergic mechanisms in inhibition of isolation-induced aggression in male mice. *Psychopharmacology*, **110**, 53–59.

Sijbesma, H., Schipper, J., De Kloet, E.R. *et al.* (1991) Postsynaptic 5-HT$_1$ receptors and offensive aggression in rats: a combined behavioural and autoradiographic study with eltoprazine. *Pharmacol. Biochem. Behav.*, **38**, 447–458.

Yen, C.Y., Stanger, R.L. and Millnam, N. (1959) A taractic suppression of isolation-induced aggressive behaviour. *Arch. Int. Pharmacodyn. Ther.*, **123**, 179–185.

Yudofsky, S.C. and Silver, J.M. (1986) The overt aggression scale for the objective rating of verbal and physical aggression. *Am. J. Psychiat.*, **143**, 35–39.

9 Analysis of Different Forms of Aggression in Male and Female Mice: Ethopharmacological Studies

P. PALANZA, R.J. RODGERS,[a] D. DELLA SETA, P.F. FERRARI AND S. PARMIGIANI

Dipartimento di Biologia e Fisiologia Generali, Università di Parma, Italy
[a]Department of Psychology, University of Leeds, UK

INTRODUCTION

Different forms of aggression have been described and classified according to the sex, physiological state and/or context in which animals attack members of the same or other species. Indeed, aggression is a heterogeneous phenomenon in terms of motivation, behavioural phenotype and presumed function (Moyer, 1968; Wittenberger, 1981). The non-unitary nature of the phenomena we encompass under the term aggression is also evinced from studies indicating that major differences exist in the neural substrates of different types of aggression (Adams, 1980). Ethologists do not consider predatory attack to be a form of aggression but to be a feeding behavioural strategy. In fact, motivation, neural substrates and functions of predation are very different from those of other forms of aggression (Adams, 1980). In functional terms, it is therefore possible to distinguish between two broad categories of aggression, one concerned with competition for resources (competitive aggression) and the other concerned with protection of self or offspring from potentially dangerous conspecifics or predators (protective aggression) (Archer, 1988).

Intraspecific competitive aggression is generally characterized by 'ritualized' or 'offensive' patterns of attacks in that animals are usually restrained in the use of the deadliest weapons at their disposal; this limits the likelihood of causing serious injuries to their rivals. Protective aggression against conspecifics (e.g. parental attack to protect offspring) may be characterized by much less ritualized or 'defensive' form of attack. For example, in rodents (such as mice and rats), offensive and defensive forms of intraspecific attack can be distinguished on the basis of the behavioural phenotypes, since only in defensive attack do animals persistently direct their bites to vulnerable regions

Ethology and Psychopharmacology. Edited by S.J. Cooper and C.A. Hendrie
© 1994 John Wiley & Sons Ltd

(head, ventrum and inguinal areas) of the opponent (Blanchard *et al.*, 1977; Brain, 1981). It is important to note that a clear-cut distinction between offensive and defensive intraspecific aggression is impossible because some forms of aggression, depending on the context and sex of interacting animals, may result in a mixture of offensive and defensive types of attack (Archer, 1988; Parmigiani, 1986).

Aggression in mice

The forms of aggression described above have been extensively investigated in the house mouse (*Mus musculus domesticus*). Consequently, this rodent species provides a useful experimental model for understanding sex differences in the expression of different forms of aggression and the relationships between functional and causal mechanisms (Brain and Parmigiani, 1990).

In fact, male and female mice show differences in the display and the timing of aggression towards adult and young conspecifics (i.e. infanticide). Males are competitive only among each other for establishing and holding territory and/or social rank and, ultimately, for mating. Since reproduction is largely confined to dominant or exclusively territorial males (Wolff, 1985; Hurst, 1986), intermale aggression can limit the reproductive potential of same-sex conspecifics and facilitate dispersion and colonization. Females become aggressive when they associate with a territory-holding male. This suggests that interfemale competition arises in relation to reproductive acitivity (Palanza *et al.*, 1994). Female mice exhibit an intense aggressive behaviour during lactation, when their young are threatened by conspecifics. This behaviour, referred to as maternal aggression, is a complex and heterogeneous phenomenon ranging in form from offensive to defensive attack and subserving a variety of functions according to the context and the characteristics of conspecific intruders (Parmigiani, 1986; Parmigiani *et al.*, 1988a). For instance, lacatating females may use aggression in competing with same-sex conspecifics to establish a social hierarchy or to space rivals (competitive aggression), and in defence of the litter from infanticidal conspecifics (Parmigiani *et al.*, 1988a).

Competitive aggression in mice is not restricted to overt fighting activity with adult conspecifics, but can also include the elimination of their offspring. Infanticide (i.e. the killing of unrelated young) has been recently acknowledged as an adaptive strategy in order to gain access to resources and prospective mates (Hrdy, 1979). In male mice, infanticide involves intraspecific competition for mates, whereas, in females, it appears to be a resource competition strategy (vom Saal and Howard, 1982; Parmigiani *et al.*, 1994).

Given this background, two important questions concerning the proximal and ultimate causation of aggression arise. (1) Is a particular function reflected in the form (i.e. the behavioural phenotype of attack and defence) of aggression which in turn may be an expression of a specific underlying motivation (i.e. neurochemical substrate) (Archer, 1988; Brain, 1981)? (2) Are functionally similar, but phenotypically different, forms of aggression modulated by similar neural substrates in the two sexes? Most of the studies on aggressive behaviour and its neurochemical basis have involved only tests on male rodents, and comparatively little is known about the regulation of female aggression (e.g. Brain and Parmigiani, 1990). In this respect, pharmacology can be used as a tool to probe the neurochemical mechanisms underlying different forms of aggression. Ethopharmacology combines ethological analysis and drug administration in an attempt to understand more fully the mechanisms which modulate and regulate behaviour (Rodgers and Randall, 1987).

This chapter describes ethopharmacological experiments on the effects of the antiaggressive drug, fluprazine (DU27716, Duphar) on different forms of aggression in Swiss albino mice (*Mus musculus domesticus*). One aim was to determine whether or not there are relationships (proximal and ultimate) between different forms of male and female aggression. The defining characteristic of the drug fluprazine (a phenylpiperazine derivative, which acts as a mixed 5-HT$_1$ receptor agonist) is its ability to decrease competitive forms of aggression in mice (Bradford *et al.*, 1984) and rats (Blanchard *et al.*, 1985; Flannelly *et al.*, 1985; Olivier *et al.*, 1984) without substantially impairing other components of the behavioural repertoire (Blanchard *et al.*, 1985; Parmigiani *et al.*, 1989b). Fluprazine does not alter predatory attack in northern grasshopper mice (*Onychomys leucogaster*) or, when the prey is small (i.e. crickets and earthworms) and incapable of retaliation, in laboratory rats (Kemble, 1989). Thus, fluprazine has proven to be an effective tool in discriminating between different forms of aggression and, albeit indirectly, their neurochemical substrates.

MALE AGGRESSION → Give Examples of male aggression

Agonistic behaviour between adult males (intermale aggression), which mostly occurs in the context of territory establishment and defence, is one of the best-studied forms of male competitive aggression. However, competitive strategies among males also include infanticide. In fact, while the proportions vary between genetic stocks, sexually naive male mice generally attack, kill and cannibalize young conspecifics. As in other mammalian species, one of the commonest natural circumstances in which male mice kill unrelated young is when they take over a reproductive area to gain access to mates (Hrdy, 1979; vom Saal and Howard, 1982). This behaviour seems to have evolved as a form of postmating competition among males (Hrdy, 1979; vom Saal and Howard, 1982). In fact, the infanticidal male eliminates a competitor's offspring and accelerates the female's return to oestrus, thus advancing his mating opportunities and increasing reproductive success (vom Saal and Howard, 1982). Thus, this form of infanticide is functionally involved in competitive strategies and may be considered a unique form of competitive intraspecific aggression (leading to the death of interacting animals). If male infanticide is a form of competitive aggression it might be expected that the neurochemical substrates involved in the control of pup killing may be similar (if not identical) to those underlying intraspecific attack towards same sex conspecifics rather than to those underlying predatory attack. To test this hypothesis, we compared the effect of fluprazine on intermale attack, infanticide and predation of male mice (Parmigiani and Palanza, 1991). Coleopteran larvae of similar body size and movement characterisitics to newborn mouse pups, but incapable of retaliation, were used as prey. The palatablity of the larvae was checked in a pilot study using non-food-deprived animals. All experimental tests were carried out on non-deprived animals to rule out possible interference between predatory and infanticidal motivation.

Males were independently preselected for aggression towards a same-sex opponent, a two-day-old pup or a larva. Approximately 70% of the males showed intermale aggression or infanticide and 55% killed the larva. Within each selected behavioural group (i.e. aggressive, infanticidal and predatory), males were randomly assigned to one of four treatment conditions: saline, 1.0, 2.0 and 5 mg/kg fluprazine. Twelve experimental groups (12–14 animals in each group) were obtained with each male tested as previously selected (i.e. aggressive males were tested for intermale aggression; infanticidal males for infanticide; predators for predation).

While all saline-treated males (controls) attacked the intruders, exhibited infanticide or killed the larvae, 1–2 mg/kg fluprazine dose-dependently reduced attacks on intruder males and pups but did not significantly alter predatory attack on the larva (Figure 1). Although males that do not attack pups generally ignore them, five males in the 2–5 mg/kg fluprazine conditions actually showed paternal behaviour (i.e. retrieved pups into the nest and crouched over them). This preliminary finding suggests that serotonergic substrates may be involved in the mechanisms which mediate the transition from infanticide to paternal behaviour in male mice. Importantly, when retested 24 h after drug treatment, all males had recovered aggressive, infanticidal and predatory responses.

A second experiment examined the effects of fluprazine (2 mg/kg) on infanticidal and predatory attack in males selected for *both* behaviours. Fluprazine significantly reduced infanticide (four out of 14 males showing the behaviour, $p < 0.005$, Fisher's exact probability test) but not predation (11 out of 14 males showing the behaviour). When retested 24 h later, all these subjects showed a full reinstatement of infanticidal or predatory behaviour. This result rules out the possibility that the behavioural selection for animals showing different forms of attack (Experiment 1) might have indirectly resulted in differential drug sensitivity between the groups, and clearly supports the hypothesis that infanticide and predation are different phenomena. Furthermore, the present data suggest that the motivational and neurochemical substrates underlying intermale aggression and pup killing may be similar to each other, but different from those which regulate predatory attack. This

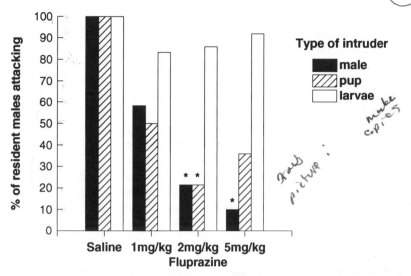

Figure 1 Effect of different doses of fluprazine on intermale, infanticidal and predatory attack by males. *Differs from corresponding saline control, $p < 0.01$, Fisher's exact probability test.

finding supports Hrdy's view that this kind of infanticide is a competitive strategy (Hrdy, 1979), providing indirect evidence that infanticide is a form of intraspecific aggression (Parmigiani and Palanza, 1991). Compared with the monotonic dose-dependent inhibition of intermale attack, it is interesting that infanticide inhibition is less clearly dose dependent. This finding suggests the possibility that the neurochemical substrates responsible for the inhibition of infanticide may vary from that underlying intermale aggression or alternatively that an overlap between predatory and infanticidal motivations may exist in some male mice.

FEMALE AGGRESSION

Female mice spend a significant portion of their adult lifespan either pregnant or lactating and these reproductive periods are associated with rapid neuroendocrine changes and significant maternal investment in the successful rearing of the young. These factors, along with the associated risk of infanticide by males, plausibly suggest that reproductively active female mice are more likely to exhibit aggressive behaviour than non-reproductive (virgin) animals (Svare, 1989). For this reason maternal aggression has been the most studied form of female aggression.

The characteristics of attack by lactating mice on male (defensive form) and female (offensive form) conspecific intruders provide a unique model for investigating the neurochemical substrates of offensive and defensive aggression in female mammals. Topographically, lactating females attack sexually naive male intruders with bites mostly directed toward the head, ventral surface and inguinal area (a defensive pattern), whereas virgin females are comparatively rarely (three to five times less than in the case of males) bitten on such vulnerable body surfaces (an offensive pattern) (Parmigiani, 1986; Parmigiani et al., 1988a). Furthermore, female intruders elicit more social investigation from lactating residents than do males, whereas males evoke more responses consistent with 'fearfulness' (i.e. the patterns of attack involve tentative thrusts and retreat, with considerable vocalization even while attacking). In this context, a study with the opioid antagonist naloxone supported the view that this dichotomy in attacking behaviours may reflect differences in the neurochemical substrate. Thus, naloxone reduced attack on females to a much greater extent than attack on males and induced more fear-related behaviour (cf. saline-injected controls) in response to male versus female intrusion (Parmigiani et al., 1988b).

Defensive aggression by lactating residents toward males (the more infanticidal gender in laboratory strains and stocks) has been interpreted as a counter-strategy to infanticide (Parmigiani, 1986), while the offensive aggression towards females may serve to establish a social hierarchy or to space rivals of the same sex (Parmigiani et al., 1988a). Indeed, several observations suggest that female aggression is not restricted to pup protection and may play an important role in social dynamics (e.g. Yasukawa et al., 1985). In fact, females appear to be largely responsible for the regulation of the reproductive potential of the deme unit (which generally consists of a dominant territorial male, one or more females and their offspring) through intrasexual aggression (intolerance of other females), inhibition of subordinate female reproduction and the killing of unrelated young (Hurst, 1987; Parmigiani et al., 1989a; Palanza et al., 1993). As in the case of males, dominant females are the most reproductively successful, and infanticidal behaviour by females has been interpreted as a resource competition strategy increasing the probability of access to food and survival of their own offspring.

Competitive (intrasexual attack and infanticide) and protective forms of aggression exhibited by female mice provide a good model for understanding their neurochemical substrates and their possible relationships with different forms of male aggression. Since fluprazine can discriminate between offensively and defensively motivated behaviours, we examined the effect of this drug on maternal attack towards intruders of either sex (Parmigiani et al., 1989b). For this purpose, 90-day-old primiparous lactating mice were injected intraperitoneally with saline, 1 mg/kg, or 5 mg/kg of fluprazine hydrochloride. Twenty minutes post injection, subjects were tested against an unfamiliar sexually naive male or a virgin female conspecific in a 10 min intruder test. The results (Table 1) showed that, compared to saline controls, the proportion of female intruders attacked was reduced by 1 mg/kg fluprazine and virtually

Table 1 Effect of fluprazine on attack by lactating mice on male and female conspecific intruders

	Proportion of attacked intruders			
Sex of intruder	Saline	Fluprazine 1 mg/kg	Fluprazine 5 mg/kg	Fluprazine 10 mg/kg
Male	10/10	13/13	10/10	3/8*
Female	7/10	6/13	1/10*	–

*Differs from corresponding saline control, $p < 0.01$ (Fisher exact probability test).

eliminated by the 5 mg/kg dose. Although 100% of males were attacked in all treatment conditions, fluprazine dose-dependently increased attack latencies in response to this type of intruder. To test whether higher doses of fluprazine could affect the defensive type of maternal attack, eight lactating females were injected with 10 mg/kg of the drug and confronted with male intruders. This treatment decreased the aggression shown by lactating females to males to a level comparable to that produced by fluprazine at 1 mg/kg against female intruders. These findings support our hypothesis concerning the non-unitary nature of the motivational substrates involved in offensive and defensive attack in lactating females. This observed dichotomy may reflect the diverse functions of attack in that males pose a much greater threat to the parental investment of the lactating resident than do females. Such an interpretation is consistent with the observation that only by substantially increasing the doses of fluprazine was a significant reduction in attack towards males observed. These findings on the differential sensitivity of different forms of attack to the inhibitory effects of fluprazine suggest that there is a continuum between offensive and defensive aggression and that elicitation of fear by external stimuli (in this case a male intruder) may be responsible for a strategic shift from an offensive to a defensive attack pattern.

Although less frequently than in Swiss males or females of wild stock, virginal Swiss female mice can kill and cannibalize unrelated young. This behaviour has been functionally interpreted as a form of competition between females (Parmigiani *et al.*, 1994). As in the case of males (see above), it may be hypothesized that in females the neurochemical mechanisms underlying intraspecific competitive aggression and infanticide may be similar to each other but different from those underlying predatory attack. Consequently, to examine relationships between intrasexual, infanticidal and predatory attack in females, and whether the neurochemical substrates of these female behaviours are similar to those in males, a preliminary study with fluprazine has been carried out.

As described above for males, adult (60 days old) virgin females were preselected for infanticide (25 out of 124) or predatory attack (40 out of 50).

Within the two selected groups, females were randomly assigned to one of four treatment conditions: saline, 1.0, 2.0 or 5.0 mg/kg fluprazine. Eight experimental groups were obtained and each female was tested as previously selected. As expected, saline-treated females exhibited infanticide (6/6) and predation (9/10). Fluprazine reduced ($p < 0.05$ versus control, Fisher exact probability test) the proportion of females showing infanticide (2/6, 1 mg/kg; 2/7, 2 mg/kg; 2/6, 5 mg/kg) but *did not* affect the proportion of females showing predation (8/10, 1 mg/kg; 8/10, 2 mg/kg and 10/10, 5 mg/kg). This result suggests that, similar to the result of studies in males, the neural substrates of infanticide and predation are different. Furthermore, although infanticide and predation were tested in virgin females while intrasexual competitive attack was tested in lactating females, the inhibitory effects of fluprazine upon both female infanticide and intrasexual maternal attack also support the hypothesis that the motivational and neurochemical substrates underlying these two behaviours may be similar to each other, in females as well as males. It is important to note that, contrary to the majority of wild female stocks, female laboratory mice show a low incidence of infanticide as virgins. However, the frequency of infanticide can vary with reproductive state and the age of the alien pup (Parmigiani *et al.*, 1994) and, as such, studies on infanticide in pregnant and lactating mice will be required to substantiate these conclusions further.

CONCLUSION

The antiaggressive drug, fluprazine, produced similar inhibitory effects on infanticide, intermale and intrasexual maternal attack (i.e. competitive forms of attack), but did not affect predatory attack in either male or female mice. This profile suggests that phenotypically different forms of aggression, such as intrasexual aggression and infanticide, which have *similar* competitive functions, may also have similar neurochemical substrates in the two sexes. More specifically, while the endocrine regulation of murine aggression appears to be gender dependent (Edwards, 1968; Svare, 1989), serotonergic regulation of such behaviour may be gender independent.

Aggression by lactating females, which is phenotypically different towards intruders of differing sex, facilitated the study of competitive (offensive) and protective (defensive) forms of attack in the same animal, the same physiological state (lactation), and the same context (nest defence). Under these test conditions, fluprazine inhibited attack on females at doses 10-fold lower than doses required to inhibit attack on males. This differential potency of fluprazine on intra- and intersexual aggression in lactating females would be consistent with the view that these behaviours (offence and defence, respectively) involve different motivational and neurochemical substrates. However, since attack against males was reduced by fluprazine, albeit at comparatively high doses, our data suggest that a continuum may exist between offensive and defensive aggression in lactating mice. Such a motivational distinction appears to have adaptive value in that males pose a much greater threat to the offspring than do females. In this case, phenotypically different forms of aggression, which have *different* functions, may have rather different neurochemical substrates.

Together, present observations emphasize the importance of an evolutionary approach to ethological analyses of the proximal mechanisms of behaviour. The ultimate causation of any phenotype (including behaviour) is the result of selective pressures that have acted upon proximal factors (e.g. neurochemical substrates). It therefore follows that it is important to consider the context and function of behaviour when studying underlying substrates. As such, etho-pharmacological studies may help to clarify not only the proximal mechanisms of a given behaviour but also its adaptive significance. This evolutionary approach to behavioural pharmacology, which distinguishes ethopharmacology from psychopharmacology, may also allow for the development of a better understanding of drug action.

Note. All experiments were performed in accordance with ASAB guidelines governing animal behaviour research (Elwood, 1991; Elwood and Parmigiani, 1992). Care was taken to minimize stress on both adult and infant mice. The number of pups used for infanticide testing was minimized by confronting test animals with a single pup. Tests were stopped as soon as a pup was harmed (infanticide and maternal aggression tests) or when fighting escalated between adults.

REFERENCES

Adams, D.B. (1980) Motivational systems of agonistic behavior in muroid rodents: a comparative review and neural model. *Aggressive Behav.*, **6**, 295–346.

Archer, J. (1988) *The Behavioural Biology of Aggression*. Cambridge University Press, Cambridge.

Blanchard, D.C., Takushi, R., Blanchard, R.J. *et al*. (1985) Fluprazine hydrochloride does not decrease defensive behaviors of wild and septal syndrome rats. *Physiol. Behav.*, **35**, 349–353.

Blanchard, R.J., Blanchard, D.C., Takahashi, T. and Kelly, M.S. (1977) Attack and defensive behavior in the albino rat. *Anim. Behav.*, **25**, 194–224.

Bradford, L.D., Olivier, B., van Dalen, D. and Schipper, J. (1984) Serenics: the pharmacology of fluprazine and DU 28412. In *Ethopharmacological Aggression Research* (eds K. Miczek, M. Kruk and B. Olivier). Liss, New York, pp. 191–207.

Brain, P.F. (1981) Differentiating types of attack and defence in rodents. In: *Multidisciplinary Approaches to Aggression Research* (eds P.F. Brain and D. Benton). Elsevier/North-Holland, Amsterdam, pp. 53–78.

Brain, P.F. and Parmigiani, S. (1990) Variation in aggressiveness in house mouse populations. *Biol. J. Linnean Soc.*, **41**, 257–269.

Edwards, D.A. (1968) Mice: fighting by neonatally androgenized females. *Science*, **161**, 1027–1028.

Elwood, R.J. (1991) Ethical implication of studies on infanticide and maternal aggression in rodents. *Anim. Behav.*, **42**, 841–849.

Elwood, R.W. and Parmigiani, S. (1992) Ethical recommendations for workers on aggression and predation in animals. *Aggressive Behav.*, **18**, 139–142.

Flannelly, K.J., Murakoa, M.Y., Blanchard, C. and Blanchard, R.J. (1985) Specific anti-aggressive effects of fluprazine hydrochloride. *Psychopharmacology*, **87**, 86–89.

Hrdy, S.B. (1979) Infanticide among animals: a review, classification, and examinations of the implications for the reproductive strategies of females. *Ethol. Sociobiol.*, **1**, 13–40.

Hurst, J.L. (1986) Mating in free living wild house mice (*Mus domesticus* Rutty). *J. Zool.*, **210**, 623–628.

Hurst, J.L. (1987) Behavioural variation in wild house mice (*Mus domesticus* Rutty): a quantitative assessment of female social organization. *Anim. Behav.*, **35**, 1864–1857.

Kemble, E.D. (1989) Some further ethoexperimental studies of the antiaggressive drug fluprazine hydrochloride. In: *Ethoexperimental Approaches to The Study of Behavior* (eds R.J. Blanchard, P.F. Brain, D.C. Blanchard and S. Parmigiani). Kluwer, Dordrecht, pp. 484–493.

Moyer, K.E. (1968) Kinds of aggression and their physiological basis. *Commun. Behav. Biol.*, **2**, 65–87.

Olivier, B., van Aken, H., Jaarsma, I. *et al.* (1984) Behavioral effects of psychoactive drugs on agonistic behaviour of male territorial rats (resident–intruder model). In: *Ethopharmacological Aggression Research* (eds K. Miczek, M. Kruk and B. Olivier). Liss, New York, pp. 137–156.

Palanza, P., Brain, P.F. and Parmigiani, S. (1993) Intraspecific aggression in mice (*Mus domesticus*): male and female strategies. In: *The Development of Sex Differences and Similarities in Behaviour* (eds M. Haung, R. Whalen, C.L. Aron and K.L. Olsen). Kluwer, Dordrecht, pp. 191–203.

Palanza, P., Parmigiani, S. and vom Saal, F. (1994) Male urinary cues induce intrasexual aggression and urine-marking in wild female mice. *Anim. Behav.* (in press).

Parmigiani, S. (1986) Rank order in pairs of communally nursing female mice and maternal aggression towards conspecific intruders of differing sex. *Aggressive Behav.*, **12**, 377–386.

Parmigiani, S. and Palanza, P. (1991) Fluprazine inhibits intermale attack and infanticide, but not predation, in male mice. *Neurosci. Biobehav. Rev.*, **15**, 511–513.

Parmigiani, S., Brain, P.F., Mainardi, D. and Brunoni W. (1988a) Different patterns of biting attack generated when lactating female mice (*Mus domesticus*) encounter male and female conspecific intruders. *J. Comp. Psychol.*, **102**, 287–293.

Parmigiani, S., Rodgers, R.J., Palanza, P. and Mainardi, M. (1988b) Naloxone differentially alters parental aggression by female mice towards conspecific intruders of differing sex. *Aggressive Behav.*, **14**, 213–224.

Parmigiani, S., Brain, P.F. and Palanza, P. (1989a) Ethoexperimental analysis of different forms of intraspecific aggression in the house mouse (*Mus domesticus*). In: *Ethoexperimental Approaches to The Study of Behavior* (eds R. Blanchard, P.F. Brain, D.C. Blanchard and S. Parmigiani). Kluwer, Dordrecht, pp. 418–431.

Parmigiani, S., Rodgers, R.J., Palanza, P. *et al.* (1989b) The inhibitory effects of fluprazine on parental aggression in female mice are dependent upon intruder sex. *Physiol. Behav.*, **46**, 455–459.

Parmigiani, S., Palanza, P., Brain, P.F. and Mainardi, D. (1994) Infanticide and protection of young in the house mouse (*Mus domesticus*): female and male strategies. In: *Infanticide and Parental Care in Animals and Man* (eds S. Parmigiani and F. vom Saal). Harwood, London (in press).

Rodgers, R.J. and Randall, J.I. (1987) Situation-dependency and differential mediation of analgesic reactions to conspecific attack in male mice. In: *Ethopharmacology and Agonistic Behaviour in Animals and Humans* (eds J. Mos, B. Olivier and P.F. Brain). Martinus Nijhoff, Amsterdam, pp. 79–82.

Svare, B. (1989) Recent advances in the study of female aggressive behaviour in mice.

In: *House Mouse Aggression: A Model for Understanding the Evolution of Social Behaviour* (eds P.F. Brain, D. Mainardi and S. Parmigiani). Harwood, New York, pp. 135–159.

vom Saal, F.S. and Howard, L.S. (1982) The regulation of infanticide and parental behavior: implication for reproductive success in male mice. *Science*, **215**, 1270–1272.

Wittenberger, J.F. (1981) *Animal Social Behavior*. Duxbury Press, Boston.

Wolff, J.O. (1985). Maternal aggression as a deterrent to infanticide in *Peromyscus leucopus* and *P. maniculatus*. *Anim. Behav.*, **33**, 117–123.

Yasukawa, N.J., Harvey, M., Leff, F.L. and Christian, J.J. (1985) Role of female behavior in controlling population growth in mice. *Aggressive Behav.*, **11**, 49–64.

10 Novel Odours Increase Defensiveness and Inhibit Attack Behaviour in Mice

ERNEST D. KEMBLE

Division of Social Sciences, University of Minnesota–Morris, Morris, Minnesota, USA

INTRODUCTION

Presentation of partial predatory stimuli such as non-contact exposure to a cat (Blanchard and Blanchard, 1990b), cat odours alone (Blanchard *et al.*, 1990b), or the recorded calls of avian predators (Hendrie, 1991; Hendrie and Neill, 1991) reliably evoke an array of species-typical fear responses collectively referred to as risk assessment behaviour (e.g. Blanchard and Blanchard, 1990a). Risk assessment is thought to represent an active investigation of potentially dangerous stimuli which is motivated by an anxiety-like state (e.g. Blanchard and Blanchard, 1990b). Generally consistent with this view is the reduction of these behaviours by treatment with benzodiazepines or ethanol (Blanchard *et al.*, 1990a, 1990b; Blanchard and Blanchard, 1990a; Zangrossi and File, 1992). Thus, presentation of predator odours and/or other partial predator stimuli would seem to offer a useful tool for pharmacological investigations.

The major impetus for the research to be reported here was curiosity about the critical stimulus features which mediate odour-induced fear. Since the subjects in the experiments described above had no previous exposure to cats or their odours, and since fear reactions to cats may be conditioned in a single trial, it has been suggested that rats and mice may recognize potentially dangerous predators without prior experience (e.g. Blanchard and Blanchard, 1971; Williams *et al.*, 1990; Williams and Scott, 1989) and respond to them with species-specific defence responses (e.g. Bolles, 1970; Curio, 1975). A substantial body of evidence is now available which is congruent with this interpretation. Some birds, for example, display an apparently innate avoidance of colour patterns characteristic of snake predators (e.g. Smith, 1975, 1977) or brightly coloured distasteful bugs (Sillen-Tullberg, 1985). Owings and Coss (1977) also report that naive ground squirrels are more likely to avoid

Ethology and Psychopharmacology. Edited by S.J. Cooper and C.A. Hendrie
© 1994 John Wiley & Sons Ltd

snakes if the habitat from which they are drawn contains venomous rattle-snakes. In addition, both fear responses and endogenous analgesia are evoked among inbred laboratory mice by the calls of predatory owls but not by those of several non-predatory species (Hendrie, 1991; Hendrie and Neill, 1991). A careful series of both pen bioassays and field studies by Sullivan and his co-workers (Sullivan et al., 1985a, 1985b, 1988, 1990) which utilized both natural and synthetic predator odours to deter feeding on various plants is of particular interest. These investigators report that the presence of anal gland, urine and/or faecal odours from mustelid and fox predators produces a sustained (38 days or more) suppression of feeding by deer, snowshoe hares and various rodents on odour-treated plants. Moreover, the effective odours seem somewhat specific for a given predator species. The odour of wolverine urine, but not faeces, for example, was a potent deterrent (Sullivan et al., 1985a) while anal gland compounds (other mustelid species) or faeces odours (fox) from other predator species seem quite effective (Sullivan et al., 1988). Finally, the presumably novel odours of deer urine or hare blood had no repellent properties (Sullivan et al., 1985a).

Although the above experiments suggest that unconditioned predator recognition may well underlie risk assessment behaviours in some cases, there is also considerable evidence that novelty is an important stimulus dimension as well. Exploration of various novel environments, for example, has been extensively validated as an index of anxiolytic and anxiogenic drug effects (e.g. Benjamin et al., 1990; Costall et al., 1989; Crawley, 1985; File, 1986; Lister, 1987). Bronson (1976) also reports that novelty is a potent elicitor of urine marking in male mice, while chickens display aerial alarm calls to a wide range of overhead predatory and non-predatory stimuli (Gyger et al., 1987). More to the point, the novel odour of citronella is known to induce, if mildly, hypoalgesia (Lester and Faneslow, 1985) and prolonged exposure to cat odours reduces later responsivity to them (Williams et al., 1990). These results argue that in some instances risk assessment evoked by predator odours may be more parsimoniously interpreted as neophobic reactions. Such generalized responses to novelty might be of considerable adaptive value if species (such as mice or rats) are preyed upon by a wide array of avian and terrestrial predators.

This contribution summarizes a series of experiments conducted over the past two to three years which explored the role of odour novelty in the evocation of fearfulness. All of the experiments to be reported employed CD-1 albino mice. This strain readily displays conspecific aggression and responds to the odours of dominant conspecifics with risk assessment behaviours (e.g. Garbe et al., 1993a).

PREFERENCE AND ANALGESIA EXPERIMENTS

In our first experiment the odours of a potential predator (unscented clay litter soiled by a domestic cat), unsoiled cat litter, sawdust bedding soiled by a conspecific, and the control odour of unsoiled sawdust were presented in a four-choice olfactory preference apparatus (Kemble and Gibson, 1992). If mice innately recognize cat odours, we reasoned, then the soiled, but not unsoiled, cat litter should be avoided. If, on the other hand, novelty is the critical stimulus dimension, both unsoiled and soiled litter should be avoided. Conspecific odours are regularly preferred in this apparatus (e.g. Rawleigh et al., 1993) and were included to determine if the test was bidirectionally sensitive to aversive and appetitive odours. The results of the experiment are summarized in Figure 1. Mice showed a strong and equivalent rejection of both soiled and unsoiled litter odours while exhibiting the expected preference for conspecific odours. Although the novel odours in this initial experiment were strongly avoided, we could not be certain that this reaction was not secondary in some way to the strong preference shown for conspecific odours. We therefore conducted a second experiment which examined responses to two additional novel odours (chocolate and cinnamon) and unsoiled bedding but with no conspecific odours present (Kemble and Gibson, 1992). The mice in this experiment displayed an emphatic rejection of both novel odours which was virtually identical to that displayed towards soiled or unsoiled cat litter.

Since exposure to predators (e.g. Kavaliers, 1988; Lester and Fanselow, 1985), novel environments (Kavaliers and Innes, 1988) or the odours of dominant conspecifics (e.g. Rodgers and Randall, 1986) evoke endogenous analgesia we next examined the possibility that the novel odours used in our initial experiments would also produce this effect. Following 5 min exposure to unsoiled litter, cinnamon or unsoiled bedding odours, flinch/jump thresholds

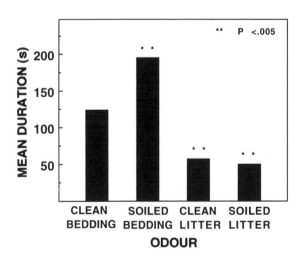

Figure 1 Mean time in compartments containing the odours of unsoiled conspecific bedding, soiled conspecific bedding, unsoiled cat litter and soiled cat litter. (Reproduced from Kemble and Gibson, 1992, by permission of *Psychological Record*.)

to electric foot shock were determined. Flinch thresholds were significantly elevated by exposure to cinnamon odour, while jump thresholds were elevated by unsoiled cat litter when compared to unsoiled bedding levels (Kemble and Gibson, 1992).

RISK ASSESSMENT AND APPETITIVE BEHAVIOURS

Although the above findings were encouraging, it must be noted that the preference/rejection paradigm did not provide direct measures of risk assessment and, thus, odour rejection may not have necessarily resulted from increased fearfulness. This point was borne home to us by a parallel series of experiments in our laboratory which examined reactivity to conspecific odours. Mice were rendered either dominant or subordinate by a series of resident–intruder encounters and their responsiveness to the odours of their familiar antagonists and unfamiliar conspecifics examined in the apparatus described above. These preference tests (Rawleigh *et al.*, 1993) revealed that both dominant and subordinate mice showed a reliable preference for the odours of their familiar antagonists (although the preference of subordinates was somewhat weaker). When these odours were presented in the subject's home cage, however, subordinates showed substantial levels of risk assessment to the odours of dominants, while these behaviours were virtually absent when dominant mice were exposed to subordinate odours (Garbe *et al.*, 1993a). A further finding of special interest, however, was that *both* subordinates and dominants in the latter study showed similar levels of approach to, and contact with, the odours of their familiar antagonist. These experiments argue that similar levels of approach to odourants ('preference') may arise from strikingly different motivational states and, hence, that the preference paradigm is not optimal for investigations of odour-induced fear.

Our next experiments therefore directly measured the effects of several novel odours on both risk assessment and appetitive behaviours. If novelty is an important contributor to the fear-inducing effects of predator odours, then increases in the former, and inhibition of the latter, behaviours might be expected. In addition, we wished to expand the range of novel odours somewhat to include those of a non-predatory mammal. Although our previous data suggested to the contrary, it seemed possible that mammalian odours, regardless of predatory status, might be particularly effective stimuli. In these experiments responsiveness to the odours of sheep wool, cat fur, chocolate, citronella and unsoiled bedding (control odour) were examined. Novel odours were without effect when testing was conducted in a straight runway similar to that employed by the Blanchards (e.g. Blanchard and Blanchard, 1990a) but when testing was carried out in the home cage clear differences in responsiveness to the odours emerged (Garbe *et al.*, 1993a). The effects of the novel odours on three risk assessment behaviours are summarized in Figure 2. It can be seen that each of the novel odours was effective in increasing at least one

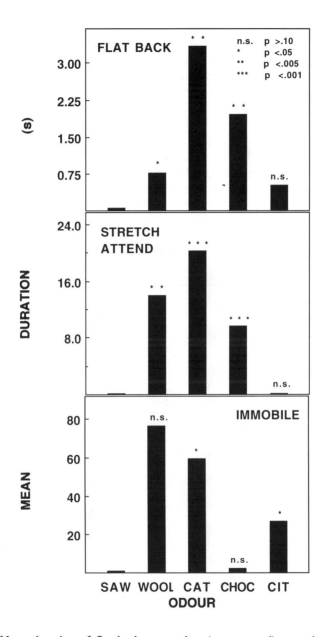

Figure 2 Mean duration of flat back approaches (upper panel), stretched attention (middle panel) and immobile (lower panel) in response to unsoiled conspecific bedding (SAW), sheep wool (WOOL), cat fur (CAT), chocolate (CHOC) or citronella (CIT) odours. All comparisons are with unsoiled bedding. (Reproduced from Garbe *et al.*, *Aggressive Behavior*, 1993, reprinted by permission of John Wiley & Sons, Inc.)

risk assessment behaviour. Cat, wool and chocolate odours also seemed somewhat more consistently effective than citronella. The effects of the odours on two appetitive behaviours are shown in Figure 3. As the figure shows, each of the novel odours suppressed rearing behaviour at least moderately and three of the four odours suppressed eating. Although cat and sheep odours evoked a somewhat wider range of behavioural effects, it should be noted that all odours altered at least three behaviours. The similar behavioural profiles evoked by sheep and cat odours also clearly indicate that predator odours are not uniquely effective fear stimuli.

We have also begun a series of experiments to assess the sensitivity of novel odour-induced fearfulness to pharmacological agents. Since benzodiazepine treatment reduces levels of risk assessment provoked by cat odours (Blanchard *et al.*, 1990b) a similar effect on novel odour reactivity might be expected after

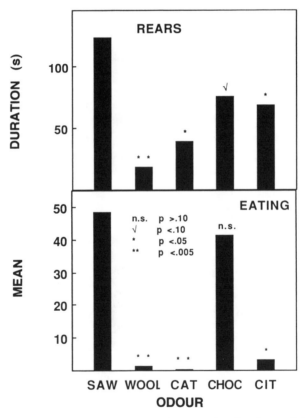

Figure 3 Mean duration of rears (upper panel) and eating (lower panel) in response to unsoiled conspecific bedding (SAW), sheep wool (WOOL), cat fur (CAT), chocolate (CHOC) or citronella (CIT) odours. All comparisons are with unsoiled bedding. (Reproduced from Garbe *et al.*, *Aggressive Behavior*, 1993, reprinted by permission of John Wiley & Sons, Inc.)

treatment with anxiolytics. Since our previous data revealed similar responses to cat fur and sheep wool, only the latter odour was used. The results of this experiment (Garbe *et al.*, 1993b) are summarized in Figure 4. Treatment with 12.0 mg/kg chlordiazepoxide, but not 2.0 or 8.0 mg/kg, significantly reduced both flat back approaches and stretch attend postures. We (Kemble and Gordon, unpublished) have also examined the effects of the adrenoceptor antagonist yohimbine on these behaviours. Since this drug displays a consistent anxiogenic profile (e.g. File and Johnston, 1987; Guy and Gardner, 1985; Harris and Newman, 1987), some elevation in risk assessment to wool odour

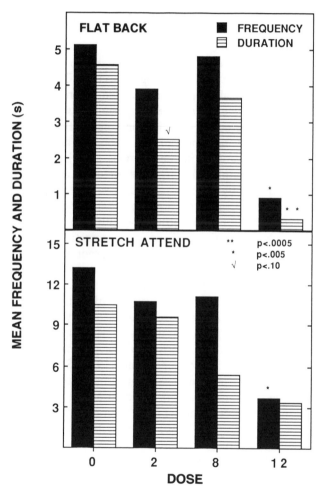

Figure 4 Mean frequency and duration of flat back approaches and stretch attends by groups receiving 0 (saline), 2.0, 8.0 and 12.0 mg/kg CDP treatments. (Reproduced from Garbe *et al.*, *Aggressive Behavior*, 1993, reprinted by permission of John Wiley & Sons, Inc.)

might be expected. Although we found no effects of 0.5 or 2.0 mg/kg yohimbine treatment on either flat back approaches or stretch attend postures, both doses significantly increased the frequency and duration of immobility and decreased the duration of rearing behaviour. We plan to explore the usefulness of this paradigm further by utilizing a wider range of anxiolytic and anxiogenic agents in the future.

CONSPECIFIC AGGRESSION

The above findings leave little doubt that odour novelty evokes some degree of fearfulness, perhaps akin to anxiety (e.g. Blanchard and Blanchard, 1990b). If so, then it seems reasonable to ask whether the effects of these manipulations extend to conspecific aggression as well. Although exposure to a cat strongly suppresses attack by residents on intruding males (e.g. Blanchard et al., 1984), it is not clear that the partial stimulation provided by predator or novel odours would be similarly effective. In our next experiments we therefore examined the effects of brief novel odour exposure on conspecific aggression. Because the odours of sheep and cat, and those of chocolate and citronella, yielded similar risk assessment profiles in the previous experiment, only sheep and chocolate odours were employed. Intermale attack (Kemble and Garbe, un-published) was induced by socially isolating resident males for a period of three weeks and introducing a slightly smaller male intruder. Sheep wool, chocolate or unsoiled bedding was sprinkled evenly over the home cage floor of the resident 5 min before testing. All agonistic interactions were then recorded for 15 min. Exposure to wool odour (Figure 5) produced a significant reduction in the frequency and duration of both lateral attack and boxing. A closely similar, and statistically significant, reduction in these behaviours by chocolate was seen in a second experiment. The apparently paradoxical inhibition of boxing by these odours appeared to be a secondary effect of substantial increases in the presumably prepotent defensive response of fleeing.

Since maternal attack differs from that of males along a number of dimensions (e.g. Erskine et al., 1978; Gandelman, 1972; Svare and Gandelman, 1973) an extension of our observations to maternal aggression also seemed of interest. When these odours were presented to 60–72 h postpartum females prior to the introduction of a smaller male, duration (but not frequency) of lunge attacks were mildly ($p < 0.10$) reduced by both novel odours, and boxing was significantly reduced by chocolate (Garbe et al., 1993b). There were no effects of the odours on other offensive or defensive behaviours. The latter data imply that maternal aggression is rather weakly inhibited by novel odours. This weak effect may have resulted from very high levels of fearfulness among the females due to the introduction of the intruding male and/or the fact that maternal attack is often launched during approach by the intruder and without initial social investigation.

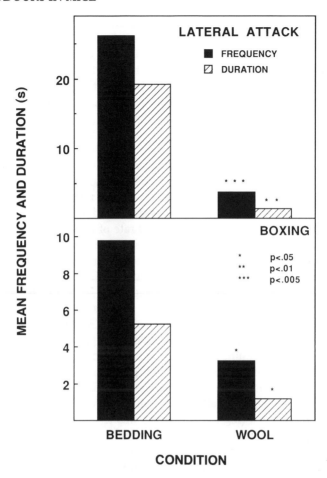

Figure 5 Mean frequency and duration of lateral attack (upper panel) and boxing (lower panel) by males exposed to the odour of unsoiled bedding or sheep wool. (Submitted for publication.)

DISCUSSION

These experiments reveal a number of close similarities in the behavioural effects of a variety of novel olfactory stimuli. The findings therefore clearly argue that stimulus novelty *per se* is an effective elicitor of fear. This, of course, does not rule out the possibility that the degree and/or form of defensive responding may be biased by unconditioned predator recognition in some cases. Although all of the novel odours thus far tested have increased at least some defensive responses, sheep wool and cat fur seem to be slightly more consistent than either chocolate or citronella in their evocation of risk assessment behaviours. This raises the possibility that some mammalian odours, though not restricted to predators, are highly potent fear-inducing stimuli. The fact that either natural or synthetic fox or mustelid odours produce avoidance which lasts for periods of weeks or months (e.g. Sullivan *et al.*, 1985a, 1990) also seems consistent with this view. If mammalian odours are, in fact, particularly effective stimuli, then identification of the responsible chemical compounds may make it possible to elevate or reduce levels of risk assessment by altering the chemical composition of odorants and/or their concentration. Such control would be of obvious value in psychopharmacological studies.

Alternatively, presentation of two or more forms of novel stimulation may prove to be more effective in elevating risk assessment. In a recent report (Evans *et al.*, 1993), for example, it was shown that rate of aerial alarm calls by chickens (evoked by overhead computer-generated raptor-like stimuli) were jointly determined by the apparent size and rate of movement of the overhead stimuli. Since freezing responses in rats are increased by the abrupt movement of both inanimate objects and potential (cat or dog) predators (Blanchard *et al.*, 1975) the use of moving stimuli in conjunction with novel odours may be a particularly effective combination. In addition, the fear-inducing properties of unfamiliar predator or gull calls (Hendrie, 1991) suggests that novel sounds may also provide useful stimuli. We (Kemble and Gordon, unpublished) have recently completed a preliminary study which suggests that this approach is indeed feasible. We examined the risk assessment behaviours evoked by wool odour in three experimental settings. One group of mice was tested in their familiar home cage with odour as the only source of novelty. A second group received odours in a novel 5-gallon glass aquarium which was otherwise barren (low novel), and a third (high novel) group was tested in a considerably larger aquarium (20 gallons) whose novelty was further enhanced by six novel objects (e.g. a ticking timer, a brown glass vial, a section of 3.9 diameter plastic tubing) scattered about the aquarium floor and a shadow which swept over the aquarium floor at 60 rpm. Mice which were tested in the high novel environment showed a significant elevation in the frequency and duration of flat back approaches to the odours and a significant suppression of both rearing and defensive burying relative to the other two groups. In future research we plan to extend the range of novel stimuli presented in conjunction with novel odours and to assess the effects of a wider range of drugs on odour-induced risk assessment.

Taken together, the findings suggest that the use of novel odours, either alone or in combination with other stimuli, holds promise as an effective tool in psychopharmacological research. Since the effects of some psychoactive drugs may be mediated in part by altered olfactory function (e.g. Dixon, 1982; Kemble and Rawleigh, 1991; Kemble *et al.*, 1986; Ostrem *et al.*, 1992; Soffie and Lamberty, 1988), drug effects on odour-induced fear, when compared to results from other novelty-based paradigms (e.g. plus-mazes), may be particularly useful in assessing the mechanisms of anxiolytic or anxiogenic drug effects. In addition, a clearer understanding of the mechanisms underlying novelty-induced fear may make it possible to experimentally control levels of risk assessment over a considerable range. Such control will require systematic investigation of the critical dimension(s) underlying odour-induced fear as well as their interaction with other sources of novelty. Such research may make it possible to design behavioural tests which are optimally sensitive for a wide range of drugs. This possibility would seem to merit further examination.

ACKNOWLEDGEMENT

I would like to thank Drs. S.J. Cooper and Colin Hendrie for their hospitality during this conference and for their helpful comments on an earlier version of this material.

REFERENCES

Benjamin, D., Lal, H. and Meyerson, L.R. (1990) The effects of 5-HT1B characterizing agents in the mouse elevated plus-maze. *Life Sci.*, **47**, 195–203.

Blanchard, R.J. and Blanchard, D.C. (1971) Defensive reactions in the albino rat. *Learning Motivation*, **2**, 351–362.

Blanchard, D.C. and Blanchard, R.J. (1990a) Effects of ethanol, benzodiazepines and serotinin compounds on ethopharmacological models of anxiety. In: *Anxiety* (eds N. McNaughton and G. Andrews). University of Otago Press, Dunedin, pp. 188–199.

Blanchard, R.J. and Blanchard, D.C. (1990b) An ethoexperimental analysis of defense, fear, and anxiety. In: *Anxiety* (eds N. McNaughton and G. Andrews). University of Otago Press, Dunedin, pp. 124–133.

Blanchard, R.J., Mast, M. and Blanchard, D.C. (1975) Stimulus control of defensive reactions in the albino rat. *J. Comp. Physiol. Psychol.*, **88**, 81–88.

Blanchard, R.J., Kleinschmidt, C.K., Flannelly, K.J. and Blanchard, D.C. (1984) Fear and aggression in the rat. *Aggressive Behav.*, **10**, 309–315.

Blanchard, D.C., Blanchard, R.J. and Rodgers, R.J. (1990a) Pharmacological and neural control of anti-predator defense in the rat. *Aggressive Behav.*, **16**, 165–175.

Blanchard, R.J., Blanchard, D.C., Weiss, S.M. and Meyer, S. (1990b) Effects of ethanol and diazepam on reactivity to predatory odors. *Pharmacol. Biochem. Behav.*, **35**, 775–780.

Bolles, R.C. (1970) Species-specific defense reactions and avoidance learning. *Psychol. Rev.*, **71**, 32–48.

Bronson, F.H. (1976) Urine marking in mice: causes and effects. In: *Mammalian Olfaction, Reproductive Processes, and Behavior* (ed. R.L. Doty). Academic Press, New York, pp. 119–141.

Costall, B., Jones, B.J., Kelly, M.E. *et al.*, (1989) Exploration of mice in the black and white box: validation as a model of anxiety. *Pharmacol. Biochem. Behav.*, **32**, 777–785.

Crawley, J.N. (1985) Exploratory behavior models of anxiety in mice. *Neurosci. Biobehav. Rev.*, **9**, 37–44.

Curio, E. (1975) The functional organization of anti-predator behaviour in the red flycatcher: a study of avian visual perception. *Anim. Behav.*, **23**, 1–115.

Dixon, A.K. (1982) A possible olfactory component in the effects of diazepam on social behavior of mice. *Psychopharmacology*, **77**, 246–252.

Erskin, M.S., Barfield, R.J. and Goldman, R. (1978) Intraspecific fighting during late pregnancy and lactation in rats and effects of litter removal. *Behav. Biol.*, **23**, 206–218.

Evans, C.S., Macedonia, J.M. and Marler, P. (1993) Effects of apparent size and speed on the response of chickens, *Gallus gallus*, to computer generated simulations of aerial predators. *Anim. Behav.*, **46**, 1–11.

File, S.E. (1986) Aversive and appetitive properties of anxiogenic and anxiolytic agents. *Behav. Brain Res.*, **21**, 189–194.

File, S.E. and Johnston, A.L. (1987) Chronic treatment with imipramine does not reverse the effects of 3 anxiogenic compounds in a test of anxiety in the rat. *Pharmacopsychiatry*, **17**, 187–192.

Gandelman, R. (1972) Postpartum aggression elicited by the presence of an intruder. *Horm. Behav.*, **3**, 23–28.

Garbe, C.M. and Kemble, E.D. (1993) Effects of novel odor exposure on maternal aggression in mice. *Bull. Psychonomic Soc.*, **31**, 571–573.

Garbe, C.M., Kemble, E.D. and Rawleigh, J.M. (1993a) Novel odors evoke risk assessment and suppress appetitive behaviors in mice. *Aggressive Behav.*, **19**, 447–454.

Garbe, C.M., Kemble, E.D. and Strunk, P. (1993b) Effects of chlordiazepoxide on odor-induced risk assessment in mice. *Bull. Psychonomic Soc.*, **31**, 314–316. (submitted to *Aggressive Behavior*)

Guy, A.P. and Gardner, C.R. (1985) Pharmacological characterization of a modified social interaction model of anxiety in the rat. *Neuropsychobiology*, **13**, 194–200.

Gyger, M., Marler, P. and Pickert, R. (1987) Semantics of an avian alarm call system: the male domestic fowl, *Gallus domesticus*. *Behaviour*, **102**, 15–40.

Harris, J.C. and Newman, J.D. (1987) Mediation of separation distress by alpha-2-adrenergic mechanisms in a nonhuman primate. *Brain Res.*, **410**, 353–356.

Hendrie, C.A. (1991) The calls of murine predators activate endogenous analgesia mechanisms in mice. *Physiol. Behav.*, **49**, 569–573.

Hendrie, C.A. and Neill, J.C. (1991) Exposure to the calls of predators of mice activates defensive mechanisms and inhibits consummatory behaviour in an inbred mouse strain. *Neurosci. Biobehav. Rev.*, **15**, 479–482.

Kavaliers, M. (1988) Brief exposure to a natural predator, the short-tail weasel, induces benzodiazepine-sensitive analgesia in white-footed mice. *Physiol. Behav.*, **43**, 187–193.

Kavaliers, M. and Innes, D.G.L. (1988) Novelty-induced analgesia in deer mice (*Peromyscus maniculatus*): sex and population differences. *Behav. Neural Biol.*, **49**, 54–60.

Kemble, E.D. and Gibson, B.M. (1992) Avoidance and hypoalgesia induced by novel odors in mice. *Psychol. Rec.*, **42**, 555–563.

Kemble, E.D. and Rawleigh, J.M. (1991) Resident–intruder paradigms and anti-aggressive drugs: some further data. *Psychol. Rec.*, **41**, 255–269.

Kemble, E.D., Schultz, L.A. and Thornton, A.E. (1986) Effects of fluprazine hydrochloride on conspecific odor preferences in rats. *Physiol. Behav.*, **37**, 53–56.

Lester, L.S. and Fanselow, M.A. (1985) Exposure to a cat produces opioid analgesia in rats. *Behav. Neurosci.*, **99**, 756–759.

Lister, R.G. (1987) The use of the plus-maze to measure anxiety in the mouse. *Psychopharmacology*, **92**, 180–185.

Ostrem, J.L., Rawleigh, J.M. and Kemble, E.D. (1991) Effects of eltoprazine hydrochloride on reactivity to conspecific or novel odors and activity. *Pharmacol. Biochem. Behav.*, **41**, 581–585.

Owings, D.H. and Coss, R.G. (1977) Snake mobbing by California ground squirrels: adaptive variation and ontogeny. *Behaviour*, **62**, 50–69.

Rawleigh, J.M., Kemble, E.D. and Ostrem, J. (1993) Differential effects of prior dominance or subordination experience on conspecific odor preferences in mice. *Physiol. Behav.*, **54**, 35–39.

Rodgers, R.J. and Randall, J.I. (1986) Resident's scent: a critical factor in acute analgesic reaction to defeat experience in male mice. *Physiol. Behav.*, **37**, 317–322.

Sillen-Tullberg, B. (1985) Higher survival of an aposematic form than of a cryptic form of a distasteful bug. *Oecologia*, **67**, 411–415.

Smith, S.M. (1975) Innate recognition of a coral snake pattern by a possible avian predator. *Science*, **187**, 759–760.

Smith, S.M. (1977) Coral snake pattern recognition and stimulus generalisation by naive great kiskadees (Aves: Tyrannidae). *Nature*, **265**, 535–536.

Soffie, M. and Lamberty, Y. (1988) Scopolamine effects on juvenile recognition in rats: possible interaction with olfactory sensitivity. *Behav. Proc.*, **17**, 181–190.

Sullivan, T.P., Nordstrom, L.O. and Sullivan, D.S. (1985a) The use of predator odors as repellents to reduce feeding damage by herbivores. I. Snowshoe hares (*Lepus americanus*). *J. Chem. Ecol.*, **11**, 903–919.

Sullivan, T.P., Nordstrom, L.O. and Sullivan, D.S. (1985b) The use of predator odors as repellents to reduce feeding damage by herbivores. II. Black-tailed deer (*Odocoileus hemionus columbianus*). *J. Chem. Ecol.*, **11**, 921–935.

Sullivan, T.P., Crump, D.R. and Sullivan, D.S. (1988) Use of predator odors as repellents to reduce feeding damage by herbivores. III. Montane and meadow voles (*Microtus montanus* and *Microtus pennsylvanicus*). *J. Chem. Ecol.*, **14**, 363–377.

Sullivan, T.P., Crump, D.R., Wieser, H. and Dixon, E.A. (1990) Response of pocket gophers (*Thomomys talpoides*) to an operational application of synthetic semiochemicals of stoat (*Mustela erminea*). *J. Chem. Ecol.*, **16**, 941–949.

Svare, B. and Gandelman, R. (1973) Postpartum aggression in mice: experimental and environmental factors. *Horm. Behav.*, **4**, 323–334.

Williams, J.L. and Scott, D.K. (1989) Influence of conspecific and predatory stressors and their associated odors on defensive burying and freezing responses. *Anim. Learning Behav.*, **17**, 383–393.

Williams, J.L., Rogers, A.G. and Adler, A.O. (1990) Prolonged exposure to conspecific and predator odors reduces fear reactions to these odors during subsequent prod shock tests. *Anim. Learning Behav.*, **18**, 453–461.

Zangrossi, H. and File, S.E. (1992) Chlordiazepoxide reduces the generalized anxiety but not the direct responses, of rats exposed to cat odor. *Pharmacol. Biochem. Behav.*, **43**, 1195–1200.

11 The Involvement of Pheromones in Offensive and Defensive Agonistic Behaviour in Laboratory Mice

P. DONÁT*, M. KRŠIAK AND A. ŠULCOVÁ[a]

Institute of Pharmacology, 3rd Medical Faculty, Charles University, Prague, Czech Republic
[a]*Department of Pharmacology, Medical Faculty of Masaryk University, Brno, Czech Republic*

INTRODUCTION

J.H. Mackintosh and E.C. Grant were among the first to study the effects of pheromones on the behaviour of mice in the laboratory. A number of investigators had previously noticed the importance of odour communication in the agonistic behaviour of rodents, which are essentially macrosmatic animals. It had been found, for example, that family recognition in mice depends on olfactory cues and that the smell of a stranger can precipitate fighting (Eibl-Eibesfeldt, 1950). Very few experimental studies, however, had been completed at this time.

Mackintosh and Grant began by rubbing a mouse from an established pair against the perineal regions of an unfamiliar mouse. They found that there was a substantial increase in the agonistic behaviour in the reassembled pair, provided that urine had been passed from the stranger to the rubbed animal. They concluded that mouse urine contains a substance or substances which give olfactory information to other members of the species as to the familiarity or unfamiliarity of the mouse in question (Mackintosh and Grant, 1966). They classed these substances as *pheromones* (Butenandt and Karlson, 1959), i.e. substances produced by an animal causing a specific response in a receiving animal of the same species.

Within a few years, the importance of pheromones in the agonistic

*deceased

Ethology and Psychopharmacology. Edited by S.J. Cooper and C.A. Hendrie
© 1994 John Wiley & Sons Ltd

behaviour of rodents was confirmed in numerous other reports, for example, in mice (Archer, 1968; Ropartz, 1968; Carr *et al.*, 1970; Haug, 1970; Mugford and Nowell, 1971a, 1971b; Stark and Hazlett, 1972), rats (Krames *et al.*, 1969; Alberts and Galef, 1973), hamsters (Devor and Murphy, 1973), etc. Although agonistic behaviour was defined as the whole complex of behaviours occurring in intraspecies conflicts (Scott and Fredericson, 1951), most investigators only focused their attention on the aggressive components. The possible involvement of olfactory cues in defensive–escape components of agonistic behaviour remained practically uninvestigated.

One of the main principles of ethology to be considered is that no one component of behaviour can be understood without reference to the structure of behaviour as a whole (Chance, 1966; Lát, 1965; Dixon, 1982). Pre-exposure of isolated mice to the soiled sawdust of the future opponents (to be encountered 10 days later) caused noticeable reduction in aggressive as well as defensive behaviour in subsequent encounters. The lack of aggressive *and* defensive behaviours suggests that the male pheromone, normally associated with the release of aggressive behaviour, influences the animal's responses in the whole spectrum of agonistic behaviours (Kimelman and Lubow, 1974). Group-housed mice avoided parts of an open field spoiled by urine of isolated or dominant males; the aversive property of the pheromone contained in the urine of these donors was accompanied by reductions in activity scores (Jones and Nowell, 1974c), which were thought to be suppressed due to an increase in fear (Kumar, 1970; Sawyer, 1977; Williams *et al.*, 1990).

Thus, the aim of this chapter is to review the effects of olfactory communication in male mice from the point of view of subjects exhibiting offensive or defensive agonistic strategies. When singly housed male mice are exposed to non-aggressive group-housed opponents some isolates attack their opponents (aggressive mice), while others show escape or defensive postures without attacks (timid mice). It should be stressed that the spontaneous nature of 'timidity' distinguishes it from the submissive behaviour that is released as a consequence of defeat. Thus the timid behaviour occurs at the beginning of the establishment of social dominance before any defeats are experienced. A body of evidence suggests that it is an alternative defensive behavioural strategy that may be applied in conflict situations with unfamiliar conspecifics. It seems to be connected with fear; its usefulness in the assessment of the anxiolytic activity of drugs has already been described (Kršiak *et al.*, 1984).

The cues eliciting timidity are not yet well understood; however, olfactory stimuli may play a very important role. The timid behaviour usually diminishes within several brief encounters with the same opponent, which occurs in conjunction with the diminishing importance of the chemosensory signals as the experience of subjects increases (Meredith, 1983; Wysocki, 1989). Comparisons between aggressive and defensive behavioural strategies provides a unique opportunity to discuss the olfactory communication in male mice from the functional point of view.

PHEROMONES AND OLFACTORY COMMUNICATION IN RODENTS

Olfactory signals are involved in almost all aspects of social communication. Brown (1979) classifies the social odours of mammals into two main groups: (a) *identifier odours*—those produced by the body's normal metabolic processes that are stable for long periods of time (individual, colony, species-typical, age-specific and sex-specific odours); (b) *emotive odours*—those produced or released only in special circumstances (rut, social status, stress, maternal odours). This classification provides an overview of the range of functions, although odours from both groups seem to be involved in the agonistic behaviour of rodents. Archer (1968) has suggested that the odour of male mice has functionally distinct components, one of which is of a general nature and elicits attacks from other males, while another, which is specific to the individual, allows its identification by other members of its species.

The production of a pheromone, which stimulates aggression and causes aversion in other males, has proved to be androgen dependent (Mugford and Nowell, 1970; Brain and Evans, 1974). The aversive effect of the urine diminished after castration and was restored after testosterone propionate treatment. A delay of five days before the exogenous androgen exerted any effect indicates that the pheromonal substance is released from an androgen-dependent tissue rather than being excreted as an androgen metabolite (Jones and Nowell, 1974c).

The preputial glands have been tentatively implicated in the production of hormone-dependent olfactory signals in male mice (McKinney and Christian, 1970; Mugford and Nowell, 1971b, 1971c; Brain and Homady, 1985a). Preputialectomy significantly reduced attacks (Mugford, 1973; Homady and Brain, 1982; Hayashi, 1987) and preputial homogenates were found to elicit attacks (Homady and Brain, 1982). A feature of preputial gland is its obvious dependence on hormonal factors (Homady and Brain, 1982; Brain and Homady, 1985a, 1985b). Castrates are less subject to conspecific attack than intact male counterparts in various rodent species (Brain and Evans, 1974; Payne, 1973; Yahr et al., 1977). The function of the preputial gland is restored by androgenic treatment (Johnston, 1981; Yahr, 1981; Homady and Brain, 1982; Kimura and Hagiwara, 1985).

Gonadectomy markedly depresses preputial sebum content (Homady and Brain, 1982) and diminishes territorial marking, as shown in mice (Wolff and Powell, 1984; Kimura and Hagiwara, 1985), gerbils (Yahr, 1981), hamsters (Johnston, 1981) and Mongolian gerbils (Probst, 1985). Dominant mice scent-mark by deposition of urine more than subordinates, and they spread marks with different spatial patterns (Desjardins et al., 1973; Wolff and Powell, 1984). The preputial glands are larger in dominant animals than in subordinates (Bronson and Marsden, 1973), and this is especially noticeable in wild mice (Barnett et al., 1980).

Excluding taste, which appears to contribute little to the perception of pheromones, there are several chemoreceptor sensory systems which can serve as potential pheromone detectors; (1) the trigeminal nerve (common chemical sense); (2) septal organ of Masera; (3) nervus terminalis; (4) fila olfactoria (the olfactory nerve); (5) the vomeronasal organ, with the exception of fish, birds and Old World primates (Wysocki, 1989; Meredith, 1983). The vomeronasal organ is connected via a single synapse in the accessory olfactory bulb to a region of the amygdala having direct connections with the hypothalamus (Scalia and Winans, 1975). The accumulated evidence indicates that it is directly involved in the perception of the species-typical responses to chemo-sensory signals modulating agonistic behaviour (Bean, 1982; Meredith, 1983). Thus, its deafferentation results in consistent reduction of agonistic behaviour towards the intruders (Bean, 1982; Wysocki, 1989) and in urine marking (Labov and Wysocki, 1989).

Each male's odour contains information about his individual identity as well as his dominance status (Brown, 1979). Dominant and subordinate animals are clearly distinguished by olfactory cues in mice (Carr et al., 1970; Parmigiani et al., 1982a), rats (Krames et al., 1969), bank voles (Clethrionomys glareolus) (Hoffmeyer, 1982) and brown lemmings (Lemmus trimucronatus) (Huck et al., 1982). In addition, familiar and unfamiliar subjects are recognized (Alberts and Galef, 1973; Krames and Shaw, 1973). The ability to distinguish individual scents has been shown in rats (Brown, 1988) and hamsters (Johnston et al., 1993). Individual recognition seems to be stored in long-term memory: male guinea-pigs were able to recognize individual female urine samples, presented for only 2 min, after seven days (Beauchamp and Wellington, 1984) and Mongolian gerbils were shown to discriminate conspecific odours up to four weeks later (Cheal et al., 1982).

Defeated rats urine-mark less over the odour of the male that defeated them, in comparison with other conspecific odours. This suggests that the rat's experience with the *particular* dominant male alters its response to the individual odour of that male (Brown, 1992), and therefore, the odour of dominance (Krames et al., 1969) may be less salient than the odour of a particular male (Halpin, 1980).

The odour can be regarded as a communication signal that is important for the exhibition of certain kinds of behaviour. In turn, the behavioural consequences may alter physiological conditions within the organism, including the production and quality of the subject's odour. For example, if losing an agonistic encounter diminishes the level of testosterone in a defeated animal, its production of androgen-dependent pheromone decreases, and perhaps changes qualitatively (Jones and Nowell, 1974c; Brain and Homady, 1985a, 1985b). Similarly, the preputialectomized mice showed no aggression towards sham-operated males, although they were recipients of preputial odours (Hayashi, 1987). The reduction of aggressivity seems to be attributable to a decline in aggressive motivation rather than a decline of aggression-inducing stimuli, as the odour recipients retained lower status than sham-operated opponents. Furthermore, the place of odour deposition has to be considered: a particular substance may have opposite effects when applied to the opponent or to the surrounding environment. The urine from highly aggressive males elicited attacks by intact males directed towards castrates scented on their body, while a substantial decline of aggression was found when the encounters were performed in cages filled with bedding soiled by highly aggressive males (Sandnabba, 1986a).

These few examples show the complexity of olfactory communication. We can expect two-way communication of information, which may exert feedback regulatory effects upon the exhibition of agonistic strategies in both participants. It is also plausible to expect that olfactory stimuli are especially important in eliciting appropriate responses in inexperienced animals and that experienced animals may be conditioned through experience to respond to input from other systems (Meredith, 1983). Because of these factors, the study of individually housed male mice showing variable behavioural strategies during the establishment of social relationships seems to be especially appropriate.

GENERAL METHODS

Albino outbred ICR mice bred at Velaz, Prague, were used throughout our experiments. The tested males were individually housed for four weeks in metal self-cleaning cages (8 × 16 × 13 cm) at the age of approximately 40 days. They were not handled except on the experimental days. This housing procedure is known to stimulate intensive agonistic behaviour in male mice. After the period of individual housing, the mice were tested in interactions with group-housed opponents of the same age and origin. The opponents were housed in groups of 10–15 in standard plastic cages (38 × 22 × 14 cm) with the floors covered with a sawdust. The group housing nearly abolishes aggression of mice towards isolated males, hence the competitive conditions during the encounter are unequal. The group-housed males behave as standard non-aggressive opponents, while the behaviour of individually housed subjects remains virtually spontaneous. All animals were housed under light:dark conditions 12:12 h (light on 07.00 h) and temperature approximately 22 °C. Food and water were supplied *ad libitum*.

Two procedures were used to alternate the involvement of pheromones in regulatory mechanisms of agonistic behaviour. (1) Since the production of pheromones is known to be gonad dependent (Mugford and Nowell, 1970), the emission of the olfactory signal by stimulus opponents was excluded by their castration. They were bilaterally gonadectomized or controls were sham operated, under ether anaesthesia, four to five weeks before the beginning of the experiments. (2) The opposite approach excluded the sensation of the olfactory signal in tested subjects by zinc sulphate anosmia.

The two experimental manipulations were required because the urine from group-housed male mice may contain pheromones of low efficiency (Jones and Nowell, 1974a) and because of uncertainty in the precise site of pheromone reception. Among various chemosensory systems existing in mammals, the vomeronasal organ seems to be the most prominent in the reception of species-specific signals (Meredith, 1983). Zinc sulphate treatment (Alberts and Galef, 1971) remains the only non-surgical lesion shown to spare vomeronasal input (Meredith, 1983); its efficacy was verified in mice (Childs and Brain, 1979; Brain et al., 1982), rats (Alberts and Galef, 1971; Flannelly and Thor, 1976), hamsters (Devor and Murphy, 1973), etc. In our experimental subjects, the anosmia was induced by inserting 0.2 μl of 4% $ZnSO_4$ (Brain et al., 1981) into the nostrils under short ether anaesthesia. The procedure was repeated three times. The efficacy of the treatment was proved by the loss of ability to discriminate female urine from distilled water by anosmic mice.

The behaviour of individually housed mice was tested in Plexiglas observation boxes (20 × 30 × 20 cm) with clean sawdust provided before each encounter. The subjects were allowed 30 min adaptation in the cage before the opponent was introduced. Then the interactions were videotaped for 4 min.

The following behavioural catalogue of acts and postures, similar to those described by Grant and Mackintosh (1963), was recorded by a trained observer: *aggressive activities*—attack, threat postures (sideways and upright); *defensive–escape activities*—defensive posture (upright), escape, alert posture; ambivalent tail rattle; *sociable activities*—social sniffing; *locomotory–exploratory activities*—walk, rear. Behavioural elements, including some spatial relationships (approach, following, leave from the opponent), were recorded on a computer with a program for ethological observations.

The individually housed males tested showed important interindividual differences in their spontaneous behaviour towards non-aggressive opponents. Some mice attack the opponents (aggressive mice), while others show spontaneous defensive postures and escapes and no attacks (timid mice). It should be emphasized that this 'timid' behaviour is spontaneously exhibited, as the opponents are non-aggressive. Results were statistically evaluated using a two-tailed non-parametric Wilcoxon matched-pairs signed-ranks test separately for aggressive and timid animals, where available (Siegel, 1956).

AGONISTIC BEHAVIOUR OF MALE MICE IN INTERACTIONS WITH VARIOUS TYPES OF OPPONENTS

Male and female mice differ in their ability to affect aggressive behaviour in conspecifics. While the scent of males is known to stimulate attacks (Mackintosh and Grant, 1966), the scent of females inhibits them (Mugford and Nowell, 1970; Dixon and Mackintosh, 1971). Both aggression-promoting effects of male urine (Mugford and Nowell, 1970; Mugford, 1974; Brain and Evans, 1974) and aggression-inhibiting effects of female urine (Mugford and Nowell, 1971b; Mugford 1973) are gonad dependent. Different types of opponents may produce variable sequences of aggressive behaviour (Brain *et al.*, 1981). The question, however, of whether the various types of opponents also affect the *defensive* components of agonistic behaviour has not been answered so far.

We have tested individually housed males showing aggressive and timid behavioural strategies in interactions with sham-operated males, castrates, sham-operated females and ovariectomized females. Each subject was tested with all types of opponents in a randomized order. The reproductive status of stimulus females was not controlled during the experiment because the urine from oestrus and dioestrus females was reported to produce similar degrees of anti-aggression activity (Mugford and Nowell, 1971b).

Among 17 individually housed males there were 12 subjects aggressive in interactions with male opponents, 10 with castrates, six with females and eight with ovariectomized females. The amounts of exhibited attacks are presented in Figure 1. The tested males attacked the sham-operated males more vigorously than all other types of opponents, although the difference between males and castrates in this particular experiment was not significant. This relatively small difference might be caused by the interference of randomized interactions with females. A similar reason could also explain the relatively high proportion of males attacking females, since some subjects first attacked the opponents introduced into the cage and only *then* differentiated them by sniffing.

In addition to the confirmation of already known effects on aggressive behaviour, we have found significant effects on defensive behaviour and on non-agonistic sociable activities. The tested subjects exhibited significantly more defensive postures towards males in comparison with either castrates or females (Figure 1) and significantly less social investigation of males than all other opponents. All tested subjects showed either an aggressive or a timid agonistic behavioural strategy towards males, while four of them exhibited no agonistic behaviour at all in interactions with castrates, eight with females and four with ovariectomized females. The occurrence of non-agonistic (sociable) behavioural strategy appeared to differ significantly according to the type of opponent ($p < 0.05$, Cochran Q-test).

The results indicate that a factor specific to male opponents stimulates both aggressive as well as defensive components of agonistic behaviour in male mice. The agonistic behaviour seems to be affected by the type of opponent as a whole and its reduction is balanced by an increase in non-agonistic sociable activities.

INHIBITION OF OPPONENT'S OLFACTORY SIGNALS ALTERS ALL COMPONENTS OF AGONISTIC BEHAVIOUR IN RECIPIENTS

The experiments with various types of opponents suggested that olfactory signals might be responsible for the stimulation of all components of agonistic

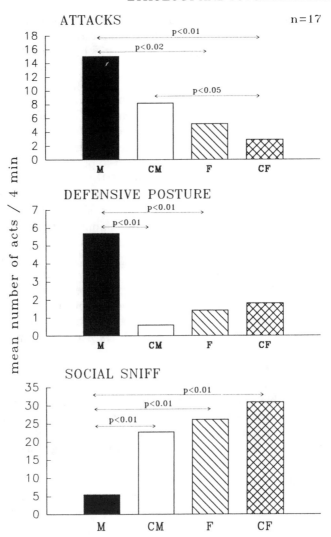

Figure 1 Agonistic behaviour of individually housed male mice in interactions with opponents of different social status. M = sham-operated males, CM = castrates, F = sham-operated females, CF = ovariectomized females. Values are given as averages from 17 males exhibiting aggressive and non-aggressive behavioural strategies. Probabilities were calculated by non-parametric Wilcoxon t-test.

behaviour in male mice. Although the importance of pheromones in offensive aggression has been extensively studied, there has been no evidence that they also exert effects on alternative defensive strategies. Indirect evidence suggests that an aversive pheromone might affect emotionality (Jones and Nowell, 1974c) through an increase in fear (Kumar, 1970). Emotionality and fear, however, have rather subjective definitions and therefore are not very suitable for experimental evaluation.

Thus we have decided to examine the behaviour of individually housed mice that spontaneously exhibit alternative aggressive and timid behavioural strategies. The gonad-dependent property of the male mice pheromones (Mugford and Nowell, 1970; Brain and Evans, 1974) allowed us to use castrates as reference subjects that do not produce an active compound in contrast to intact males.

The effect of reducing aggressive behaviour by castration of opponents was confirmed in an experiment involving 25 aggressive individually housed males that attacked sham-operated males significantly more than castrates (Figure 2). This effect was accompanied by a similar decrease in the number of tail rattles and balanced by a significant increase in sociable activities in interactions with castrates, i.e. social sniffing and following ($p < 0.01$). There were no obvious effects on defensive activities, since they were almost absent in aggressive animals.

Almost half of the experimental subjects tested in experiments with castrates exhibited a timid behavioural strategy in control interactions with sham-operated opponents. The timid males ($n = 23$) exhibited significantly less defensive postures towards castrates compared to sham-operated males (Figure 2). The significant decrease in fear-related activities was accompanied by an increase in sociable and aggressive activities, although this was non-significant. The observed increase in the number of attacks may be explained, in part, by reduced fear of the opponent when the typical male scent was absent, but it may also be due to the experience gained in previous non-aggressive encounters.

The analysis of behavioural strategies suggests that there is a good positive correlation between the presence of pheromone and agonistic behaviour. Among 95 tested animals, there were 71 males exhibiting agonistic (either offensive or defensive) behavioural strategies in interactions with males. In contrast, the number of males exhibiting non-aggressive strategy increased from 24 to 41 in interactions with castrates. This effect was highly significant ($\chi^2 = 12.36$; $p < 0.01$ McNemar test).

Athough the abolition of aggression-inducing pheromonal effects by castration has been demonstrated in various rodent species (Mugford and Nowell, 1970; Payne, 1973; Yahr, 1981), a serious question can be raised about the quality of the odour produced by intact stimulus males. The urine from dominant and subordinate individuals is differentiated by other males or oestrous females, as described in mice (Carr et al., 1970, 1982; Jones and Nowell, 1974b; Parmigiani et al., 1982a, 1982b), rats (Krames et al., 1969; Taylor et al., 1982) and brown lemmings (Huck et al., 1981). For example, the urine from dominant and isolated males, but not that of group-housed males, was found to exert aversive effects in tested group-housed subjects and this aversive property was lost after regrouping of isolated donors (Jones and

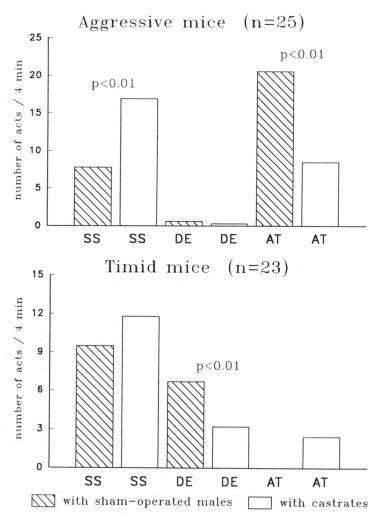

Figure 2 Behaviour of individually housed males in interactions with sham-operated and castrated group-housed males. The subjects were classified as *aggressive* or *timid* according to the behavioural strategy exhibited in interactions with sham-operated males. Decisive activities (SS = social sniffing, DE = defensive posture, AT = attack) are presented as average values per observation. Statistical comparisons were evaluated by non-parametric Wilcoxon test.

Nowell, 1974a). The lack of aversion to the urine from group-housed males, however, does not indicate an inability to discriminate the odour because the motivation for preferring one odour to another is intrinsic to the test animal. No preference may indicate simply a lack of motivation for choosing between odours or that two odours are equally attractive (Brown, 1979).

Regardless of the reported dependence of odour quality on the donor's social status, our results demonstrate that the individually housed males responded to group-housed opponents, performing both offensive as well as defensive behavioural strategies. Nevertheless, the excitatory effects upon agonistic behaviour might also be mediated by systems other than olfaction. The specific involvement of olfaction was further explored using experimentally induced anosmia in tested subjects.

ANOSMIA AFFECTS BOTH AGGRESSIVE AND DEFENSIVE AGONISTIC BEHAVIOUR IN MICE

The vomeronasal organ seems to be especially important in sensation of species-typical chemosensory signals (Meredith, 1983; Wysocki, 1989). Surgical olfactory bulbectomy completely abolishes aggression (Ropartz, 1968; Bean, 1982), although the lesions are accompanied by non-specific destruction of other neural systems. A perfusion of the olfactory epithelium with zinc sulphate solution almost certainly damages the olfactory epithelium; however, not all receptors are necessarily destroyed by the treatment and there is usually some regeneration. With these considerations in mind, we have used control groups for comparisons of the effects of anosmia, as well as comparisons before and after treatment.

After anosmia, a significant reduction in the number of attacks was found in aggressive males ($n = 9$), which was accompanied by a significant increase in social investigation (Figure 3). No significant changes were detected in a simultaneously tested group of untreated animals. The defensive activities were practically absent in both groups of aggressive animals. The similar numbers of males exhibiting aggressive behaviour before and after the treatment suggests that anosmia reduced the frequency of aggressive acts rather than the selection of offensive aggressive strategy.

The effects of anosmia on defensive agonistic behaviour was tested in a group of timid mice ($n = 8$) that exhibited a highly significant decrease in the number of defensive postures (Figure 4) and an increase in social sniffing. No differences were found in a group of control animals. A small increase in attacks was detected in both experimental and control groups which may be accounted for in terms of non-olfactory factors. Out of eight males showing the timid behavioural strategy before anosmia, there remained only one after the treatment. This difference suggests, in contrast to the aggressive mice, that the timid behavioural strategy may be less frequently selected by anosmic animals.

In summary, our results confirmed the importance of olfactory signals in the modulation of aggression. Furthermore, the significant reduction of defensive behaviour in timid males clearly indicates that the involvement of olfactory signals is not restricted to aggression but is also involved in the whole complex of agonistic behaviour, i.e. offensive aggressive as well as defensive–escape components. This finding is also supported by an increase in non-agonistic

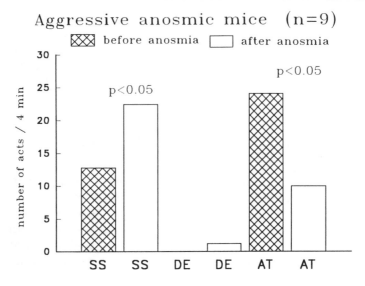

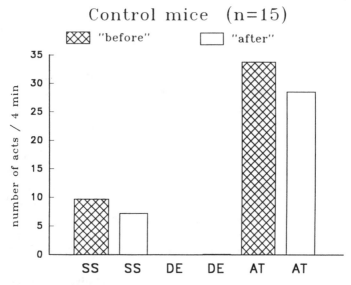

Figure 3 Effects of anosmia on behaviour of aggressive individually housed males in interactions with group-housed opponents. The subjects were classified as *aggressive* according to the behavioural strategy exhibited before treatment. Columns represent the decisive activities (SS = social sniffing, DE = defensive posture, AT = attack) as average per observation. Statistical comparisons were evaluated by non-parametric Wilcoxon tests.

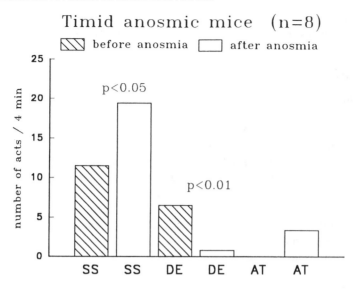

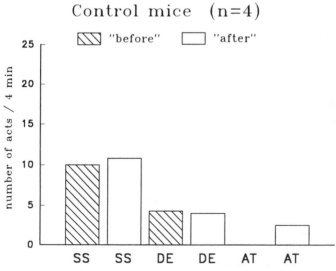

Figure 4 Effects of anosmia on behaviour of timid individually housed males in interactions with group-housed opponents. The subjects were classified as *timid* according to the behavioural strategy exhibited before treatment. Columns represent the decisive activities (SS = social sniffing, DE = defensive posture, AT = attack) as averages per observation. Statistical comparisons were evaluated by non-parametric Wilcoxon test.

social investigation which was observed in both aggressive and timid mice when their agonistic responsiveness was reduced by anosmia.

GENERAL DISCUSSION

The experiments, involving animals which exhibit alternative behavioural strategies in intraspecies conflicts, indicate that the motivation for agonistic behaviour was affected rather than a specific behavioural component, i.e. aggression. A basic principle in ethology stresses the importance of theoretical approaches using fundamentally different levels of analysis: 'how questions', about the *proximate causes* of the behaviour (they ask *how* mechanisms within an animal operate, enabling the creature to behave in a certain way) and '*why* questions', about the *ultimate causes* (they ask what is the purpose, the function, and why the animal has evolved the proximate mechanisms that cause it to perform an activity) (Alcock, 1993). From the evolutionary point of view, a trend towards increasing aggression seems to be unlikely. In contrast, a trend towards increasing agonistic motivation seems more feasible, if agonistic behaviour is understood as a competitive behaviour to acquire access to limited resources (such as territory or females) which are necessary for the reproductive success of a particular individual. This goal is achieved in mutual encounters with conspecifics through an offensive form of aggression. Each agonistic conflict, however, is coupled with the potential danger of loss and injury and that is why the function for the defensive subsystem in agonistic behaviour is fully comprehensive. Some animals may prefer to avoid a potentially dangerous combat; differences between aggressive and non-aggressive wild male mice have been interpreted in terms of fundamentally different behaviour strategies adopted in response to social interaction (Benus *et al.*, 1992).

The energetic costs and the risk of injury in agonistic encounters can be reduced by prior assessment of opponents in scent-marking. Brown (1979) explains the hypothesis originally raised by Gosling (1982) that the intruder first learns the odour of the resident from his scent marks. Then, when the intruder meets the resident, he compares the scent of the resident with the odour which has previously been encountered, and 'when these scents match then the resident is identified and the intruder responds appropriately, usually by withdrawal'. Since owners of territory are generally high-quality animals, it will pay the owner to escalate and the intruder to give up early. In our experiments, the relationship between different odour quality and responding was obvious from the virtually non-aggressive behaviour of group-housed opponents to the highly agonistic behaviour of individually housed subjects. The extensive urine-marking in wild mice (Barnett *et al.*, 1980), quantity of marks deposited by aggressive males (Taylor *et al.*, 1988), and the differences in urinary patterns between dominant and subordinate mice (Desjardins *et al.*, 1973) further strengthen the plausibility of the hypothesis about scent-marking under laboratory conditions.

Urine from highly aggressive males, when applied to castrates, stimulated attacks in moderately aggressive males, while the bedding soiled by highly aggressive males suppressed their aggressiveness (Sandnabba, 1986a). The differential effects of pheromonal substances deposited in the environment or over the body of the opponent support the theory of odour comparisons described above.

The pattern of olfactory learning and behavioural change may be different from the dominant and subordinate males. The dominant male may increase his scent-marking in response to the odour of the subordinate male, while the subordinate male may show reduced aggression when he encounters the resident's odour (Brown, 1992). Subjecting castrates to training that resulted in an aversive response to male odours, which was similar to the avoidance exhibited by intact males, did not result in 'intact-like' agonistic behaviour of castrates. A possible explanation for the failure to influence the agonistic behaviour of castrate subjects concerns what might be labelled the social significance of urine odours. Desensitizing the brain mechanisms via removal of the hormone could presumably alter spontaneous social responsiveness to various stimuli without affecting an animal's ability to learn responses to such stimuli. While the avoidance training was able to replace the aversiveness of the odour to the castrate, it was not able to replace the social significance of the odours, and hence could not replace the agonistic behaviour (Sawyer, 1981).

The responses to olfactory signals are significantly altered by previous social and sexual experience (our unpublished results; Haug, 1970; Wysocki, 1989; Labov and Wysocki, 1989), previous exposure to the odour (Williams et al., 1990), activity of the stimulus subject (Connor and Lynds, 1977), rearing conditions (Brown, 1991), and may be either hereditarily determined or acquired through learning (Sandnabba, 1986b), as shown in rats and mice. The high variability of the recipient's responses to olfactory stimuli raises doubts about the specific chemical structure of a single active compound. Brown (1979) argues that the specific dominance odour may be less salient than individual odours. Indeed, the identification of sex, social status, familiarity, and even individual recognition of the encountered opponent may be better explained, perhaps, by the perception of a mixture of compounds that are released, under particular physiological conditions, from the organism. Although the high correlation between physiological markers and behavioural effects might exist in group data, the links may not necessarily have to be observed at an individual level (Probst, 1985).

The ensuing behaviour is not 'released' by the odour; rather, the odour may provide information that leads to a certain response (Vandenbergh, 1975). Isolated mice that proved to win during the subsequent agonistic encounters showed no aversion to the urine from prospective losers or winners. In contrast, the subjects that subsequently lost the encounters exhibited aversion to the urine from donors that later proved to win the encounters. Thus, differential responsiveness to urine odours may influence the outcome of the encounter between two mice (Sawyer, 1977). Unfortunately, very little is known about the olfactory signal characteristics of stress induced by electric shock or physical defeat (Carr *et al.*, 1970) and 'fear scent' (*Angstgeruch*) elicited by frightened mice (Müller-Velten, 1966). Such stress-related odours may either distinguish the donor's social status and/or reduce his motivation for agonistic competition. Therefore, the specific dominance odour, if it exists, should be distinguished by means other than aggressive responses of recipients, for example, by a chemical separation and subsequent discrimination of an active compound (Nishimura *et al.*, 1989).

In conclusion, research has led to many new questions since the term 'pheromone' was applied to the aggressive behaviour in mice (Mackintosh and Grant, 1966). While the chemical structure of olfactory signals remains unclear, we have shown that olfactory cues affect both aggressive and defensive components of agonistic behaviour. Although the effects of a species-typical chemical substance ('pheromone') could be linked to 'agonistic' instead of 'aggressive' behaviour, such a conclusion would be suspicious because of differential responding of the tested subjects, the complexity of the response and the modulation by experience. Thus, the proximate causes of agonistic behaviour have to be further examined.

In contrast, the ultimate causes for the involvement of olfactory signals in the whole complex of agonistic behaviour seem to be rather convincingly explained by a functional insight which emphasizes the costs and benefits of an encounter to both the territory owner and the intruder (Gosling, 1982). Despite this, the olfactory signals should be regarded as the means of two-way communication. They provide the opponent with an assessment of the quality of the donor and give important information to the recipient which leads to the decision (Payne *et al.*, 1992) regarding the appropriate behavioural strategy under prevailing social and environmental circumstances.

ACKNOWLEDGEMENTS

Parts of our work described here were supported by grants from the Ministry of Health of Czech Republic (No. 0865-3) and Charles University (No. 225). The authors acknowledge the receipt of a Wellcome Trust Travel Grant.

REFERENCES

Alberts, J.R. and Galef B.G. (1971) Acute anosmia in the rat: a behavioural test of a peripherally induced olfactory deficit. *Physiol. Behav.*, 6, 619–621.

Alberts, J.R. and Galef, B.G. (1973) Olfactory cues and movement: stimuli mediating intraspecific aggression in the wild Norway rat. *J. Comp. Physiol. Psychol.*, 85, 233–242.

Alcock, J. (1993) *Animal Behavior*, 5th edn. Sinauer Associates, Sunderland, MA.

Archer, J. (1968) The effects of strange male odours on aggressive behaviour in male mice. *J. Mammal.*, 49, 572–575.

Barnett, S.A., Dickson, R.G. and Warth, K.G. (1980) Social status, activity and preputial glands of wild and domestic house mice. *Zool. J. Linnean Soc.*, **70**, 421–430.

Bean, N.J. (1982) Modulation of agonistic behavior by the dual olfactory system in male mice. *Physiol. Behav.*, **29**, 433–437.

Beauchamp, G.K. and Wellington, J.L. (1984) Habituation to individual odours occurs following brief, widely-spaced presentations, *Physiol. Behav.*, **32**, 511–514.

Benus, R.F., Koolhaas, J.M. and van Oortmerssen, G.A. (1992) Individual strategies of aggressive and non-aggressive male mice in encounters with trained aggressive residents. *Anim. Behav.*, **43**, 531–540.

Brain, P.F. and Evans, C.M. (1974) Influences of two naturally occurring androgens on the attack directed by 'trained fighter' to strain mice towards castrated mice of three different strains. *IRCS Res. Endocrinology*, **2**, 1672.

Brain, P.F. and Homady, M.H. (1985a) Effects of sex steroids on structure and activity of the preputial gland in long-term castrated mice: I. Testosterone. *IRCS Med. Sci.*, **13**, 238–239.

Brain, P.F. and Homady, M.H. (1985b) Effects of sex steroids on structure and activity of the preputial gland in long-term castrated mice: II. 5-alpha dihydrotestosterone. *IRCS Med. Sci.*, **13**, 240–241.

Brain, P.F., Benton, D., Childs, G. and Parmigiani, S. (1981) The effect of the type of opponent in tests by murine aggression. *Behav. Proc.*, **6**, 319–327.

Brain, P.F., Goldsmith, J.F., Parmigiani, S. and Mainardi, M. (1982) Involvement of various senses in responses to individual housing in laboratory albino mice: 1. The olfactory sense. *Boll. Zool.*, **49**, 213–222.

Bronson, F.H. and Marsden, H.M. (1973) The preputial gland as an indicator of social dominance in male mice. *Behav. Biol.*, **9**, 625–628.

Brown, R.E. (1979) Mammalian social odours: a critical review. In: *Advances in the Study of Behavior*. Academic Press, New York, pp. 103–162.

Brown, R.E. (1988) Individual odours of rats are discriminable independently of changes in gonadal hormone levels. *Physiol. Behav.*, **43**, 359–363.

Brown, R.E. (1991) Effects of rearing condition, gender, and sexual experience on odour preferences and urine marking in Long–Evans rats. *Anim. Learning Behav.*, **19**, 18–28.

Brown, R.E. (1992) Responses of dominant and subordinate male rats to the odours of male and female conspecifics. *Aggressive Behav.*, **18**, 129–138.

Butenandt, A. and Karlson, P. (1959) Pheromones (ectohormones) in insects. *Annu. Rev. Ent.*, **4**, 39–58.

Carr, W.J., Martorano, R.D. and Krames, L. (1970) Responses of mice to odours associated with stress. *J. Comp. Physiol. Psychol.*, **71**, 223–228.

Carr, W.J., Kimmel, K.R., Anthony, S.L. and Schlocker, D.E. (1982) Female rats prefer to mate with dominant rather than subordinate males. *Bull. Psychonomic Soc.*, **20**, 89–91.

Chance, M.R.A. (1966) Resolution of social conflict in animals and man. In: *Ciba Foundation Symposium on Conflict in Society* (eds A.V.S. de Reuck and J. Knight). Churchill JA, London, pp. 16–35.

Cheal, M., Klestzick, J. and Domesick, V.B. (1982) Attention and habituation: odour preferences, long-term memory, and multiple sensory cues of novel stimuli. *J. Comp. Physiol. Psychol.*, **96**, 47–60.

Childs, G. and Brain, P.F. (1979) A videotape analysis of behavioural strategies of attacked anosmic mice in encounters with three different types of conspecific. *IRCS Med. Sci.*, **7**, 80.

Connor, J.L. and Lynds, P.G. (1977) Mouse aggression and the intruder-familiarity effect: evidence for multiple-factor determination. *J. Comp. Physiol. Psychol.*, **91**, 270–280.

Desjardins, C., Maruniak, J.A. and Bronson, F.H. (1973) Social rank in house mice: differentiation revealed by ultraviolet visualization of urinary marking patterns. *Science*, **182**, 939–941.

Devor, M. and Murphy, M.R. (1973) The effect of peripheral olfactory blockade on the social behaviour of the male golden hamster. *Behav. Biol.*, **9**, 31–42.

Dixon, A.K. (1982) Ethopharmacologie: ein neuer Weg zur Untersuchung des Einflusses von Medikamenten auf das Verhalten. *Triangel*, **21**, 95–105.

Dixon, A.K. and Mackintosh, J.H. (1971) Effects of female urine upon the social behaviour of adult male mice. *Anim. Behav.*, **19**, 138–140.

Eibl-Eibesfeldt, I. (1950) Beiträge zur Biologie der Haus- und der Ährenmaus nebst einigen Beobactungen an anderen Nagern. *Z. Tierpsychol.*, **7**, 558–587.

Flannelly, K.J. and Thor, D.H. (1976) Territorial behavior of laboratory rats under condition of peripheral anosmia. *Anim. Learning Behav.*, **4**, 337–340.

Gosling, L.M. (1982) A reassessment of the function of scent marking in territories. *Z. Tierpsychol.*, **60**, 89–118.

Grant, E.C. and Mackintosh, J.H. (1963) Comparison of the social postures of some laboratory rodents. *Behaviour*, **21**, 246–259.

Halpin, Z.T. (1980) Individual odours and individual recognition: review and commentary. *Biol. Behav.*, **5**, 233–248.

Haug, M. (1970) Mise en évidence de deux odeurs aux effets opposés de facilitation et d'inhibition des conduits agressives chez la souris male. *CR Acad. Sci. Paris*, **271**, 1567–1570.

Hayashi, S. (1987) The effects of preputialectomy on aggression in male mice. *Zool. Sci.*, **4**, 551–555.

Hoffmeyer, I. (1982) Responses of female bank voles (*Clethrionomys glareolus*) to dominant vs subordinate conspecific males and to urine odours from dominant vs subordinate males. *Behav. Neural Biol.*, **36**, 178–188.

Homady, M.H. and Brain, P.F. (1982) Effects of marking with preputial gland material on the attack directed towards long-term castrates by isolated males. *Aggressive Behav.*, **8**, 137–140.

Huck, U.W., Banks, E.M. and Wang, S.C. (1982) Olfactory discrimination of social status in the brown lemming. *Behav. Neural Biol.*, **33**, 364–371.

Johnston, R.E. (1981) Testosterone dependence of scent marking by male hamsters (*Mesocricetus auratus*). *Behav. Neural Biol.*, **31**, 96–99.

Johnston, R.E., Derzie, A., Chiang, G. *et al.* (1993) Individual scent signatures in golden hamsters: evidence for specialization of function. *Anim. Behav.*, **45**, 1061–1070.

Jones, R.B. and Nowell, N.W. (1974a) The urinary aversive pheromone of mice: species, strain and grouping effects. *Anim. Behav.*, **22**, 187–191.

Jones, R.B. and Nowell, N.W. (1974b) A comparison of the aversive and female attractant properties of urine from dominant and subordinate male mice. *Anim. Learning Behav.*, **2**, 141–144.

Jones, R.B. and Nowell, N.W. (1974c) Effects of androgen on the aversive properties of male mouse urine. *J. Endocrinol.*, **60**, 19–25.

Kimelman, B.R. and Lubow, R.E. (1974) The inhibitory effect of preexposed olfactory cues on intermale aggression in mice. *Physiol. Behav.*, **12**, 919–922.

Kimura, T. and Hagiwara, Y. (1985) Regulation of urine marking in male and female mice: effects of sex steroids. *Horm. Behav.*, **19**, 64–70.

Krames, L. and Shaw, B. (1973) Role of previous experience in the male rats reaction to odours from group and alien conspecifics. *J. Comp. Physiol. Psychol.*, **82**, 444–448.

Krames, L., Carr, W.J. and Bergman, B. (1969) A pheromone associated with social dominance among male rats. *Psychonomic Sci.*, **16**, 11–12.

Kršiak, M., Šulcová, A., Donát, P. *et al.* (1984). Can social and agonistic interaction be used to detect anxiolytic activity of drugs?. In: *Ethopharmacological Aggression Research* (eds K.A. Miczek, M.R. Kruk and B. Olivier). Liss, New York, pp. 93–114.

Kumar, R. (1970) Effects of fear on exploratory behaviour in rats. *Q. J. Exp. Psychol.*, **22**, 205–214.

Labov, J.B. and Wysocki, C.J. (1989) Vomeronasal organ and social factors affect urine marking by male mice. *Physiol. Behav.*, **45**, 443–447.

Lát, J. (1965) The spontaneous exploratory reactions as a tool for psychopharmacological studies: a contribution towards a theory of contradictory results in psychopharmacology. In *Pharmacology of Conditioning, Learning and Retention* (eds M.Y. Mikhelson, V.G. Longo and Z. Votava). Pergamon Press, Oxford; Czechoslovak Medical Press, Praha, pp. 47–66.

Mackintosh, J.H. and Grant, E.C. (1966) The effect of olfactory stimuli on the agonistic behaviour of laboratory mice. *Z. Tierpsychol.*, **23**, 584–587.

McKinney, E.D. and Christian, J.J. (1970) Effect of preputialectomy on fighting behavior in mice. *Proc. Soc. Exp. Biol. Med.*, **134**, 291–293.

Meredith, M. (1983) Sensory physiology of pheromone communication. In: *Pheromones and Reproduction in Mammals*. Academic Press, New York, pp. 199–252.

Mugford, R.A. (1973) Intermale fighting affected by home-cage odours of male and female mice. *J. Comp. Physiol. Psychol.*, **84**, 289–295.

Mugford, R.A. (1974) Androgenic stimulation of aggression eliciting cues in adult opponent mice castrated at birth, weaning, or maturity. *Horm. Behav.*, **5**, 93–102.

Mugford, R.A. and Nowell, N.W. (1970) The aggression of male mice against androgenized females. *Psychonomic Sci.*, **20**, 191–192.

Mugford, R.A. and Nowell, N.W. (1971a) The relationship between endocrine status of female opponents and aggressive behaviour of male mice. *Anim. Behav.*, **19**, 153–155.

Mugford, R.A. and Nowell, N.W. (1971b) Endocrine control over production and activity of the anti-aggression pheromone from female mice. *J. Endocrinol.*, **49**, 225–232.

Mugford, R.A. and Nowell, M.W. (1971c) The preputial glands as a source of aggression-promoting odours in mice. *Physiol. Behav.*, **6**, 247–249.

Müller-Velten, H. (1966) Über den Angstgeruch bei der Hausmaus (*Mus musculus*). *Z. Vergl. Physiol.*, **52**, 401–429.

Nishimura, K., Utsumi, K., Yuhara, M. *et al.* (1989) Identification of puberty-accelerating pheromones in male mouse urine. *J. Exp. Zool.*, **251**, 300–305.

Parmigiani, S., Brunoni V. and Pasquali, A. (1982a) Behavioural influences of dominant, isolated and subordinated male mice on female socio-sexual preferences. *Bool. Zool.*, **49**, 31–35.

Parmigiani, S., Brunoni, V. and Pasquli, A. (1982b) Socio-sexual preferences of female mice (*Mus musculus domesticus*): the influence of social aggressive capacities of isolated or grouped males. *Bool. Zool.*, **49**, 73–78.

Payne, A.P. (1973) The aggressive behaviour of isolated male golden hamsters towards individuals of differing hormonal status. *Acta Endocrinol.*, **177**, 287.

Payne, J.W., Bettman, J.R. and Johnson, E.J. (1992) Behavioral decision research: a constructive processing perspective. *Annu. Rev. Psychol.*, **43**, 87–131.

Probst, B. (1985) Individual marking activities not reflected by respective testosterone levels in male gerbils. *Physiol. Behav.*, **34**, 363–367.

Ropartz, P. (1968) The relation between olfactory stimulation and aggressive behaviour in mice. *Anim. Behav.*, **16**, 97–100.

Sandnabba, K.N. (1986a) Differences between two strains of mice, selectively bred for high and low aggressiveness, in the capacity of male odours to affect aggressive behaviour. *Aggressive Behav.*, **12**, 103–110.

Sandnabba, K.N. (1986b) Changes in male odours and urinary marking patterns due to inhibition of aggression in male mice. *Behav. Proc.*, **12**, 349–361.

Sawyer, T.F. (1977) Aversive odours of male mice: experiential and castration effects and the preditability of the outcomes of agonistic encounters. *Aggressive Behav.*, **4**, 263–275.

Sawyer, T.F. (1981) Learned aversion to the odours of male mice: effects on agonistic behaviour. *Physiol. Behav.*, **27**, 19–25.

Scalia, F. and Winans, S.S. (1975) The differential projections of the olfactory bulb and accessory olfactory bulb in mammals. *J. Comp. Neurol.*, **161**, 31–56.

Scott, J.P. and Fredericson, E. (1951) The causes of fighting in mice and rats. *Physiol. Zool.*, **24**, 273–309.

Siegel, S. (1956) *Nonparametric Statistics for the Behavioral Sciences.* McGraw-Hill, New York.

Stark, B. and Hazlett, B.A. (1972) Effect of olfactory experience on aggression in *Mus musculus* and *Peromyscus maniculatus. Behav. Biol.*, **7**, 262–269.

Taylor, G.T., Haller, J. and Regan, D. (1982) Female rats prefer an area vacated by a high testosterone male. *Physiol. Behav.*, **28**, 953–958.

Taylor, G.T., Griffin, M. and Rupich, R. (1988) Conspecific urine marking in male rats (*Rattus norvegicus*) selected for relative aggressiveness. *J. Comp. Psychol.*, **102**, 72–77.

Vandenbergh, J.G. (1975) Hormones, pheromones and behavior. In: *Hormonal Correlates of Behavior. Vol. 2: An Organismic View* (eds B.E. Eleftheriou and R.L. Sprott). Plenum, New York, pp. 551–584.

Williams, J.L. and Barber, R.G. (1990) Effects of cat exposure and cat odours on subsequent amphetamine-induced stereotypy. *Pharmacol. Biochem. Behav.*, **36**, 375–380.

Williams, J.L., Rogers,, A.G. and Adler, A.P. (1990) Prolonged exposure to conspecific and predator odours reduces fear reactions to these odours during subsequent prod-shock tests. *Anim. Learning Behav.*, **18**, 453–461.

Wolff, P.R. and Powell, A.J. (1984) Urine patterns in mice: an analysis of male/female counter-marking. *Anim. Behav.*, **32**, 1185–1191.

Wysocki, C.J. (1989) Vomeronasal chemoreception: its role in reproductive fitness and physiology. In: *Neural Control of Reproductive Function* (eds J.M. Lakoski and R.J. Perez-Polo). Liss, New York, pp. 545–566.

Yahr, P. (1981) Scent marking, sexual behavior and aggression in male gerbils: comparative. *Am. Zool.*, **21**, 143–151.

Yahr, P., Coquelin, A., Martin, A. and Scouten, C.W. (1977) Effects of castration on aggression between male Mongolian gerbils. *Behav. Biol.*, **19**, 189–205.

12 An Ethopharmacological Approach to Behavioural Teratology

PAUL F. BRAIN, HELENA KURISHINGAL, KAREN
WHITING AND COLIN J. RESTALL
School of Biological Sciences, University of Wales, Swansea, UK

INTRODUCTION

Behaviour is largely the output of the central nervous system (CNS)—an organ system that is one of the first to differentiate embryologically (around day 9 post fertilization in the mouse) but is also one of the last structures to be completed (major changes occur up to the 15th postnatal day in the mouse). A wide variety of chemicals (ranging from dietary factors, through heavy metals, vitamins, hormones, psychoactive drugs and somatic drugs) influence both the developing brain and consequent behavioural output (e.g. Abel, 1978; Ewert and Cutler, 1979; Grimm, 1984; Swaab and Mirmiran, 1984) in rodents. These studies parallel growing concerns about potential actions of such factors in human neonates (e.g. Anandan *et al.*, 1980; Ferrier *et al.*, 1973; Solomon *et al.*, 1990). Chemical influences on the developing brain are clearly rather diverse and complex but animal models facilitate exploration of the possibilities within this area. Behaviour is the most sensitive indicator of such influences, generating the subspecialism of 'behavioural teratology' (Yanai, 1984). Early studies tended to assess drug actions on learning tasks (Gai and Grimm, 1982) but Grant and Mackintosh's (1963) rodent posture analysis lends itself to investigating the likely effects of early exposure to hormones and psychoactive drugs on later *social* behaviour in animals and humans. This review essentially looks at the link between ethology and behavioural teratology, provides an overview of our studies in this area and illustrates directions for new research, especially those concerned with identifying neural mechanisms for recorded actions.

ETHOLOGY AND PSYCHOPHARMACOLOGY

Ethology plays two basic roles in attempting to understand the lasting behavioural consequences of exposing developing organisms to psychoactive drugs. These are: selecting test situations and analysing complex interactions.

Ethology and Psychopharmacology. Edited by S.J. Cooper and C.A. Hendrie
© 1994 John Wiley & Sons Ltd

An understanding of the functions of natural behaviour enables one to devise laboratory-based tests which reflect the potentials of the particular species studied. For example, Brain (1992) has advocated that an understanding of the behaviours of wild rodents and lagomorphs can actually help one to design optimal living conditions for common laboratory animals in which they can express a wide range of activities. This approach for ethopharmacology has been recently highlighted in Blanchard *et al*. (1989) and Brain *et al*. (1991). In particular, one can draw on our understanding of behaviours in developing neonates to assess if the drugs are accelerating or slowing the onset of appearance of particular elements. This is the basis on which studies looking at dates of eye opening, development of fur, 'rooting' behaviour (an activity in groups of neonates where animals attempt to burrow to the centre of the group), the righting reflex (where animals, placed on their backs, right themselves), the cliff avoidance response (where animals back away from clear perspex areas placed over a visual 'cliff') and the ultrasonic distress calling (a sound produced by isolated neonates that normally stimulates retrieval by the mother) are performed.

The use of videotape techniques (often assisted by computers) has been strongly advocated by many workers investigating the impact of psychoactive drugs on social behaviour. This area has been recently reviewed by Brain *et al*. (1989, 1991, 1992). Briefly, the semi-permanent videotape record of behavioural interactions between rats or mice are beneficial as:

1. social (especially agonistic) encounters involve rapid, complex movements of at least two participants;
2. encounters involve the complete range of subtle acts and postures described initially by Grant and Mackintosh (1963);
3. attention spans of human observers are limited and one can use the technique to assess observer reliability;
4. technology enables one to record with minimal disturbance to the animals, often involving the use of subdued lighting, the absence of the experimenters from the roof and electronically screened equipment (to eliminate extraneous ultrasound);
5. records enable one to assess the precise function of particular elements and postures in a given strain of mouse in a particular test (see Jones and Brain, 1985); and
6. this technique enables one to look at the full spectrum of behaviour, a necessary requirement when one is uncertain what the precise impact of early exposure to a drug or hormone might be (it is also obvious that 'traditional' responses such as a reduction in 'aggression' could be achieved in a variety of very different ways, e.g. an antihostility effect, by increasing 'fearfulness', via sedation or suppressing motor activity).

Although the vast majority of ethological descriptions of social interactions in rats and mice are based on the pioneering work of Grant and Mackintosh (1963), there is rather too much variation in the schemes used in the literature and more aggreement should be negotiated.

The level of ethological analysis employed in studies of psychoactive drugs can also be quite variable. It is not always appropriate or economical to study the frequency and total duration of each behavioural element (particularly in routine screening operations) and a number of workers have traditionally combined elements which seem to serve broadly the same function (this is the approach most common in behavioural teratology). Broad functional categories are created, e.g. 'non-social investigation', 'social investigation', 'care of body surface', 'attack' and 'threat'. It seems advisable in many cases to validate the inclusion of particular elements constituting categories (by sequence analysis?) as the precise function of elements seems to change with test situation or the strain employed. A variety of microcomputer-based, data-logging and analysis methods for ethopharmacology have been described (Brain *et al.*, 1989; Hendrie and Rodgers, 1990; Olivier and Mos, 1986).

Simple sequence analysis can also be used to study the effects of drugs on behaviour. In such analyses, the acts and postures may be used to a positional, agglomerative hierarchical cluster analysis (Brain *et al.*, 1989; Jones and Brain, 1985) to generate a 'dendrogram'. Sequence analysis can also be examined using semi-Markov chains (Meelis *et al.*, 1990) or by survivor plots (Bressers *et al.*, 1990). All these approaches give the experimenter a more precise indication of the 'structure' of behaviour rather than simply the time devoted to broad behavioural categories or the number of acts and postures (which may be very variable in terms of bout length). Sequence analysis and other techniques can be used to study which elements are eliminated or added as a result of the application of a particular drug as well as changes in the relationships between particular elements and postures. These approaches are of particular utility in the early stages of examining the potential broad-spectrum actions of novel compounds.

PERINATAL EXPOSURE TO HORMONES AND SUBSEQUENT BEHAVIOURAL POTENTIAL IN A RANGE OF MAMMALS

Non-primates

Sex differences in aggressiveness have been noted in a variety of situations (see Brain, 1979) and seemingly reflect differences in the early patterns of endogenous sex steroid secretion and/or adult production of hormones. Androgens have effects on neural processes in perinatal life, altering the capacities of the animals to react aggressively in adulthood (Leshner, 1981). An appropriate androgen titre in adult animals is also a necessary prerequisite for some forms of this behaviour. Dixson (1980) opined that the neural mechanisms mediating patterns of sexual and aggressive behaviour in rodents are profoundly 'masculinized' and 'defeminized' by androgenic influences on the developing brain

(NB: masculinization and defeminization are *different* processes). Male and genetically female rats (*Rattus norvegicus*) which have been androgenized not only need higher oestrogen doses to produce female-typical sexual responses (e.g. lordosis) than non-masculinized females (van de Poll and van Dis, 1977), but are also non-reponsive to testosterone, which induces this behaviour in females (van de Poll *et al.*, 1978). Most studies relating neonatal hormone applications to adult aggressive behaviour have used 'aromatizable' androgens (i.e. those which can be converted to oestrogens by enzymes in target tissues, including the CNS). Male rats and house mice (*Mus musculus domesticus*) have a greater potential for aggressiveness than female counterparts in certain tests because endogenous hormone secretion in the testis occurs earlier than that in the ovary. The earlier surge of testosterone in males was said in rodents to 'create' the neural circuitry of that sex from the 'undifferentiated' (female) condition. Recently revealed complications in this process are detailed by Aron *et al.* (1991), Brain and Haug (1991) and Goy and Roy (1991).

Testosterone propionate treatment of neonatally castrated male (vom Saal *et al.*, 1976) and female (Mugford, 1974) mice increases the incidence of fighting in adulthood in such animals compared with control injected counterparts. It seems likely that (in rodents at least) testosterone plays an important role in producing the mechanism for expressing and maintaining some varieties of aggressive behaviour. One should note, however, that in certain species and situations no sex differences in testosterone-mediated aggression are evident. This is certainly true of same-sex encounters in particular strains of rats (van de Poll *et al.*, 1981).

Early exposure to testosterone (and other aromatizable androgens) increases some forms of aggressiveness in a wide range of non-human species. There are, however, considerable species differences in the precise roles of hormones influencing the prepubertal onset of aggressive behaviour (Brain, 1978), with available evidence suggesting that fishes, reptiles and rodents are more likely to show 'hormonal dependence' than animals such as dogs and primates. Although this may be interpreted as a phylogenetic influence, the longer life-spans of the less 'hormonally dependent' species may be crucial here. Primates, in particular, are likely to acquire a range of social experiences before castration and/or steroid hormone treatment whereas these are often lacking in rats and mice.

Intriguing studies on the intrauterine location phenomenon have added greatly to our knowledge of how early exposure to hormones influence subsequent behavioural potential (vom Saal, 1991). The fetus' position during intrauterine development alters the precise hormonal titres to which developing male and female rats and mice are subjected. Vom Saal and Bronson (1980) found that on the 17th day of gestation male mouse fetuses produce three times the level of circulating testosterone evident in female counterparts. Consequently, intrauterine position in relation to male and female peers, probably by changing early sex steroid exposure, consequently influences the potential for particular types of 'sexually dimorphic' behaviour in adult mice (vom Saal, 1983). Indeed, 2M female mice (those developing between two males) are aggressive towards and establish dominance over OM (those developing between two females) counterparts (Vom Saal and Bronson, 1978). Indeed, intrauterine location also influences the propensity for infanticidal behaviour in females of three strains of mice (Yousif et al., 1989). Further, 2M female rats, after treatment in adulthood with testosterone, exhibited more mounting of receptive females than did OM counterparts (Clemens et al., 1978).

The impact of castration on aggression is less evident in experienced fighter rodents, suggesting that learning overrides hormonal influences even in such species (Brain et al., 1983). Having said this, there is also some evidence from studies on mice that stimulation of gondal function (e.g. by breeding activity) *without* the opportunity to fight reduces the ease with which the propensity for fighting can be suppressed by castration. Perhaps some of the androgen-induced changes in aggressiveness in adults are relatively persistent once generated?

Early exposure to 'stress' (perhaps including the hormones of the pituitary–adrenocortical axis) also modifies adult behavioural potentials for aggressive and 'emotional' activities in rats and mice (reviewed in Chevins, 1990).

Non-human primates

Goy (1968) examined the effects of exposing non-human primates to testosterone in early life. Prenatal exposure to testosterone propionate caused the external genitalia of female rhesus monkeys to be masculinized and they increased their 'rough and tumble' and chasing play—features regarded as more typical of the male. Augmented aggression was still evident in ovariectomized/androgen-treated female adults who had been exposed neonatally to testosterone (Eaton et al., 1973). Dixson (1980) reviewed available data on such studies and concluded that 'androgen administered prenatally has important consequences for behaviour, including aggressive responses, in female rhesus monkeys'. It seemed to him that testosterone (a major androgen in the circulation of fetal rhesus monkeys), present in much higher concentrations in males than females (Resko, 1974), influences brain development. Progesterone, which is present in higher concentrations in female rhesus monkeys, may protect the female's developing brain from masculinization. Dixson (1980) argues (not unreasonably) that it is important (given the variability *within* the order) to assess whether these relationships hold in other primate species.

Humans

Meyer-Bahlburg (1980) and Meyer-Bahlburg and Ehrhardt (1982) produced detailed reviews of the impact of variations in early hormone exposure on subsequent human aggressiveness. These are largely based on data involving endocrine syndromes (e.g. partial androgen insensitivity and congenital adrenal hyperplasia) or treatment with hormones of pregnant women (generally to reduce the probability of miscarriage). There are few reliable data on the incidences of such conditions in particular populations (they are also quite variable in their severity) but their importance is *not* as potential *causes* of problems in society but in providing information concerning the normal biological mechanisms which influence 'sexually dimorphic' behaviours. The 5α-reductase deficiency syndrome (where testosterone cannot be converted to 5α-dihydrostestosterone the metabolite which normally influences body hair growth and masculine 'form') is very rare, being associated with 38 hermaphroditic individuals born to 23 interrelated families in two mountain villages in the Dominican Republic where inbreeding was common. It does suggest, however, that important processes influencing dimorphic behaviours in which pregnant females are given androgen involve metabolites of testosterone in our species.

Small sample sizes are a serious problem in analysing the literature but Meyer-Bahlburg (1980) claims that exogenous sex hormones that slightly increase aggressiveness in female offspring always produce some degree of genital masculinization. He felt that the data resulting from treating toxaemic pregnancies with progesterone were inconsistent. Boys from diabetic pregnancies exposed to progestogen–oestrogen combinations and boys *and* girls from pregnancies treated with medroxyprogesterone acetate (MPA) did show some reduction in subsequent aggressiveness. It is, of course, uncertain precisely how such behavioural effects are generated, as features such as parental rearing styles, degree of exercise and changes in the musculoskeletal system are clearly involved in creating the 'dimorphisms' *and* are likely to be influenced (directly or indirectly) by early hormonal factors.

Early exposure to androgens seems to modify temperament, increasing 'impetuous and active' styles of acting. Olweus (1984) has suggested that this factor has a weak direct action on the potential for aggression in boys but may also have a stronger indirect action on this potential by increasing parental permissiveness of aggression.

Although this section has concentrated on clearly sexually dimorphic behaviours such as sexual aggressive activities, it is very likely that early hormone exposures influence other categories of behaviour such as exploration and social investigation.

PERINATAL EXPOSURE TO PSYCHOACTIVE DRUGS AND SUBSEQUENT SOCIAL BEHAVIOUR IN MICE

One of our earliest studies (Grimm *et al.*, 1984) assessed the utility of the posture analysis in mice to increase our understanding of how pre- and early postnatal exposure to psychoactive drugs influences later social interactions. The study involved the benzodiazepine diazepam, which has been clinically associated with the 'floppy infant syndrome', where a high incidence of hypothermia, hyperbilirubinaemia, hypotonia, asphyxia, respiratory complications and poor suckling responses are seen in the newborn infant (McAllister, 1980). Briefly, female albino mice were injected subcutaneously (s.c.) each day with vehicle or 2.5 mg/kg of diazepam (TEVA Pharmaceutical Industries Ltd, Tel Aviv, Israel) over the last one to six days of pregnancy and for four days post partum. Male offspring were weaned at 22 days of age then individually housed for 14 days in standard caging. Twelve mice in each treatment category then had a docile anosmic male 'standard opponent' introduced for 10 min into its previously cleaned cage. The resulting encounter was videotaped under white lighting in the 'dark' portion of the animal's light/dark cycle and the incidences of 43 behavioural elements were recorded (procedures fully described in Brain et al., 1989). Although there were few dramatic changes in behaviour, diazepam-exposed males showed a significant increase in sideways offensive element compared with controls. Obvious problems of such studies include its being unclear whether the drug:

1. acts prenatally or postnatally (or both);
2. influences the brain of the fetus or simply changes maternal behaviour or lactation;
3. is transmitted in the milk to the neonate;
4. interferes with key developmental processes or behavioural experiences.

Brain et al. (1986) tried to answer some of these questions by applying a range of materials to pregnant mice pre and post partum, post partum only and pre partum only with cross-fostering of the offspring to untreated mothers. Diazepam did not influence broad behavioural categories of social exploration, defence, threat and attack (formed by summing particular behavioural elements) in any of the treatments. It seems likely that the early influences of this compound are mainly limited to influences on learning ability (Benton et al., 1985). In contrast, ethanol modified all categories in the pre- and post-partum application and depressed defensive behaviour was still evident if the offspring were cross-fostered. The fetal alcohol syndrome is a well-known phenomenon (Volk, 1984) of considerable clinical importance. Treatment of pregnant rodents with low doses of ethanol results in their offspring being hyperaggressive in adult life, whereas higher doses seemingly suppress threat and attack (Yanai and Ginsburg, 1977). Brain et al. (1987) carried out a re-evaluation of these effects in albino mice using the treatment regimes described earlier (Brain et al., 1986). Giving mothers 1, 2 or 4 g/kg of ethanol each day reduced defence in their male offspring compared with controls. Two and 4 g/kg also increased social investigation and 2 g/kg increased threat and attack. Giving the same materials in early post-partum life had no discernible effects on the behaviours of male offspring and only ethanol-exposed offspring cross-fostered to ethanol-treated mothers showed significant influences on behaviour. It appears that the pre-natal period is important *and* there is a maternal influence in such phenomena.

Pankaj and Brain (1991a, 1991b, 1991c) tried to answer some of the questions raised by studies with prenatal exposure to benzodiazepines on early development and subsequent adult social behaviour in mice. Daily treatment of pregnant mothers was limited to the period 9–10 days before parturition and *all* neonates were cross-fostered to untreated mothers to eliminate maternal effects. The benzodiazepine agonists chlordiazepoxide and midazolam (both Roche Products Ltd, Welwyn Garden City) were used at doses of 10 or 20 mg/kg and 2.5 or 5.0 mg/kg respectively. Both drugs retarded growth in both male and female offspring. There was also some evidence that the exposures impaired the development of the righting reflex in both sexes but had little effect on the day of eye opening. Both compounds modified social behaviour but the influences of midazolam were more striking. The posture changes suggested that anxiety was increased in males but reduced in females by this exposure. Working with the benzodiazepine antagonists flumazenil (Hoffmann La-Roche, Basle) and CGS 8216 (Ciba-Geigy Corporation, Suffern, New York) at doses of 10 or 20 mg/kg, it was found that growth was inhibited by flumazenil in both sexes but only changed by the higher dose of CGS 8216 from around day 8. The date of eye opening was relatively little changed by either drug exposure but flumazenil produced some improvements in the righting reflex, whereas CGS 8216 sometimes impaired the response. There was some evidence of increased attack and threat in male offspring exposed to these drugs and the higher dose of CGS 8216 decreased defensive/submissive behaviour in female progeny. The inverse agonists DMCM (Schering AG, Berlin) and FG 7142 (Research Biochemicals Inc., Natick, Maryland) were given at doses of 0.5 or 1 mg/kg and 7.5 or 15 mg/kg respectively. Growth was increased by 0.5 mg/kg of DMCM but impaired by 1.0 mg/kg of this material. FG 7142 suppressed later growth. DMCM accelerated the day of eye opening whereas the higher dose of FG 7142 suppressed this indicator and the lower accelerated it. DMCM produced some impairments of the righting reflex but FG 7142 did not influence this measure. DMCM increased threat in male offspring but FG 7142 had no significant effects. Taken together, the data clearly reveal that prenatal exposures to particular benzodiazepine drugs modify development and change adult social behaviour even in cross-fostered mice. Changes were evident in both sexes but particular classes of drugs did not always generate the same picture.

Kurishingal *et al.* (1992) examined the impact of exposure to chlordiazepoxide further by looking at the righting reflex, cliff avoidance and the rooting reflex (an activity of neonates designed to maintain body temperature) in the offspring of mothers given daily injections of 10 or 20 mg/kg of the agonist. They also looked at ultrasonic distress calls over the first five postnatal days (cf. Benton and Nastiti, 1988) at 36 °C, which has been used as an indicator of anxiety (see also later). Drug treatment retarded postnatal body growth and delayed the righting reflex (confirming Pankaj and Brain, 1991a). It also impaired cliff avoidance, augmented rooting behaviour and generally increased ultrasonic calling (except in the early stages at the higher dose, when it depressed calling). Broadly speaking, the results can be interpreted as the drug exposure in fetal life retarding motor development and physical maturation and producing a sedative/anxiolytic action (especially at higher doses).

Ajarem and Ahmad (1991) found that consumption of instant coffee (1, 2 or 4 ml/kg) by female mice before and after parturition or pre partum only reduced non-social investigation, defence and displacement but increased threat and attack in male offspring tested in opponent tests after 14 days of individual housing (commencing at 22 days of age). Interestingly, exposure to instant coffee also substantially increased the levels of acetylcholinesterase in the brains of these male progeny. That particular study did not utilize cross-fostering and employed ingested *instant* coffee. Ajarem and Brain (1993) used 10 and 40 mg/kg of pure caffeine (Reidel-de Haan, Germany) injected s.c. and used a cross-fostering design. In comparable social tests with male offspring, the higher dose significantly *reduced* threat, attack and displacement. It is uncertain whether the change in aggressive behaviour is related to the purity of the compound, the route of administration or the existence of a strong maternal effect in the initial study.

STUDIES ON THE POSSIBLE PHYSIOLOGICAL MECHANISMS UNDERPINNING THE LASTING BEHAVIOURAL INFLUENCES OF EARLY CHEMICAL EXPOSURE

Receptor ligands

It is naturally assumed that the lasting influences of perinatal exposure to psychoactive drugs or hormones on subsequent behavioural potential involve modifications in the receptors for these materials. There is certainly good evidence that hormonal titres can influence the numbers of neural receptors for these factors (Brain, 1978, 1979). Although we have not performed studies on the numbers or affinities of receptors, many investigations have used a wide range of agonists and antagonists to examine the roles of neurotransmitter systems in ultrasonic distress calling of mouse neonates (Benton, 1989; Benton and Brain, 1988; Benton and Nastiti, 1988; Brain et al., 1991; Nastiti et al., 1991) at 20 °C (for high rates) and 37 °C (for low rates). *No* receptor system in the mouse brain is fully established at birth and the various synapses only become fully functional between postnatal days 12 and 28. Broadly speaking, benzodiazepine and GABAergic agonists reduced ultrasonic calling. Serotonergic antagonists and a limited number of noradrenergic and dopaminergic antagonists also had this effect. In contrast, inverse benzodiazepine agonists and a limited number of dopaminergic agonists increased 'distress calling'. These results are broadly in line with the known anxiolytic and anxiogenic actions of the psychoactive drugs. Indeed, using the production of these calls as a 'screen' for anxiety seems more reliable than the black/white box, the elevated plus-maze and the social interaction tests (Lee, 1990).

Membrane fluidity changes

Steroids and some of the psychoactive compounds used here (e.g. diazepam) are lipid-soluble drugs that might be expected to influence the membranes surrounding neuronal elements. Indeed, alcohol (which does not have a major action via a specific receptor) may induce many of its actions by influencing membrane fluidity (Brain *et al.*, 1987). The possibility thus exists that some of the lasting early influences of hormones and psychoactive drugs on behaviour involve fluidity changes in neuronal membranes rather than receptor alterations.

Lipid bilayer membranes were created by dispersing egg yolk phosphatidyl-choline in 200 mM Tris–Cl at a pH of 7.2 followed by sonication to produce unilamellar liposomes. Membrane fluidity was measured by the steady-state fluorescence polarization method using 1,6-diphenyl-1,3,5-hexatriene (DPH) as a fluorophore (Shinitzky and Barenholz, 1978). The fluorescence anisotropy of DPH (or the rotational relaxation time) indicates the mobility of the probe and thus reflects the ordering of the membrane core. Treatment of the membrane with progesterone at a concentration of $2-10$ μM brought about an increase in the ordering of the membrane. Testosterone ($2-10$ μM) had no detectable effect on membrane fluidity. Testosterone is, however, aromatized in the brain to 17β-oestradiol and the latter metabolite increases membrane fluidity. These data cast some doubt on the previous claims of Deliconstantinos (1988, 1990) concerning the effects of testosterone on synaptosomal plasma membranes (which may be capable of aromatizing the androgen).

The previously mentioned lipophilic nature of the benzodiazepines enables them to interact with the hydrophobic region of the membrane in a way that might influence their pharmacological activity. Studies conducted in our laboratory using the model system show that benzodiazepines:

1. increase the lipid fluidity of membranes in a way that reflects their therapeutic potency;
2. are less effective at fluidizing membranes that are initially more ordered, such as those in which the cholesterol/phospholipid ratio has been increased.

Benzodiazepines may thus produce differential effects according to the *in vivo* fluidity of the membrane. Indeed, changes in membrane fluidity may increase the accessibility of the receptor and hence its affinity for ligands. Our studies have shown that the antagonist flumazenil fluidizes the membrane more effectively than the agonists. This effect (due to similar molecular shapes?) could explain the behavioural similarities frequently recorded between flumazenil and agonists that cannot be explained by simple interaction between the GABA–receptor complex, e.g. influencing defensive–submissive behaviour in mice (Pankaj and Brain, 1991b), inducing escape deficit by an uncontrollable stress (Theibot, 1983), and inhibiting maternal aggression in the rat (Mos and Olivier, 1987, 1989).

Even small changes in membrane fluidity have considerable effects on neuronal function, e.g. transport of impulses and regulation of enzymatic activities. Changes in fluidity could explain the development of tolerance and even withdrawal symptoms seen in patients. There is suggestive evidence that such membrane-mediated effects are important in explaining particular effects of the benzodiazepines and may prove to be useful in understanding some of their less well-known therapeutic effects.

CONCLUSIONS

It is clear that the vast array of chemicals (including hormones and psychoactive drugs) that perinatally influence subsequent behavioural potential in mammals exert their actions in a variety of ways (see Figure 1). Some

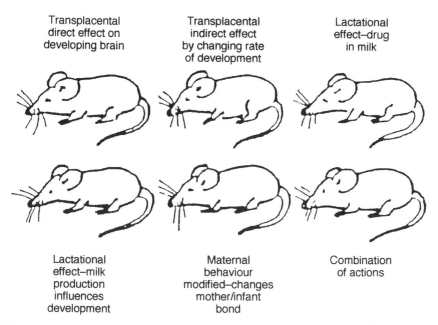

Transplacental
direct effect on
developing brain

Transplacental
indirect effect
by changing rate
of development

Lactational
effect–drug
in milk

Lactational
effect–milk
production
influences
development

Maternal
behaviour
modified–changes
mother/infant
bond

Combination
of actions

Figure 1 Some of the ways in which perinatal exposure to psychoactive drugs or hormones can influence later behaviour in rodents.

compounds influence the architecture and/or physiology of the developing brain after placental transfer, others simply interfere with development (perhaps causing animals to be deficient in certain crucial experiences) and yet others are actively transported in the mother's milk. Certain exposures will modify the efficiency of maternal lactation and/or interfere with maternal care—factors which can also influence development. Naturally, some compounds will combine several of these actions. The precise ways in which hormones and psychoactive drugs mediate direct effects on the developing brain also appear varied, including influencing receptor populations and modifying the fluidity of neuronal membranes.

REFERENCES

Abel, E.L. (1978) Effects of ethanol on pregnant rats and their offspring. *Psychopharmacology*, 57, 5–11.

Ajarem, J.S. and Ahmad, M. (1991) Behavioural and biochemical consequences of perinatal exposure of mice to instant coffee: a correlative evaluation. *Pharmacol. Biochem. Behav.*, 40, 847–852.

Ajarem, J.S. and Brain, P.F. (1993) Prenatal caffeine modifies behavioural responses in mice. *Behav. Pharmacol.*, 4, 541–544.

Anandan, N., Felegi, W. and Stern, J.M. (1980) In utero alcohol heightens juvenile reactivity. *Pharmacol. Biochem. Behav.*, 13, 531–535.

Aron, C., Chateau, D., Schaeffer, C. and Roos, J. (1991) Heterotypical sexual behaviour in male mammals: the rat as an experimental model. In: *Heterotypical Behaviour in Man and Animals* (eds M. Haug, P.F. Brain and C. Aron). Chapman & Hall, London, pp. 98–126.

Benton, D. (1989) Models of mother infant interactions: their use to screen for psychotropic activity. In: *Ethoexperimental Approaches to the Study of Behavior* (eds R.J. Blanchard, P.F. Brain, C. Blanchard and S. Parmigiani). Kluwer, Dordrecht, pp. 508–524.

Benton, D. and Brain, P.F. (1988) The role of opioid mechanisms in social interaction and attachment. In: *Endorphins, Opiates and Behavioural Processes* (eds R.J. Rodgers and S.J. Cooper). Wiley, Chichester, pp. 217–235.

Benton, D. and Nastiti, K. (1988) The influence of psychoactive drugs on the ultrasonic calling of mouse pups. *Psychopharmacology*, 95, 99–102.

Benton, D., Dalrymple-Alford, J.C., Brain, P.F. and Grimm, V. (1985) Prenatal administration of diazepam improves radial maze learning in mice. *Comp. Biochem. Physiol.*, 80C, 273–275.

Blanchard, R.J., Brain, P.F., Blanchard, C. and Parmigiani, S. (1989) *Ethoexperimental Approaches to the Study of Behavior*. Kluwer, Dordrecht.

Brain, P.F. (1978) *Hormones and Aggression, Vol. 2*. Eden Press, Montreal.

Brain, P.F. (1979) *Hormones and Aggression, Vol. 3*. Eden Press, Montreal.

Brain, P.F. (1992) Understanding the behaviours of feral species may facilitate design of optimal living conditions for common laboratory rodents. *Anim. Technol.*, 43, 99–105.

Brain, P.F. and Haug, M. (1991) Are behaviours specific to animals of particular sex? In: *Heterotypical Behaviour in Man and Animals* (eds M. Haug, P.F. Brain and C. Aron). Chapman & Hall, London, pp. 1–15.

Brain, P.F., Haug, M. and Alias bin Kamis (1983) Hormones and different tests for 'aggression' with particular reference to the effects of testosterone metabolites. In:

Hormones and Behaviour in Higher Vertebrates (eds. J. Balthazart, E. Prove and R. Gilles). Springer-Verlag, Berlin, pp. 290–304.

Brain, P.F., Ajarem, J.S. and Petkov, V.V. (1986) The application of ethopharmacological techniques to behavioural teratology: preliminary investigations. *Acta Physiol. Pharmac. Bull.*, **12**, 3–11.

Brain, P.F., Ajarem, J.S. and Petkov, V.V. (1987) The utility of ethological assessments of murine agonistic interactions in behavioural teratology: the foetal alcohol syndrome. In: *Ethopharmacology of Agonistic Behaviour in Animals and Humans* (eds B. Olivier, J. Mos and P.F. Brain). Martinus Nijhoff, Dordrecht, pp. 110–121.

Brain, P.F., McAllister, K.H. and Walmsley, S.V (1989) Drug effects on social behaviour: methods in ethopharmacology. In: *Neuromethods, Vol. 13: Psychopharmacology* (eds A.A. Boulton, G.B. Baker and A.J. Greenshaw). Humana Press, Clifton, NJ, pp. 689–739.

Brain, P.F., Nastiti Kusumorini and Benton, D. (1991) 'Anxiety' in laboratory rodents: a brief review of some recent behavioural developments. *Behav. Proc.*, **25**, 71–80.

Brain, P.F., Cerezo, A.L. and Haug, M. (1992) Ethopharmacological approaches for studying the properties of psychoactive drugs: a review. *Rev. Neurosci.*, **3**, 307–324.

Bressers, M., Meelis, E., Haccou, P. and Kruk, M. (1991) When did it really start or stop: the impact of censored observations on the analysis of duration. *Behav. Processes*, **23**, 1–20.

Chevins, P.F.D. (1990) Early environmental influences on fear and defence in rodents. In: *Fear and Defence* (eds P.F. Brain, S. Parmigiani, D. Mainardi and R.J. Blanchard). Harwood Academic Press, Chur, pp. 269–288.

Clemens, L.G., Gladue, B.A. and Coniglio, L.F. (1978) Prenatal endogenous androgenic influences on masculine sexual behavior and genital morphology in male and female rats. *Horm. Behav.*, **10**, 40–53.

Deliconstantinos, G. (1988) Structure activity relationship of cholesterol and steroid hormones with respect to their effects on the Ca^{2+}-stimulated ATPase and lipid fluidity of synaptosomal plasma membranes from dog and rabbit brain. *Comp. Biochem. Physiol.*, **89B**, 585–594.

Deliconstantinos, G. (1990) Effects of prostaglandin E_2 and progesterone on rat brain synaptosomal plasma membranes: steroids and neuronal activity. *Ciba Found. Symp.*, **153**, 190–205.

Dixson, A.F. (1980) Androgens and aggressive behavior in primates: a review. *Aggressive Behav.*, **6**, 37–67.

Eaton, G.G., Goy, R.W. and Phoenix, C.H. (1973) Effects of testosterone treatment in adulthood on sexual behaviour of female pseudo-hermaphrodite rhesus monkeys. *Nature (Lond.)*, **242**, 119–120.

Ewert, F.G. and Cutler, M.G. (1979) Effects of ethyl alcohol on development and social behaviour in the offspring of laboratory mice. *Psychopharmacology*, **62**, 247–251.

Ferrier, P.E., Nicol, I. and Ferrier, S. (1973) Foetal alcohol syndrome. *Lancet*, 21496.

Gai, N. and Grimm, V.E. (1982) The effect of prenatal exposure to diazepam on aspects of postnatal development and behaviour in rats. *Psychopharmacology*, **78**, 225–229.

Goy, R.W. (1968) Organizing effects of androgen on the behaviour of rhesus monkeys. In: *Endocrinology and Human Behaviour* (ed. R.P. Michael). Oxford University Press, Oxford, pp. 12–31.

Goy, R.W. and Roy, M. (1991) Heterotypic behaviour in female mammals. In: *Heterotypical Behaviour in Man and Animals* (eds M. Haug, P.F. Brain and C. Aron), Chapman & Hall, London, pp. 71–97.

Grant, E.C. and Mackintosh, J.H. (1963) A comparison of social postures of some common laboratory rodents. *Behaviour*, **21**, 246–259.

Grimm, V.E. (1984) A review of diazepam and other benzodiazepines in pregnancy. In: *Neurobehavioural Teratology* (ed. J. Yanai), Elsevier, Amsterdam, pp. 158–162.

Grimm, V.E., McAllister, K.H., Brain, P.F. and Benton, D. (1984) An ethological analysis of the influence of perinatally-administered diazepam on murine behaviour. *Comp. Biochem. Physiol.*, **79C**, 291–293.

Hendrie, C. and Rodgers, R.J. (1990) Microcomputer-based data logging and analysis in pharmacoethology. In *Microcomputers, Psychology and Medicine* (eds R. West, M. Christie and J. Weinman). Wiley, Chichester, pp. 187–201.

Jones, S.E. and Brain, P.F. (1985) An illustration of simple sequence analysis with reference to the agonistic behaviour of four strains of laboratory mouse. *Behav. Proc.*, **11**, 365–388.

Kurishingal, H., Palanza, P. and Brain, P.F. (1992) Effects of exposure of pregnant mice to chlordiazepoxide (CDP) on the development and ultrasound production of their offspring. *Gen. Pharmacol.*, **23**, 49–53.

Lee, C. (1990) *Behavioural and Neurohumoral Mechanisms of Environmental Analgesia in Mus musculus*. PhD dissertation, University of Bradford.

Leshner, A.I. (1981) The role of hormones in the control of submissiveness. In: *Multidisciplinary Approaches to Aggression Research* (eds P.F. Brain and D. Benton). Elsevier, Amsterdam, pp. 309–322.

McAllister, C.B. (1980) Placental transfer and neonatal effects of diazepam when adminstered to women just before delivery. *Br. J. Anaethesiol.*, **52**, 423–427.

Meelis, E., Haccou, P. and Bressers, M. (1990) Detection of time inhomogeneity in behavioural processes: tests for multiple abrupt changes in bout lengths. *Behav. Proc.*, **22**, 121–132.

Meyer-Bahlburg, H.F.L. (1980) Androgens and human aggression. In: *The Biology of Aggression* (eds P.F. Brain and D. Benton). Sijthoff & Noordhoff, Alphen aan den Rijn, pp. 263–290.

Meyer-Bahlburg, H.F.L. and Ehrhardt, A.A. (1982) Prenatal sex hormone and human aggression: a review and new data on progestogen effects. *Aggressive Behav.*, **8**, 39–62.

Mos, J. and Olivier, B. (1987) Pro-aggressive actions of benzodiazepines. In: *Ethopharmacology of Agonistic Behaviour in Animals and Humans* (eds B. Olivier, J. Mos and P.F. Brain). Martinus Nijhoff, Dordrecht, pp. 187–206.

Mos, J. and Oliver, B. (1989) Qualitative and comparative analyses of pro-aggressive actions of benzodiazepines in maternal aggression in rats. *Psychopharmacology*, **97**, 152–153.

Mugford, R.A. (1974) Androgenic stimulation of aggression eliciting cues in adult opponent mice castrated at birth, weaning or maturity. *Horm. Behav.*, **5**, 93–102.

Nastiti, K., Benton, D., Brain, P.F. and Haug, M. (1991) The effects of 5-HT receptor ligands on ultrasonic calling in mouse pups. *Neurosci. Biobehav. Rev.* **15**, 483–487.

Olivier, B. and Mos, J. (1986) A female aggression paradigm for use in psychopharmacology: material agonistic behaviour in rats. In *Cross-disciplinary Studies on Aggression* (eds P.F. Brain and J.M. Ramirez). University of Seville Press, Seville, pp. 73–111.

Olweus, D. (1984) Development of stable aggressive reaction patterns in males. In: *Advances in the Study of Aggression*, Vol. 1 (eds R.J. Blanchard and D.C. Blanchard). Academic Press, Orlando, FL, pp. 103–137.

Pankaj, V. and Brain, P.F. (1991a) Effects of prenatal exposure to benzodiazepine-related drugs on early development and adult social behaviour in Swiss mice: I. Agonists. *Gen. Pharmacol.*, **22**, 33–41.

Pankaj, V. and Brain, P.F. (1991b) Effects of prenatal exposure to benzodiazepine-related drugs on early development and adult social behaviour in Swiss mice: II. Antagonists. *Gen. Pharmacol.*, **22**, 43–51.

Pankaj, V. and Brain, P.F. (1991c) Effects of prenatal exposure to benzodiazepine-related drugs on early development and adult social behaviour in Swiss mice: III. Inverse agonists. *Gen. Pharmacol.*, **22**, 53–60.

Resko, J.A. (1974) The relationship between fetal hormones and the differentiation of the central nervous system in primates. In: *Reproductive Behavior* (eds W. Montagna and W.A. Sadler). Plenum, New York, pp. 211–222.

Shinitzky, M. and Barenholz, Y. (1978) Fluidity parameters of lipid regions determined by fluorescence polarization. *Biochem. Biophys. Acta*, **515**, 367–394.

Solomon, E.D., Schmidt, R.R. and Adragna, P.J. (1990) *Human Anatomy and Physiology*. Saunders College Publishing, Philadelphia.

Swaab, D.F. and Mirmiran, M. (1984) Possible mechanism underlying the teratogenic effects of medicines on the developing brain. In: *Neurobehavioural Teratology* (ed. J. Yanai). Elsevier, Amsterdam, pp. 55–71.

Theibot, M.H. (1983) Behavioural models of anxiety in animals. *Encephale*, **9**, 167B–176B.

Van de Poll, N.E. and Van Dis, H. (1977) Hormone induced lordosis and its relation to masculine sexual activity in male rats. *Horm. Behav.*, **8**, 1–7.

Van de Poll, N.E., de Brulin, J.P.C., Van Dis, H. and Van Oyen, H.G. (1978) Gonadal hormones and the differentiation of sexual and aggressive behaviour and learning in the rat. In: *Progress in Brain Research*, Vol. 48. (eds M. Corner *et al.*) Elsevier, Amsterdam, pp. 309–327.

Van de Poll, N.E., de Jonge, F., van Oyen, H.G. *et al.* (1981) Failure to find sex differences in testosterone activated aggression in two strains of rats. *Horm. Behav.*, **15**, 94–105.

Volk, B. (1984) Neurohistological and neurobiological aspects of fetal alcohol syndrome in the rat. In: *Neurobehavioural Teratology* (ed. J. Yanai). Elsevier, Amsterdam, pp. 163–193.

Vom Saal, F.S. (1983) Models of early hormonal effects on intrasex aggression in mice. In: *Hormones and Aggressive Behavior* (ed. B.B. Svare) Plenum Press, New York, pp. 197–222.

Vom Saal, F.S. (1991) Prenatal gonadal influences on mouse sociosexual behaviours. In: *Heterotypical Behaviour in Man and Animals* (eds M. Haug, P.F. Brain and C. Aron). Chapman & Hall, London, pp. 42–70.

Vom Saal, F.S. and Bronson, F.H. (1978) In utero proximity of female mouse fetuses to males: effect on reproductive performance in later life. *Biol. Reprod.*, **19**, 842–853.

Vom Saal, F.S. and Bronson, F.H. (1980) Sexual characteristics of adult female mice are correlated with their blood testosterone levels during prenatal development. *Science (New York)*, **208**, 597–599.

Vom Saal, F.S., Svare, B.B. and Gandelman, R. (1976) Time of neonatal androgen exposure influences length of testosterone treatment required to induce aggression in adult male and female mice. *Behav. Biol.*, **17**, 391–397.

Yanai, J. (1984) *Neurobehavioural Teratology*. Elsevier, Amsterdam.

Yanai, J. and Ginsburg, B.E. (1977) A developmental study of ethanol's effect on behavioural and physical development in mice. *Alcoholism*, **1**, 325–333.

Yousif, Y.Y., Brain, P.F., Parmigiani, S. and Mainardi, M. (1989) Effects of genotype and intrauterine location on the propensity for infanticide by primiparous female mice. *Ethol. Ecol. Evol.*, **1**, 283–290.

13 Amphetamine-induced Stereotypy in Rats: Its Morphogenesis in Locale Space from Normal Exploration

DAVID EILAM AND ILAN GOLANI
Department of Zoology, Tel-Aviv University, Ramat-Aviv, Israel

INTRODUCTION

Although stereotyped behaviour, both in captivity (Cronin and Wiepkema, 1984; Cronin, 1985; Hediger, 1964; Stevenson, 1983), and with psychoactive drugs (Cooper and Dourish, 1990; Lyon and Robbins, 1975; Schiorring, 1971), clearly evolves in time out of normal behaviour, few attempts have been made to characterize the morphology of the transition from one to the other. Drug-induced stereotypy, for example, is commonly divided into locomotor stereotypies, characterized by repetitive pacing on the same routes (Eilam *et al.*, 1989; Geyer, 1982; Muller *et al.*, 1989; Randrup and Munkvad, 1970; Schiorring, 1979; Szechtman *et al.*, 1993), and in-place stereotypies characterized by the absence of locomotion and by repetitive head movements and intense sniffing, licking or biting of a highly restricted area (Arnt *et al.*, 1987, 1988; Brodi and Meller, 1989; Costall and Naylor, 1975; Fray *et al.*, 1980; Kelly, 1977). There are several studies which characterize the morphogenesis of in-place stereotypy from normal behaviour via locomotor stereotypy (Adani *et al.*, 1991; Eilam, 1987; Eilam *et al.*, 1991; Golani, 1992; Szechtman *et al.*, 1985). In these studies, the transition has been described in terms of the relations and changes of relation between the parts of the body (motor behaviour). In the present study, we describe the morphology of the transition in relation to places in the environment, i.e. in relation to *locale space*.

Studies of locomotor stereotypies in locale space typically represent the paths traced by the rat by drawing them on paper within a rectangle representing the testing environment, thereby conveying the confinement of the rat to a restricted part of the rectangle (Eilam *et al.*, 1989, 1991; Flicker and Geyer, 1982; Geyer *et al.*, 1986a, 1986b). Various methods discriminate between locomotor stereotypies under different drugs (Eilam *et al.*, 1991, 1992; Geyer,

Ethology and Psychopharmacology. Edited by S.J. Cooper and C.A. Hendrie
© 1994 John Wiley & Sons Ltd

1982), assess qualitative aspects of locomotor stereotypy (Muller et al., 1989), establish when a repetition of a route is indeed a replication of the previous one (Paulus and Geyer, 1991) and describe the regular appearance of parameters of stereotypy (Szechtman et al., 1993). These methods provide measures for quantifying locomotor stereotypy. They do not address, however, the question of how locomotor stereotypy arises from normal behaviour, and more specifically, what is the natural source of repetitive locomotion along the same paths.

In the present chapter we describe how incessant repetition of the same path is gradually derived from normal exploratory locomotion in rats. The database for this study was obtained from studies of 31 tamed wild rats (Rattus norvegicus) exploring an open field (1.6 × 1.6 m glass platform without walls) for a 1 h period. Each of the animals was videotaped with and without (+)-amphetamine (s.c. in the nape at concentrations of 0.5, 1, 2.5 and 5 mg/kg; $n = 8$ in three groups, $n = 7$ in one group). The animals, the observation platform, the experimental procedure and the methods of data acquisition are described in Eilam and Golani (1989, 1990).

When placed in a novel environment, a normal rat alternates between progressing and stopping; it locomotes forward, stops, performs lateral and/or vertical scanning movements while staying in place, locomotes again, stops in a new place, etc. Its behaviour thus consists of intervals of 'stops' or 'visits' to places, the movements performed during these intervals, and the paths of locomotion between the places of stopping. Our testing environment was divided into 25 squares (Figure 2), and whenever a rat stopped, the location, timing and duration of stopping was recorded (for a detailed exposition of criteria and method see Golani et al., 1993). Since rats tend to locomote in a relatively straight path between two stopping places, the sequence of stopping places provides a reasonable approximation of the rat's path.

When a rat explores a novel environment there are one or two places where it stays for a significantly longer cumulative time than in all the other places, and where it typically stops for the highest number of times. In this place, the values of these measures are of a higher order of magnitude compared to the respective values scored in all the other places. In it, the rat also shows a high and often the highest incidence of grooming—significantly higher in proportion compared to that expected by the proportion of time spent there. Finally, this place is also marked by the highest incidence of rearing, and by crouching and pivoting around the forelegs—two behaviours which are exclusive for this place. This place, which can be readily identified by any observer using the above criteria, has been termed a home base (Eilam and Golani, 1989).

From the home base the rat performs excursions into the environment. Excursions consist of round trips which start and end at the same home base, and, in the case of rats which establish two home bases, also trips which start at one base and end in the other. It has been shown that: (i) the way out from base is relatively slow and interrupted with stops in several places, whereas the way back to base is relatively rapid, including fewer stops (Eilam and Golani,

1989); (ii) there is an intrinsic upper bound on the number of times a rat stops during an excursion (Golani *et al.*, 1993); and (iii) the session's upper bound on the number of stops per excursion does not increase with the size of the explored area (Golani *et al.*, 1993).

What happens to this organization with psychoactive drugs? With (+)-amphetamine, for example, home-base behaviour is preserved (Eilam and Golani, 1990). This leads to the question of what happens to excursions when locomotor stereotypies develop after treatment with the drug. In this chapter we describe how amphetamine-induced stereotyped locomotion is derived from normal exploration through processes of reduction in the number of stops per excursion and sequencing of stopping places into a few relatively rigid routes, each constituting an excursion from (and back to) base.

Figure 1 represents the paths traced by a rat in the course of the first hour after treatment with 5 mg/kg amphetamine. In this rat's session the home base

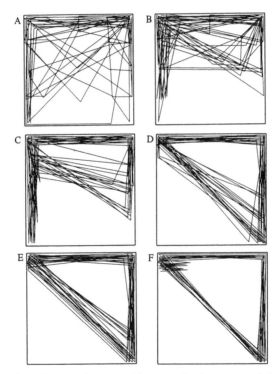

Figure 1 The paths of locomotion traced by a rat in the course of the first hour after injection of 5 mg/kg amphetamine. Blocks A–F represent the first 20 excursions performed during each of successive non-overlapping 10 min intervals. As shown, the paths became gradually more stereotyped, culminating in a repetition of one and the same path in E. Towards the end of the hour locomotion became confined to the left far corner (block F).

was located in the upper right corner. To avoid cluttering, only the first 20 excursions of six successive intervals of 10 min each are represented. The same paths, together with all the other paths performed by that rat in that session, are represented in Figure 2 in terms of symbols designating the rat's stopping places. These are written from left to right and from top to bottom in the order of their occurrence. Each line describes an excursion performed from 1, the rat's home base. In this type of representation, one can readily discern three processes: (i) the maximal number of stops per excursion is reduced in the transition from block A to block E from nine to two (excluding the home base itself); (ii) the order of stopping places becomes increasingly fixed; and (iii) the number of different routes is reduced (while each two successive excursion paths in block A are different, all excursions paths in block E follow a single route).

In the following we will show how the three processes illustrated in Figure 2 together with two additional processes—a dramatic increase in the incidence of excursions, and a change in the number of home bases—account for the establishment of amphetamine-induced stereotypy.

The case represented in Figure 2 is an example of the behaviour of all the rats treated with amphetamine: the sequence of stops is partitioned into excursions (defined below), each of which starts with a stop at the home base. As the behaviour becomes more stereotyped, the distinction between a stop at a home base and a stop elsewhere becomes increasingly difficult or even impossible to draw on the basis of the criteria established by us (Eilam and Golani, 1989, 1990). Nevertheless, as we will show, even the most stereotyped excursion following amphetamine includes a visit to what had been, at the beginning of the session, a home base location.

Figure 2 A symbolic representation of the paths of locomotion performed in the same session already presented in Figure 1. A numeral designates each of the 25 places on the platform. A map of the places on the platform is provided in block G; places in the central area are designated by large bold characters. The numerals in blocks A–F represent the places in which the rat stopped in the order of their occurrence, from left to right and from top to bottom, within each block. The blocks represent successive periods of behaviour. All stopping places in the session are presented. Each row in blocks A–F represents one excursion, starting at the home base, which is located in this rat session in the right far corner of the platform, and is designated by 1. Blocks A and B represent the first few minutes after injection, when the only apparent regularity was the frequent return to the home base, 1, and the limited number of stops per excursion. In the first excursion the rat leaves the home base, 1, and locomotes along the far edge of the platform, stopping at $0'$, then at 0, then leaves the edge, stops at **0**, proceeds to the near left corner of the platform, 5, stops there, then proceeds to $5'$, and returns to the home base, 1, from where it starts a new excursion to $0'$, 2, $2'$ . . . etc. Note that as the number of stops per excursion decreases from A to E, the variety of stopping locations decreases, stopping in the central area of the platform is eliminated, and the sequence of stopping places becomes fully predictable. Finally, the rat stays in the far left corner, engaging in side-to-side head movements.

A	B	C	D	E	F
10'0055'	11'77'	1756'C5'7	12'6'7	1 37	1 377'
10'22'366'7	11'767	15'	1 3 7	12' 7	1 37
11'22'330'	112C77'	125	1 6'7	12' 7	1 37'
10'654'43'	11'26'	15'	1 36'7	12' 7	1 377'
10'076'	100767	126'70	1 3 7	12' 7	1 37
11'0	11'276'67	16'	1 7	1 37	1 377'
11'21	127	15'	12' 7	12' 7	1 377'
1077'	11'2765'7'	126'65'57	12' 7	1 37	12'3 77'
10'07'765	17	1267	12' 7	1 37	11' 377'
10'07'76'65'65'1'	11'2767	126'5'	1 3 7	1 37	11' 377'
10'76'5'55'0	11'765'7	11'5'	1 3	1 37	11'3 77'
177'	11'227657'	11'67	12' 7	1 37	11' 377'
10'66'5'5	1167	12'6'	1 3 7	1 37	77'
1766577	1265'	122'7	1 3	1 37	77'
1226'70	176'	11'6'57'	1 7	1 37	
11'1C7	16'5'7	16'77'	1 3 7	1 37	
146'77'	176'5'7	12'765'5	1 7	1 37	
122'6'7	126'7	16'5'7'	1 36'7	1 37	
11'165'56'7	1265'	16'57		1 37	
12'76'7	11'5	167		1 37	
11'16'	15'	137		1 37	
10'07	11'25'	126'57		1 37	
11'77'06677'0	11'5'			1 37	
10	125'51			1 37	
11'276'70C57	1C5'7			1 37	
12	126'7			1 37	
11'1C77'				1 37	
16'6570C6'5'				1 37	

G

1		
7	0	0'
7	0	1'
6	C	1'
6	C	2
5'	4	2'
5	4	3
4'	4	3'
		3

EXCURSION, PATH AND ROUTE

A home base is defined in the present study in terms of the statistical properties of the behaviours performed in it. An *excursion* is defined as a trip taking place between two successive stops at a home base. A particular excursion is characterized by the path taken by the rat, and by the places along this path where the rat stopped. A *path* is thus defined as the line traced by a rat during its progression in the environment in the course of a single specific excursion from home base and back to it. A *route* is defined as a *class* of paths taking more or less the same course in the environment.

Following treatment with amphetamine, the behaviour of an individual rat varies in terms of the number of stops per excursion, the degree of maximal observed stereotypy of routes, the number of different routes and the number of bases visited by the rat. After illustrating amphetamine's effects on each of these aspects of stereotyped behaviour separately, we will examine some of these effects in relation to dose and the time-course of drug action.

ASPECTS OF STEREOTYPY IN LOCALE SPACE AFFECTED BY AMPHETAMINE

Rats perform fewer stops per excursion after amphetamine

As shown in more detail elsewhere (Golani and Eilam, 1994), with amphetamine (0.5–5 mg/kg), there was a large increase in the overall number of stops (Figure 3A), and in the number of excursions made in the course of the hour (Figure 3B). The ratio between these two means yields the mean number of stops per excursion (Figure 3C). The mean of normal rats, i.e. 6.5 stops, was reduced to a mean of three to four stops per excursion. This degree of reduction did not vary across dose. The reduction in the mean number of stops per excursion was mainly due to an increase in the percentage of excursions with few stops, so that with the drug 90% of the excursions included up to six stops. We have shown that the reduction in the mean number of stops per excursion was not a mere by-product of amphetamine's effects on several other parameters of the excursion. Thus, while amphetamine's effects on excursion length and interstop distance was variable in individual animals, it reduced the mean number of stops per excursion in almost all rats (Golani and Eilam, 1994). We could not establish a causal relationship between the increased speed observed in amphetamine-treated rats and the decrease in the number of stops (Golani and Eilam, 1994).

The degree of stereotypy of routes and of stopping locations after amphetamine

With amphetamine treatment, routes may be classified into three types.

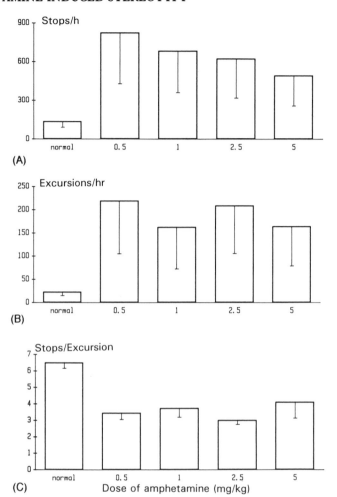

Figure 3 Means (− s.e.m.) of the overall number of stops (A), the number of excursions (B), and the number of stops per excursion (C), during an hour of exploration in normal and amphetamine-treated rats. While the difference between normal and drugged behaviour is apparent, there is no such difference among the drug groups.

A rigid route (no variability across paths and across sequences of stopping locations in different excursions)

During successive excursions the rat follows the same route in the same direction, stopping in the same places (Figure 2, block E). Figure 4 presents an example of the whole morphogenetic process, which consists of a gradual transition to a fully predictable route and a subsequent reduction in predictability.

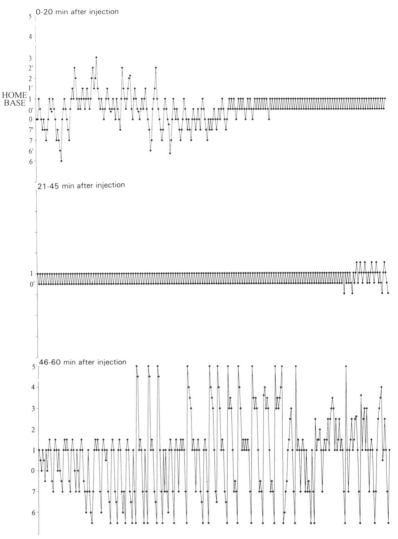

Figure 4 The morphogenesis of a rigid route in relation to a single home base is represented as a temporal series of stopping places. The y-axis represents the places on the platform (1 designates the home base; the places located in a clockwise direction in relation to it are arranged on the y-axis, on top of it, in their proper spatial order. The places located in a counterclockwise direction are similarly arranged below and away from the home base). The x-axis represents successive stops; data points designate places of stopping. The graph represents all the 912 successive stopping places (partitioned into three successive sections of 304 stops each), performed by a rat after 2.5 mg/kg amphetamine. As shown, after some 150 stops, the route became constrained to a performance of the sequence 1,0' (see Figure 2G) which was repeated about 200 times. Then, both clockwise and counterclockwise excursions reappeared, growing in length to encompass the whole perimeter of the platform, with a relatively small number of stops per excursion.

A fixed route (no variability across paths, variable stopping places across excursions)

This is the same as above, but the rat stops irregularly in different places along the fixed route. Such a route is illustrated in Figure 5, where the rat locomoted for 57 (out of 60) min along one and the same edge of the platform, stopping irregularly at different places along this edge.

A flexible route (variability across paths and stopping places)

Such a route is illustrated in Figure 6 which represents a sequence of successive excursions of a rat treated with 2.5 mg/kg. In all excursions the rat departed from the home base, which was located in the right-hand corner, 1, to the centre of the platform, stopped anywhere in the central area, then progressed to the left hand corner, 7 or nearby, and returned along the far (top) edge to the right-hand corner, performing one or two stops somewhere along the edge.

Rats have one to four routes after amphetamine

A decrease in the number of stops per excursion does not imply a stereotyped route. Given the 25 predefined places on the platform, the rats could execute a

```
   A              B              C              D
 7  6   5'        6  5'       7  6   5'          6'
 7  6      5    7  6            6'          6   5'  5
      6' 5'  5   7            7  6'                5'
 7  6   5'          6            6 6'        6 6' 5'  5
      6         7  6   5'     7  6   5'            5'  5
 7  6   5'      7  6         7  6 6'               5'
 7  6   5'  5   7  6   5'        6                 6'
      6'        7  6         7  6            6   5'  5  4'
 7  6   5'  5   7  6   5'     7  6   5'            5'
 7   6'         7  6   5'  5     6'                6'
      6  5'            5'     7  6   5'            5'  5
 7  6   5'  5   7  6   5'  5     6'                6'
 7  6   5'  5         5'         6  5'  5     7       5'
 7  6   5'  5   7  6   5'  5     6'                6'
         5'          6  5'  5 7  6   5'        6   5'  5
 7  6   5'      7  6   5'  5     6' 5'        7  6 6'
 7  6   5'  5   7  6   5'  5     6'           7  6 6'
 7   6'         7  6 6'          6  5'  5     7  6   5'  5
```

Figure 5 A fixed route is illustrated by a sequence of 72 successive excursions performed by a rat, 20 min after injection of 2.5 mg/kg amphetamine. Sequence should be read from left to right and from top to bottom, in each of the columns A–D. This rat had two home bases, in 7 and in 5' (see Figure 2G). Locomotion was confined to one edge of the platform, where stopping places varied from one excursion to the next.

EXIT	CENTRE	RETURN
1	**1**	0'
1		7' 7
1 0'		7 0 0'
1 0'		7 7' 0
1 1'		
1		7 0 0'
1 1'	**1 0**	
1 0'	**0** 0'	7 7' 0'
1 0'	**1 2 1**	7' 7 0 0'
1 1'		
1 1'	**1 0 C**	7 0'
1 0'	**1** 0' **0**	7 0'
1 0'		
1	**4 C 7**	7 0'
1	0 **0 7**	7 0'
1	**2 1 C**	0'
1	1' **0**	7 7' 0'
1	**0 2**	0
1 0'	**1**	7 7' 0'
1 0'	0	7'
1		7' 7 7' 0'
1	**1 3**	
1	**1 2**	
1 0'	**C 7**	0
1	2	
1	**2 3**	7 7' 0'
1	**1 0** 7' 6'	7 7' 0
1 0'	**1 C** 4'	7 7' 0'
1 0'	**1** 7 0	7 7' 0'
1 1'	2 1' **1 0**	7 7'
1 0'	**C 7**	7' 0'
1 1'		
1	**C**	7' 0'
1	**1 7** 7' 0	7 7' 0 0'
1	2	
1	**1 2 C** 5' **7**	7' 0'
1	**1 C 6**	7' 0'
1	**2 4 7**	7' 0 0'
1		7' 7 7' 0'
1 0'	4 4' **4**	0 0'
1	2' 1' **1 0**	
1 0'	**0**	7' 7 7' 0'

Figure 6 A flexible route is illustrated by a sequence of 42 successive excursions performed by a rat 20 min after injection of 2.5 mg/kg amphetamine. In these excursions the exit and the return portions of the route were fixed, whereas the centre part was variable in path, in the repertoire of stopping places of each path, and in the sequencing of stopping places.

wide variety of sequences of stopping places even within a range of three to four stops per excursion. Nevertheless, in the particular environment used by us, each of the drugged rats performed between one and four routes.

A single route

Rats with a single route had a rigid (Figures 2 and 4), a fixed (Figure 5) or a flexible route (Figure 6).

Two routes

Rats with more than one route had only fixed or flexible routes. The behaviour of a rat with two (fixed) routes is presented in Figure 7. The rat performed two fixed routes from its home base in 1 (at the far right corner): one along the far edge, and another along the right edge. Each of the routes consisted of a fixed path and a flexible sequence of stops. The order of performance of these routes appears to be unpredictable: once the rat was at base, it was impossible to predict which of the two routes it would follow next.

Three or four routes

When a rat had three or four routes, the routes were always flexible. As with the performance of two routes, so here the order of routes could not be predicted (Figure 8, block III). Note that if the routes are presented in the order of their performance (Figure 8, block I), it is difficult to discern a regularity in the identity of places of stopping and in their sequencing. Such regularity is highlighted once the paths are sorted into routes (Figure 8, block II).

No discernible routes

The paths of locomotion of an individual intact rat are illustrated in Figure 9. There is not enough similarity between the excursions to allow classification into routes. Each stopping place is an elementary building block of behaviour in locale space, and the combinations between these building blocks are unpredictable.

Rats may have one or two bases with amphetamine

Locomotion with reference to one base across the session

All the excursions of the rats described so far were organized in reference to a single home base. In the course of the first exposure to a novel environment, both normal (Eilam and Golani, 1989) and amphetamine-treated rats (Eilam and Golani, 1990) may, however, have more than a single base, but rarely more than two bases.

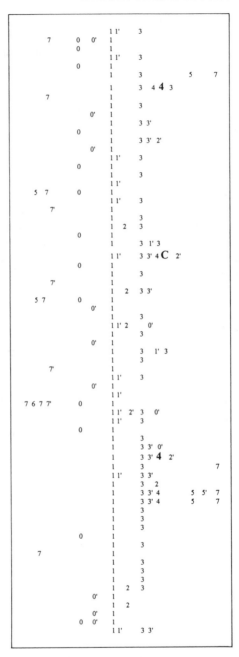

Figure 7 Two fixed routes are illustrated by 69 successive excursions performed by a rat 20 min after injection of 5 mg/kg amphetamine. The numeral representing the home base, 1, is aligned in the central column, and the stopping places along the two routes are shown in proper order on both of its sides. The route which was performed on the

Locomotion in reference to two bases across the session

When there are two home bases, they are visited in two different temporal modes. (i) Each of the two bases was used as a single base for a specific interval of time. In this way, each excursion included a stop at only one of the bases, but the cumulative record of excursions across the session included excursions organized around either of the two bases. (ii) Both bases were visited during the same excursion, so that excursions, including stops at both bases, were performed repeatedly for extended periods.

When two bases were visited at separate times (first mode), a rat typically performed a series of relatively short excursions in reference to one corner, and then switched to another corner and performed short excursions in reference to it. The rat thus had two bases (in two corners), but at a given time interval it was moving in reference to only one of them (Figure 10).

In two bases per excursion (second mode), a relatively long path connected the two bases (which were often located at two far ends of the platform). In Figure 11, the rat locomoted around the platform's perimeter in a counter-clockwise direction with a certain flexibility in the sequence of stopping places, yet it rarely skipped a stop in 5 and in 7, which were used as its home bases.

TIME-COURSE OF DRUG ACTION

Number of stops per excursion and excursion rate

Figure 12 presents the frequency distribution of excursion types (in terms of the number of stops included in them), in the course of an hour. Graphs are presented for each of four rats, first without (left), and then with (right) amphetamine. Excursions are classified on the x-axis, in terms of the number of stops included in them; frequency per 5 min bins is plotted on the vertical, z-axis. Time, in 5 min bins, is presented on the y-axis, from top to bottom across the hour.

With amphetamine, the early portion of the hour was similar to that observed in normal rats during peak activity. Then, excursions with a large number of stops were eliminated, and excursions with a small number of stops were performed at exceedingly high rates throughout the hour (note change of frequency scale in three of the right-hand graphs). The reduction in the number of stops per excursion with amphetamine was accompanied by an increase in the rate of excursions.

---

table's edge clockwise is shown on the right of the home base numeral, and the counterclockwise one, on its left; the rat visited the places shown in the figure, from top to bottom, in the following order: 1,1',3,1,0',0,7,1,0,1,1',3 ... etc. As shown, the rat switched, in what appears to be an irregular order, between the two fixed routes, but each route had a 'fixed' structure.

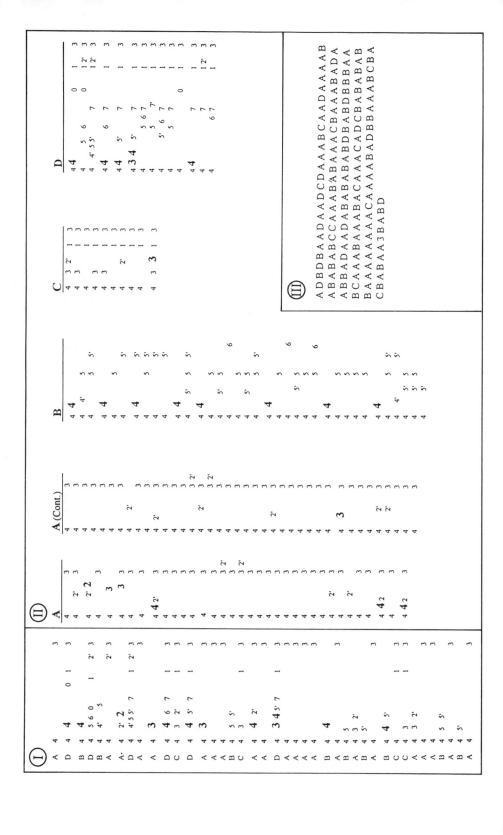

```
7  6'
7  7'  2  4   4  4'  5
7  6'
7  6   5  4   3  2'  2  1  7'
7  7'  0' 1   2  3   5  C
7  7'  6' 5   4' 4   3' 3  0
7  6   5  C   2  1
7  5   4  3
7  7'  0' 1
7  7'  0  C   4  4  3'
7  C   4  2'  1  0'
7  6   5'
7  7'  5  5'  6
7  1   2' 3   3' 4  7'
7
```

Figure 9 The temporal sequence of stopping places, partitioned into excursions, performed by an intact rat in the course of 1 h after being introduced to the platform. The rat was placed in the centre of the platform, and performed three stops (not shown) before arriving at the home base, 7, for the first time. It then performed 14 excursions and settled for the rest of the hour in the home base.

Mean number of stops across the session

We have already shown that when examined cumulatively for the whole hour, there was no effect of dose on the number of stops per excursion (Figure 3). Figure 13(A) presents the means (+ s.e.m.) of the number of stops per excursion in 20 min bins, across the hour. As shown, all four doses reduced these measurements, without a dose-dependent effect.

Figure 8 A repertoire of four routes is illustrated in the sequence of excursions performed by a rat after injection of 0.5 mg/kg amphetamine. In each block, numerals represent the order of stopping, from left to right and from top to bottom (the mapping of the platform is presented in Figure 2G). Block I represents the first 41 excursions in the session, in the original order of their performance; the column on the left classifies the excursions into routes. Block II presents sorted lists of each of the four routes. The routes are presented within each list in the order of their performance, so that stereotypy versus variability in stopping locations can be examined visually across the session. The home base 4 is located in the middle of the near edge of the platform; A and B are, respectively, routes to the nearest left and nearest right corner (and back to base): C is a route to the far right corner (and back); and D is a clockwise route around the platform's perimeter. Block III represents the sequence of routes performed by the rat throughout the session.

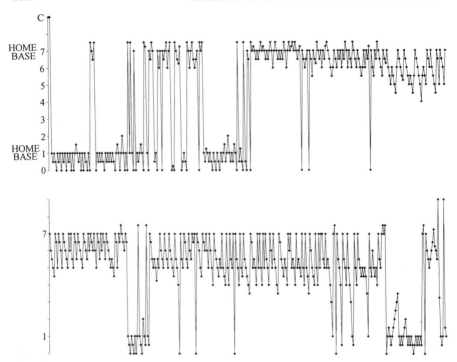

Figure 10 Locomotion with reference to two bases, separated in time. The *y*-axis represents the places on the platform's perimeter (for a map see Figure 2G). The *x*-axis represents the temporal order of stops. Each data point thus represents a stopping place. In this rat session, the home bases were located in 1 and in 7. This rat, treated with 5 mg/kg amphetamine, performed 756 stops during the hour. It started to perform excursions in reference to base 1 (beginning of top section), then, after several occasional visits to 7 and its vicinity, switched to perform excursions in reference to 7, now visiting the first home base, 1, occasionally (second half of the upper section, and most of the lower section).

Number of routes

Figure 13(C) presents the mean number of routes followed by a rat, in 20 min bins, across the session. The bin size is too large to show the initial reduction in the number of different routes, illustrated in Figure 2. This process of restriction in the number of routes was observed only in the rats which were active from the start of the session and was often completed within the first few minutes after injection. Rats that were inactive in the first few minutes started with few routes with the onset of locomotion. Figure 13(C) does show, however, that there is a distinction between low (0.5–1 mg/kg) and high (2.5–5 mg/kg) doses in the mean number of routes.

5	5'	6	6'	7	7'	0	0'	1	1'	3	3'	2'
				7		0	0'	1				
				7								
5		6		7		0		1		3		
			6'	7				1				
				7	7'			1				2'
		6		7	7'			1		3		
	5'											
5	5'		6'		7'			1		3		
			6'	7				1		3		
5		6										
5	5'		6'	7				1	1'		3'	
5			6'									
		6										
5	5'		6'	7				1		3	3'	
5	5'	6'										
5		6	6'	7				1		3		
5		6	6'	7				1		3		
5	5'											
5		6	6'									
5		6										
5			6'									
5			6'									
5	5'		6'									
5	5'											
5			6'									
5			6'	7				1		3		
5			6'									
5			6'	7				1	1'	3		
5			6'									
5			6'	7				1				
5			6'	7				1		3		
5			6'	7				1				
5			6'	7				1		3		
5			6'	7				1		3		
5			6'	7				1		3		
5		6		7				1				
5				7				1				
5		6	6'	7				1				
5				7				1				
5		6		7				1				
5	5'	6	6'	7				1				
5		6										
5		6		7				1				
5		6	6'	7						1		
5	5'											
5		6										
5				7				1				
5	5'											
5			6'	7				1				
	5'	6										
5			6'	7				1				
	5'	6	6'	7				1				
	5'	6		7				1				
	5'	6		7				1		3		

Figure 11 A single route traverses two home bases during successive excursions of a rat, 20 min after injection of 5 mg/kg amphetamine. Except for two short periods during which the rat moved in reference to only one of the bases, it traversed both bases in the same excursion, for most of the time.

258

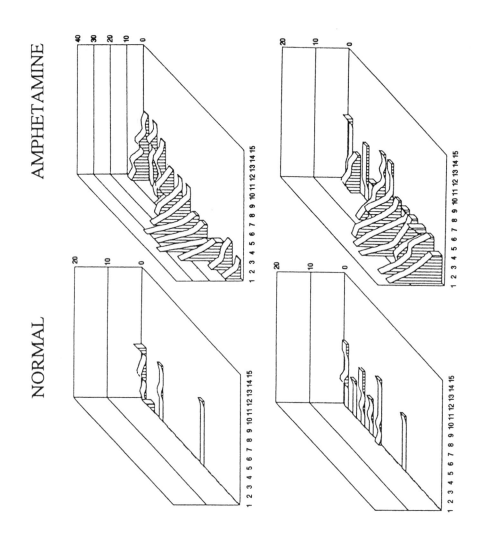

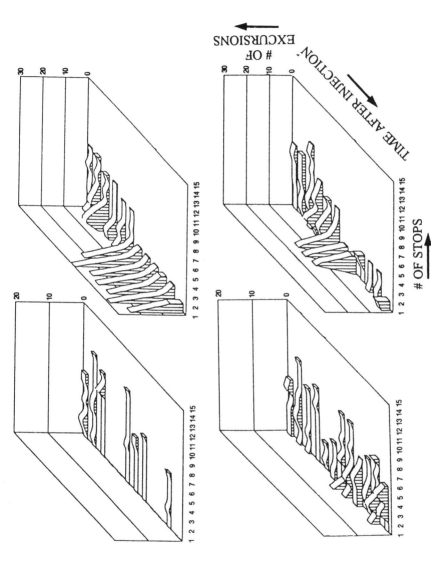

Figure 12 The effect of amphetamine on the frequency distribution of excursions with different numbers of stops, across the session; four individual examples (0.5 mg/kg, top row; 1 mg/kg, second row; 2.5 mg/kg, third row; 5 mg/kg, bottom row). Data are presented in 5 min bins. Each row represents the same rat as normal (left) and with amphetamine (right). x-axis: number of stops per excursion; y-axis: time z-axis: frequency of excursions.

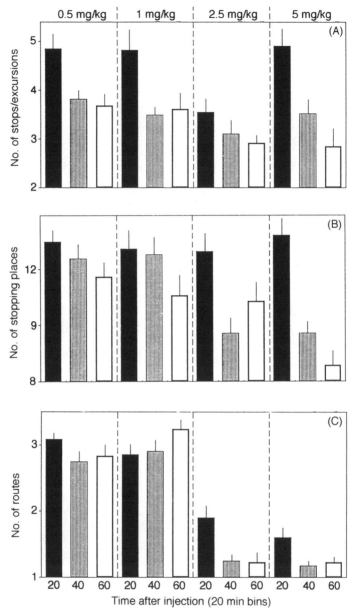

Figure 13 Changes in the mean (+ s.e.m.) number of stops per excursion (A), the mean (+ s.e.m.) number of different stopping places (B), and the mean (+ s.e.m.) number of different routes (C), in three successive 20 min time bins, over the course of drug action. For each measure, the four dose groups are represented, separated by vertical dashed lines. To facilitate comparison both across the session and across parallel time intervals with different doses, measures for the first 20 min after injection are depicted by solid bars, for the next interval of 21–40 min are depicted by hatched bars,

Table 1 Dose of amphetamine, number of bases, and the degree of stereotypy of routes. Numerals in the dose columns indicate the number of rats which exhibited the specified type of route

Type of route	Number of bases	Dose of amphetamine (mg/kg)			
		0.5	1	2.5	5
Flexible route	1	8	6	1	–
	2	–	1	–	–
Fixed route	1	–	–	–	1
	2	–	–	5	1
Rigid route	1	–	–	1	1
	2	–	–	1	4

EFFECTS OF DOSE ON THE DEGREE OF STEREOTYPY OF EXCURSIONS AND NUMBER OF BASES

Table 1 relates the amphetamine dose to the degree of stereotypy of routes at the time when the rat's behaviour is most restricted, and to the number of the rat's bases. The table suggests a dose-dependent tendency to reduce the flexibility of routes from flexible (the low doses), through fixed, to rigid (the higher doses), and increases the number of bases from one to two (with increasing dose, the ratio of two-base rats is 0/8, 1/7, 6/8 and 5/7).

EPILOGUE: 'PACKAGES' OF PLACES OF STOPPING

In summary, the rat's behaviour was organized with reference to home base over the whole range of amphetamine doses which we examined. Therefore, it is an appropriate reference place for the measurement of the drug's action (Eilam and Golani, 1990). Stopping at this reference place divides the flow of both normal and amphetamine-induced behaviour into natural morphogenetic units called *excursions* (Golani *et al.*, 1993). In the present report, we provide a first-approximation description of the morphogenesis of excursions with amphetamine in locale space. The process appears to be characterized by the shaping of routes, by a dose-dependent reduction in the number of routes, by an increase in the rigidity of routes, by a decrease in the mean number of stops per excursion compared to the normal, and by an increase in the number of bases.

Examination of the individual records reveals that during most of the session, except for the first few minutes, the drug also reduced the maximum

and for the 41–60 min interval are depicted by empty bars. (A) In all groups there was a decrease in the mean number of stops per excursion. (B) The number of different places in which the rat stopped decreased in the course of drug action. A marked decrease was observed with 2.5 and 5 mg/kg after 20 min. (C) A low mean number of roughly three routes characterizes the two lower doses. The mean was further decreased to less than two routes with the two higher doses.

number of stops per excursion (e.g. Figures 2, 3 and 12). To evaluate this process quantitatively, however, it would be necessary to establish the type(s) of the distribution of the number of stops per excursion dose dependently, using similar statistical tools to those used in the examination of normal stopping behaviour (Golani et al., 1993).

Examination of the individual records also reveals that with the higher doses there is a gradual reduction in the number of different visited places across excursions and an increase in the rigidity of their sequencing (i.e. during successive excursions the rat tends to stop in the same places, and in the same order; Figures 2, 3, 7 and 8). Figure 13(B) presents the number of different stopping places in 20 min bins across the session. As it shows, there was a marked decrease in this measure with the two high doses. To examine this phenomenon further quantitatively, it would be necessary to establish a formal method for the classification of routes. In the absence of a formal definition, we presently define routes intuitively, in much the same way that classical ethologists define 'behaviour patterns' (Barlow, 1977).

We may now re-examine the transition from normal behaviour to drug-induced stereotypies. Normal exploratory behaviour is constrained by the existence of a home base whose attraction increases after each stop performed by the rat. This is expressed by the existence of an upper bound on the number of stops per excursion. Within this bound, however, the rat appears to have relatively direct access to all the places in the environment: the location of the next place of stopping cannot be predicted on the basis of knowledge of the previous place(s) of stopping.

A low dose reduces the mean number of stops per excursion and also the maximum number of stops per excursion. It also partitions the list of all places in the environment into three to four 'packages' (Hultsch and Todt, 1989). Each package includes several specific places in which the rat has a relatively high probability of stopping. These are the flexible routes described above.

With a high dose the number of packages is reduced, the list of visited places is shorter and the sequencing of these places becomes increasingly more fixed. As with normal behaviour, the flow still consists of repeated performance of excursions, but the variety of routes, and the variability of stopping places within them, is gradually reduced. In its most extreme form, behaviour becomes consolidated into one or two packages, each consisting of the same few places in which the rat stops in a fixed order. Direct free access to places in the environment is lost; the packages are executed *en bloc*; once started, the rat proceeds in a fixed order through the full sequence of places included in this package (see Figure 2). The package, and not the individual place, now becomes both the elementary building block and the highest recognizable unit of organization of topographically specific behaviour in locale space.

This consolidation of exploratory behaviour into packages of stopping places is reminiscent of similar processes of chunking taking place during learning in humans (Miller, 1957), and in the formation of packages of songs in nightingales, during song acquisition in ontogeny (Hultsch and Todt, 1989). Chunking has been considered a strategy for coping with an increasing load on information-processing capacity, in the context of the establishment of habits, and in the consolidation of memory (DeGroot, 1965; Moats and Schumacher, 1980; Murdock, 1961; Simon, 1974). The establishment of spatiotemporal packages under amphetamine could also be explained in terms of a hypothetical mechanism for coping with a drug-induced reduction in information-processing capacity. At the present stage of knowledge, however, it might be more fruitful to continue with the study of morphogenesis of behaviour in locale space at the level of observables.

ACKNOWLEDGEMENTS

We thank the staff of the Meir Segals Garden for Zoological Research for their help in keeping and filming the animals. This research was supported by the Israel Institute for Psychobiology, Charles E. Smith Foundation, Grant 6-92 to D.E., and by the Israel Science Foundation, administered by the Israel Academy of Sciences and Humanities to I.G.

REFERENCES

Adani, N., Kiryati, N. and Golani, I. (1991) The description of rat drug-induced behaviour: kinematics versus response categories. *Neurosci. Biobehav. Rev.*, 15, 455–460.

Arnt, J., Hytell, J. and Perregaad, J. (1987) Dopamine D_1 receptor agonists combined with the selective D_2 agonist quinpirole facilitate the expression of oral stereotyped behaviour in rats. *Eur. J. Pharmacol.*, 133, 137–145.

Arnt, J., Bogeso, K.P., Hytell, J. and Meier, E. (1988) Relative dopamine D_1 and D_2 receptor affinity and efficacy determine whether dopamine agonists induce hyperactivity or oral stereotypy in rats. *Pharmacol. Toxicol.*, 62, 121–130.

Barlow, G.W. (1977) Modal action patterns. In: *How Animals Communicate* (ed. T.A. Sebeok). Indiana University Press.

Brodi, F. and Meller, E. (1989) Enhanced behavioural stereotypies elicited by injection of D_1 and D_2 dopamine agonists in intact rats. *Brain Res.*, 504, 276–283.

Cooper, S.J. and Dourish, C.T. (1990) *The Neurobiology of Stereotyped Behaviour*. Oxford Science Publications, Oxford.

Costall, B. and Naylor, R.J. (1975) Actions of dopaminergic agonists on motor function, *Adv. Neurol.*, 9, 285–297.

Cronin, G.M. (1985) *The Development and Significance of Abnormal Stereotyped Behaviour in Tethered Sows*. PhD thesis, Agricultural University of Wagening, The Netherlands.

Cronin, G.M. and Wiepkema, P.R. (1984) The development and significance of abnormal stereotyped behaviours in tethered sows. *Ann. Rech. Vet.*, 15, 263–270.

De Groot, A.D. (1965) *Thought and Choice in Chess*. Mouton, The Hauge.

Eilam, D. (1987) *Exploratory Behaviour in Norway Rats (Rattus norvegicus): Normal Behaviour and the Behaviour under the Psychoactive Drug Amphetamine*. Doctoral dissertation, Tel-Aviv University, Ramat-Aviv, Israel.

Eilam, D. and Golani, I. (1989) Home base behaviour of tame wild rats (*Rattus norvegicus*) in a novel laboratory environment. *Behav. Brain Res.*, **34**, 199–211.

Eilam, D. and Golani, I. (1990) Home base behaviour of tame wild rats (*Rattus norvegicus*) injected with amphetamine. *Behav. Brain Res.*, **36**, 161–170.

Eilam, D., Golani, I. and Szechtman, H. (1989) D-2 agonist quinpirole induces perseveration of routes and hyperactivity but no perseveration of movements. *Brain Res.*, **460**, 255–267.

Eilam, D., Clements, K.V.A. and Szechtman, H. (1991) Differential effects of D1 and D2 dopamine agonists on stereotyped locomotion. *Behav. Brain Res.*, **45**, 117–124.

Eilam, D., Talangayan, H., Canaran, G. and Szechtman, H. (1992) Dopaminergic control of locomotion, mouthing, snout contact, and grooming, opposing roles of D1 and D2 receptors. *Psychopharmacology*, **106**, 447–454.

Flicker, C. and Geyer, M.A. (1982) Behaviour during hippocampal microinfusions: I. Norepinephrine and diversive exploration. *Brain Res. Rev.*, **44**, 79–103.

Fray, P.J., Sahakian, B.J., Robbins, T.W. *et al.* (1980) An observational method for quantifying the behavioural effects of dopamine agonists. Contrasting effects of *d*-amphetamine and apomorphine. *Psychopharmacology*, **69**, 253–259.

Geyer, M.A. (1982) Variational and probabilistic aspects of exploratory behaviour in space: four stimulant styles. *Psychopharmacol. Bull.*, **18**, 48–51.

Geyer, M.A., Russo, P.V. and Masten, V.L. (1986a) Multivariate assessment of locomotor behaviour: pharmacological and behavioural analyses. *Pharmacol. Biochem. Behav.*, **25**, 277–288.

Geyer, M.A., Russo, P.V., Segal, D.S. and Kuczenski, R. (1986b) Effects of apomorphine and amphetamine on patterns of locomotor and investigatory behaviour in rats. *Pharmacol. Biochem. Behav.*, **28**, 393–399.

Golani, I. (1992) A mobility gradient in the organization of vertebrate movement: the perception of movement through symbolic language. *Behav. Brain Sci.*, **15**, 249–308.

Golani, I. and Eilam, D. (1994) Amphetamine constrains stopping behaviour in rats (*Rattus norvegicus*) during exploration. *Behav. Pharmacol.* (submitted).

Golani, I., Benjamini, Y. and Eilam, D. (1993) Stopping behaviour: constraints on exploration in rats (*Rattus norvegicus*). *Behav. Brain Res.*, **3**, 21–33.

Hediger, H. (1964) *Wild Animals in Captivity*, Dover Publications, New York.

Hultsch, H. and Todt, D. (1989) Memorization and reproduction of songs in nightingales (*Luscinia megarhynchus*): evidence for package formation. *J. Comp. Physiol. A*, **165**, 197–203.

Kelly, P.H. (1977) Drug-induced motor behaviour. in: *Handbook of Psychopharmacology*, Vol. 8 (eds L.L. Iversen, S.D. Iversen and S.H. Snyder). Plenum Press, New York, pp. 295–331.

Lyon, M. and Robbins, T.W. (1975) The action of central nervous system stimulant drugs: a general theory concerning amphetamine effects. In: *Current Developments in Psychopharmacology*, Vol. 2 (eds W. Essman and L. Valzelli). Spectrum, New York, pp. 89–163.

Miller, G.A. (1956) The magic number seven plus or minus two: some limits on our capacity for processing information. *Psychol. Rev.*, **63**, 81–97.

Moats, D.R. and Schumacher, G.M. (1980) *An Introduction to Cognitive Psychology*. Wadsworth, Belmont, CA.

Muller, K., Hollingsworth, E.M. and Cross, D.R. (1989) Another look at amphetamine-induced stereotyped locomotor activity in rats using a new statistic to measure locomotor stereotypy. *Psychopharmacology*, **97**, 74–79.

Murdock, B.B., Jr (1961) The retention of individual items. *J. Exp. Psychol.*, **62**, 618–675.

Paulus, M.P. and Geyer, M.A. (1991) Temporal and spatial scaling hypothesis for the behavioural effects of psychostimulants. *Psychopharmacology*, **104**, 6–10.

Randrup, A. and Munkvad, I. (1970) Biochemical, anatomical and psychological investigations of stereotyped behaviour induced by amphetamines. In: *Amphetamines and Related Compounds*. (eds E. Costa and S. Garattini). Raven Press, New York, pp. 695–713.

Schiorring, E. (1971) Amphetamine induced selective stimulation on certain behaviour items with concurrent inhibition of others in an open field test with rats. *Behaviour*, **39**, 1–17.

Schiorring, E. (1979) An open field study of stereotyped locomotor activity in amphetamine-treated rats. *Psychopharmacology*, **66**, 281–287.

Simon, H.A. (1974) How big is a chunk? *Science*, **183**, 482–488.

Stevenson, M.F. (1983) The captive environment: its effects on exploratory and related behavioural responses in wild animals. In: *Exploration* (eds J. Archer and L. Birke). Van Nostrand Reinhold, UK, pp. 176–197.

Szechtman, H., Ornstein, K., Teitelbaum, P. and Golani, I. (1985) The morphogenesis of stereotyped behaviour induced by the dopamine receptor agonist apomorphine in the laboratory rat. *Neuroscience*, **14**, 783–798.

Szechtman, H., Talangbayan, H., Canaran, G. *et al.* (1994) Dynamics of behavioural sensitization induced by the dopamine agonist quinpirole and a proposed central energy control mechanism. *Psychopharmacology* (in press).

14   Psychopharmacology of Behavioural Variability

CHARLES H.M. BECK,[a] STEVEN J. COOPER[b] AND LINDA J. CARTER[a]

[a]*Department of Psychology, University of Alberta, Edmonton, Alberta, Canada,*
[b]*Department of Psychology, University of Durham, UK*

INTRODUCTION

In the rat, behavioural variability or variation, defined as unpredictable fluctuations in behaviour, has many manifestations. Behavioural variability is observable in investigative reactions to the introduction of novelty (Widgiz and Beck, 1990), in reactions to alternative choices, e.g. in spontaneous alternation (Dember and Fowler, 1958), and in matching behaviour in contrast to maximizing (Mackintosh, 1969). In the latter example, an animal faced with a two-choice probability learning task may select stimuli over trials so as to match the probability of reinforcement. In this case, the choice the animal makes on a particular trial varies unpredictably. On the other hand, the animal may follow a maximizing strategy by always choosing the more frequently reinforced stimulus. In this instance the animal's choices are completely predictable.

During the initial stages of acquisition of a learning task the rat varies its sampling of the environment (Beck and Kalynchuk, 1992) and emits a variety of responses and response strategies (Beck and Kalynchuk, 1992). Although behavioural variability typically declines as an instrumental response is acquired, behavioural variability may be reinforced as an operant (Page and Neuringer, 1985). Tasks involving changes in reinforcement contingency evoke increases in behavioural variability. Examples of such tasks include negative behavioural contrast (Vogel and Principi, 1971), frustrative non-reward (Amsel and Roussel, 1952), delay of reward (Thiebot *et al.*, 1985), extinction in conditioning studies (Beck and Loh, 1990) and resource depletion in foraging studies (Mellgren *et al.*, 1984). Even in an apparently unchanging environment, variability intrudes during the habitual performance of repetitive tasks, e.g. exploratory behaviours interrupt a learned bar press (Crow, 1970),

Ethology and Psychopharmacology. Edited by S.J. Cooper and C.A. Hendrie

appear as 'errors' in discrimination (Beck and Kalynchuk, 1992) or as unpredictable arm entries in radial maze performance (Loh and Beck, 1989). Given its ubiquity, variability appears to be an intrusive intrinsic property of behavioural output.

We shall argue that what appears to be an animal's errant or incorrect performance under experimental conditions is appropriate and indeed necessary for survival in the face of evolutionary selection pressures. The natural environment is, of course, continually changing, as for example in diurnal and seasonal fluctuations in food and water supply, in predation and in weather. Thus it is plausible to envisage the adaptive advantages of behavioural variability as providing the spontaneous fluctuations in behaviour necessary for the acquiring and updating of information about environmental changes, learning new responses, reassessing accustomed modes of sampling of cues, modifying habitual response strategies, and checking for vestigial and superstitious behavioural elements (Devenport, 1989; Staddon, 1976).

The analogy has been drawn between the role of variation in the gene pool for the survival of the genome, the significance of trophic proliferation of neuronal contacts for the formation of neuronal assemblies, and the necessity of behavioural variation for the selection of strategies for sampling and manipulating the environment (Edelman, 1987; Staddon, 1976; Pringle, 1951; Russell, 1962). Thus adaptation of a species to its ecological niche, of a neurone to its target tissue, or of an organism to a particular learning situation, involves the transmission of information about changing conditions from the environment to a reproducing unit. This transmission occurs via selection by the environment from among a pool of phenotypic, synaptic and behavioural variants. Genetic evolution, neuronal plasticity and organismic learning result from two opposing forces: variation and selection-induced redundancy. As an example of the latter, the effects of selective reinforcement are commonly thought of as having the effect of increasing the probability of specific behaviours reoccurring, i.e. of inducing behavioural redundancy. Studies of readiness, exploration and extinction have provided a limited perspective of the neural mechanisms of behavioural variability (Corey, 1978; Devenport, 1983; Klemm, 1990). Much more is known about mechanisms of redundancy generation, i.e. reinforcement, sensitization and habituation, as any textbook will attest (e.g. Cotman and McGaugh, 1980).

The aim of this chapter is to describe research into three apparently disparate pharmacologically induced instances of the interaction between variability and redundancy in the hope of identifying behavioural processes common to all three. The paradigms which we have chosen are: first, the effects of benzodiazepines on fearful behaviour and learning; second, the sensitizing effects of amphetamine and schedule induction on behaviour; third, a comparison of the natural behaviour of rat pups with that of adult male rats treated with apomorphine.

BENZODIAZEPINES AND THE VARIABILITY OF BEHAVIOUR

The conventional view of the fundamental behavioural effects of benzodiazepine tranquillizers is that they reduce fear, induce amnesia and cause sedation (Hommer et al., 1987). The principal support for the hypothesis that benzodiazepines reduce fear in animals derives from findings of benzodiozepine-induced reduced fear of punishment (Koob et al., 1986), less freezing and more exploration in a frightening unfamiliar environment (Pellow and File, 1986), and decreased burying of a noxious object (Treit et al., 1981). In all of these cases benzodiazepines decrease defensive behaviours, e.g. staying next to a wall, freezing and burying. However, these tests involve competition between the fear-induced defensive behaviours and an alternative behaviour, e.g. food ingestion in the punishment test and exploration in the other two tests. If benzodiazepines had the general effect of reducing the variability of behaviour, then an animal so treated would be expected more readily to resolve the conflict in favour of one of the alternative behaviours, e.g. to keep on drinking or exploring in fearful situations. This hypothesis may also account for the finding that benzodiazepines decrease resistance to extinction of appetitive responses (Buckland et al., 1986).

Experiment 1: Diazepam selectively reduces variability in extinction

We tested the hypothesis in an extinction paradigm with the expectation that benzodiazepine treatment would reduce the variability of the operant and its competing responses (Beck and Loh, 1990). In a radial maze, saline-treated rats reinforced for many sessions with food for entering arms soon give up doing so when the operant response, arm entry, is extinguished. As expected, rats that had been injected with diazepam (1.5, 3.0, 6.0 mg/kg, i.p.) persisted in performing the arm entry response in extinction. Detailed coding of behaviour by a trained observer showed that in extinction diazepam dose-dependently increased the rate of the operant and that this was possible because diazepam reduced the number and variability of responses competing with the operant, e.g. there was less rearing and investigation. However, contrary to the hypothesis that in extinction diazepam would increase the variability of behaviour generally, diazepam increased the variability of the operant, i.e. increased the variability of arm-entry sequences, decreased the proportion of arm re-entries, and increased the variation of angle of turn between successive arms entered. The variability of arm-entry sequences was computed with the uncertainty measure (Frick and Miller, 1951) and angle of turn was measured as the angle between successive arms entered.

If diazepam acted generally to reduce behavioural variability then all manifestations of variability should have been inhibited. This did not occur because only the variability of competing responses was reduced. If diazepam acted by impairing memory, it is not clear why memory for the reinforced response remained intact. Even if the definition of fear is stretched to include apprehension about the unavailability of food in extinction, the fear-reduction hypothesis of benzodiazepine action would be hard pressed to encompass the observed selective changes in variability.

Experiment 2: Diazepam selectively reduces the variability of a well-learned operant response

If the effects of diazepam on variability are independent of anxiolytic action, then the effects of diazepam treatment on behavioural variation should be observable in a situation in which there are no aversive consequences, including withholding of reward. This was tested in a study in which food-deprived rats were treated chronically with diazepam (1.5, 3.0, 6.0 mg/kg, i.p.) for 18 sessions (Loh and Beck, 1989). During each session an entry into any arm of a radial maze was reinforced with food. Administration of diazepam compared to saline increased the predictability of the choice of arms entered. The predictability of the sequential choice of arms was defined by the uncertainty measure (Frick and Miller, 1951). The variability of right–left turn sequences between arm entries and of the frequency of entry into specific arms was not different in the experimental and control animals. Thus preference for right or left turns or for particular arms could not explain the observed effect. However, diazepam-induced potentiation of predictability was related to an increased tendency to re-enter arms, which in turn was related to a predilection for making obtuse angle turns between arms. Since mazes with enclosed alleys and no doors, such as the maze used in this study, induce modest angle-of-turn preferences in untreated animals (Mazmanian and Roberts, 1983; Pico and Davis, 1984), it is plausible that the effect of diazepam on sequential arm choices is an exaggeration of this normal tendency. Finally, the diazepam-treated rats exhibited a greater commitment to food procurement in having shorter times between arm choices, in spending a greater proportion of their time in locomoting to the food and in eating, and less time in exploring, rearing and grooming.

The results of Experiment 2 are difficult to interpret as diazepam-induced anxiolysis since the response was a thoroughly trained food-reinforced operant. Similarly, amnesic action seems improbable because memory for angle of turn was intact, as was memory for an efficient procedure of food procurement. Nor do the results fit the model of a general reduction in behavioural variability by diazepam since the decrease in variability was selective.

Diazepam potentiates prepotent behaviour

An alternative hypothesis is that diazepam increases the probability of occurrence of prepotent responses, whether species characteristic or learned. Prepotent responses are defined as behavioural biases of an individual that have a high likelihood of occurring in a given situation, whether as a result of the species' history or the individual's history. The effects of an individual's behaviour on the interaction of such behavioural biases have been well documented (Bolles, 1970; Seligman, 1970). Significantly, certain drugs, e.g. amphetamine and ethanol, have been described as being capable of enhancing an individual's prepotent behaviour (Lyons and Robbins, 1975; Steele and Southwick, 1985).

Applying this hypothesis to the action of diazepam in Experiments 1 and 2 suggests that diazepam potentiated prepotent behaviours and that this was related to a selective reduction in behavioural variability. Thus, in Experiment 1, the diazepam-induced increase in resistance to extinction of the operant, arm entry, was related to the selective decrease in the variability of the competing responses, e.g. rearing and investigation. Similarly, in Experiment 2, in asymptotically performing animals in a radial maze, a diazepam-induced increase in time devoted to food procurement was related to a decline in the variability of investigative behaviour. Finally, an increase in preference for a particular angle of turn between arm entries, a prepotent response in that apparatus, was related to the greater predictability of arm-entry choices. Predictive validity, lacking in these experiments, was supplied in two other studies.

Experiment 3: Diazepam potentiates exploration and habituation

According to the fear-reduction hypothesis, benzodiazepines increase time spent in the unwalled or open arm of an unfamiliar elevated maze by reducing the rat's fear of exposure and high places. It follows from this that repeated sessions in the maze should reduce the fear and induce exploration of the open arms by untreated animals in a manner similar to that seen in a benzodiazepine-treated naive rat. Detailed coding of behaviour by a trained observer revealed that, as expected, naive rats treated with diazepam (2.0 mg/kg, i.p.) increased investigative behaviours selectively in the open area of a novel maze (Widgiz and Beck, 1990). Unexpectedly, however, untreated animals, familiarized with the maze by repeated exposures to it, never increased their exploration of the open area. Thus, reduced fear through familiarization with the maze does not provide a good model.

Considering the maze as an interesting place to explore, an alternative model for diazepam's enhancement of exploration in the elevated plus maze is that benzodiazepines enhance the attractiveness of the maze for exploration. Effectively, this would be potentiating a behaviour which was prepotent due to incentive motivation (Robinson and Berridge, 1993). Confirming this, in a second test, the topography of the exploratory behaviour of diazepam-treated rats (2.0 mg/kg, i.p.) was closely approximated by untreated rats which were placed on the maze to explore a patch of litter marked with urine from a female rat (Widgiz and Beck, 1990).

The natural time-course of exploration of an attractive environment involves investigation followed by habituation. If diazepam is capable of potenting behaviours selectively, then depending on the familiarity of the animal with the maze, diazepam should potentiate either exploration or habituation. In the third test, this was found to be the case in the similarity of diazepam-treated rats (2.0 mg/kg, i.p.) to saline-treated rats on detailed measures of exploration and resting (Widgiz and Beck, 1990). This effect of diazepam was anticipated in the observations of biphasic locomotor effects of benzodiazepines, i.e. increased and then decreased locomotion at non-sedating doses (Davies and Steinberg, 1984; Itoh and Takaori, 1968). The effect on habituation is important because it permits a dissociation of diazepam's action specifically from a purely proexploratory effect and more generally from a rewarding effect.

Defining rewarding effects as those which elicit approach (White, 1989), it is apparent that benzodiazepines have a variety of effects that may be construed as rewarding, e.g. increasing amphetamine-induced locomotion (Rushton and Steinberg, 1966), potentiating intracranial self-stimulation (Olds, 1966), supporting intravenous self-administration (Naruse and Asami, 1987), pro-ingestive effects (Cooper, 1980), enhancing palatability responses (Berridge and Treit, 1986), conditioning place preference (Spyraki et al., 1985) and potentiating mesolimbic rewarding effects (Spyraki and Fibiger, 1988). Significantly, these rewarding effects of benzodiazepines can all be explained as the enhancement of behavioural biases sustained by reward. The latter would appear to be the preferred model since proreward action cannot explain the diazepam-induced selective decrease in behavioural variability in Experiments 1 and 2 or the habituation effect in Experiment 3.

Experiment 4: Diazepam potentiates fearful behaviour

The dissociation of the diazepam effect on prepotent behaviours from a proexploratory effect raises the possibility that the same dissociation can be demonstrated with fear. If fear is the prepotent response in a situation, then according to the prepotency hypothesis benzodiazepine treatment should enhance the fear response. To test this, 32 rats were exposed to three 30 min sessions of unsignalled inescapable foot shock trains (0.5 mA, five 1 s pulses per 10 s train) delivered on a variable-time 60 s schedule (Beck and Fibiger, 1992). A final fourth session in the same apparatus, presented without shock, was preceded 40 min earlier by either a saline injection or one of three doses of diazepam (2.5, 5.0, or 10.0 mg/kg, i.p.) to four groups of rats ($n = 8$). Behaviour was coded continuously during the session on a microprocessor which also recorded the time of each code entry. The behaviours coded included locomote, sniff, rear, groom, crouch, oral, jump, turn and immobile.

Crouch was distinguished from immobile in that during crouching the animal maintained a flattened posture, whereas immobile involved a resting posture. To indicate the time-course of an effect, the session was divided into six 5 min periods. Two-way analysis of variance (ANOVA) of groups by periods revealed significant group main effect and group by period (G × P) interaction for the percentage of time spent in locomote, for groups $F(3, 28) = 6.81$, $P < 0.01$, and for G × P $F(15, 140) = 2.05$, $P < 0.5$; sniff, for groups $F(3, 28) = 5.37$, $P < 0.01$ and for G × P $F(15, 140) = 2.17$, $P < 0.05$; crouch, for groups $F(3, 28) = 3.27$, $P < 0.05$, for G × P $F(15, 140) = 2.60$, $P < 0.05$; oral, for groups $F(3, 28) = 5.2$, $P < 0.01$. The effects for rear, groom, jump, turn and immobile were not significant. Follow-up Newman–Keuls analysis of individual group differences showed that the saline group decreased their crouching and increased their locomoting and sniffing earlier than did the diazepam-treated rats (Figure 1). It is unlikely that the group differences reflected a non-specific sedation effect induced by diazepam because crouching differentiated the groups whereas immobility did not, and because there was a dose-dependent increase in biting at the floor bars. In saline-treated rats such activity was interpreted as escape behaviour because it occurred only in the first session. Nevertheless, it would be important to replicate these findings with minimally sedating anxiolytics.

With due regard to these caveats, it is fair to say that the benzodiazepine treatment prolonged the effects of fear and retarded the return to normal behaviour. This is in contrast to reports of benzodiazepines reducing crouching induced by prior shock (Conti et al., 1990; Fanselow and Helmstetter, 1988). In those studies the animals were subjected to shorter sessions, e.g. 6 min versus 30 min sessions, and to fewer shocks, e.g. two versus 150 shocks per session, presumably providing the rats with a more balanced conflict between opposing exploration and defence. In sum, the results support the view that benzodiazepines potentiate prepotent behaviours even if that means making the organism more fearful. It would be important to assess this conjecture with physiological measures of autonomic function.

Benzodiazepines may potentiate the stronger of two conflicting responses

The idea that the relative strength of conflicting tendencies is an important determinant of drug effects has been employed with some predictive success in studies of the effects of alcohol on the behaviour of humans (Steele and Southwick, 1985). Applying this analysis to animal experimentation on benzodiazepine effects would help clarify the operational meaning of prepotent. The literature describing the similarities between the effects of ethanol and benzodiazepines on behaviour lends credence to this suggestion (cf. Beck and Loh, 1990).

An analysis of the relative strengths of conflicting tendencies might resolve the disagreement over the effect of benzodiazepine treatment on agonistic

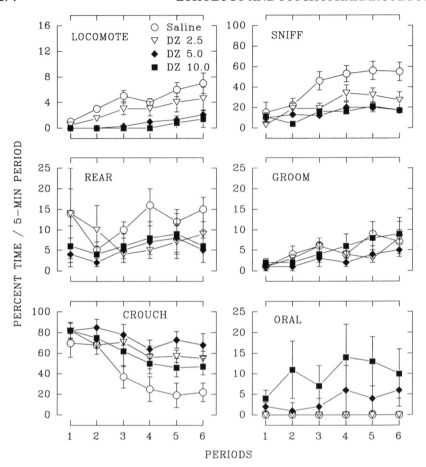

Figure 1 Mean percentage time and s.e.m.s across six 5 min periods in four groups ($n = 8$) of rats injected with saline (open circles), or diazepam 2.5 mg/kg i.p., ×1, −40 min (open triangles), 5.0 mg/kg (filled diamonds), or 10.0 mg/kg (filled squares) for six behaviours: locomote, sniff, rear, groom, crouch and oral.

social behaviour. At non-sedating doses, acute treatment with benzodiazepines have been found to decrease aggression (Olivier *et al.*, 1984), increase aggression (Miczek, 1974; Beck and Cooper, 1986b) or have no effect on aggression (File, 1982). However, a review of these studies suggests that benzodiazepine treatment increased aggression only when animals were likely to engage in agonistic behaviour, whether as a result of predisposition or environmental circumstance. This leads to the working hypothesis that benzodiazepines potentiate aggression only when it is the prepotent response and suggests that the hypothesis deserves formal testing on social behaviour generally. It also raises the interesting possibility of demonstrating that anxiogenic agents such as the benzodiazepine receptor inverse agonist, FG 7142, might have the opposite effect, namely that of decreasing prepotent behavioural biases (Beck and Cooper 1986a).

Experiment 5: Errors in a memory test by diazepam-treated rats are related to enhancement of behaviours characteristic of initial learning

If enhancement of prepotent responses can be used to explain benzodiazepine anxiolytic effects, it may also permit reinterpretation of benzodiazepine amnesic effects. To study amnesic effects we used the delayed non-matching-to-sample (NMTS) task, which permits delaying the opportunity to recognize the novel object by a variable delay interval (Kalynchuk and Beck, 1992). NMTS has the advantage that a benzodiazepine-induced amnesic effect cannot be attributed to anxiolytic action, as is the case in avoidance tests (Broekkamp et al., 1984). Nor can the deficit be ascribed to diminished neophobia because the animals are thoroughly familiarized with the testing arrangement through protracted training. Critically, manipulation of the delay intervals permits the experimenter to dissociate errors related to the duration of the delays, i.e. forgetting, from errors occurring independently of delay duration, i.e. performance effects. The only other study on the effect of benzodiazepines (nitrazepam, diazepam, flurazepam) on animals performing NMTS found a delay-related deficit (Nicholson and Wright, 1974). However, the results were less than conclusive because each animal was tested with several other drugs in addition to benzodiazepines.

To clarify further the nature of the expected benzodiazepine deficit in NMTS, we coded the ongoing behaviour of the animals during asymptotic performance under the influence of the drug diazepam (2.0 mg/kg, i.p.) or saline administered 30 min before testing. The observed diazepam-induced errors in discrimination were significantly greater than those in control rats but the increase was not related to the duration of the delay interval (Kalynchuk and Beck, 1992). This finding was congruent with other reports of failure to observe delay-dependent deficits following benzodiazepine treatment in discrimination tasks in rats (Tan et al., 1990), pigeons (Poling et al., 1986) and humans (Rodrigo and Lusiardo, 1988). Taken together, the data support the conclusion that benzodiazepine-induced amnesia involves making errors, not in forgetting but in performance.

Ethological analysis of the errors in our study (Kalynchuk and Beck, 1992) revealed that the drugged animals were not making errors because of a benzodiazepine-induced reward effect. Parenthetically, the NMTS task involved choosing the test object which matched two identical sample objects. Contrary to the reward hypothesis, diazepam-treated rats did not exhibit an increased frequency of sample object displacement, nor a decreased latency to displace test objects, nor an increase in gross overall activity, nor did they exhibit preferences for particular objects. Instead, the analysis showed that the benzodiazepine-treated rats broke implicit procedural rules, such as those to avoid object and apparatus side preferences and to investigate objects thoroughly before choosing one. Their errors occurred on those trials in which they failed to investigate both test objects, failed to investigate the objects for a long enough period of time, and chose the object on the preferred side of the apparatus (Kalynchuk and Beck, 1992). In short, the diazepam-treated rats were violating implicit rules of task performance which were independent of variations in the delay duration. The rats learned to follow the rules during predelay training. The benzodiazepine-treated rats were, in effect, behaving like naive rats (Beck and Kalynchuk, 1992). Thus diazepam reasserted the undiscriminating behaviours prepotent in the repertoire of the naive rat.

In summary, these results suggest that the reduction of behavioural variability induced by benzodiazepines may be best seen as an enhancement of learned and unlearned prepotent tendencies and may account for some of the anxiolytic and amnesic effects of these drugs. The effects may be behaviourally excitatory as in the case of promoting resistance to extinction, increasing errors in learning skills or enhancing exploration. Alternatively, they may appear as behavioural inhibition, as in the case of the prohabituation effect and the prolongation of fear-induced crouching.

AMPHETAMINE, SENSITIZATION AND POLYDIPSIA

If we view benzodiazepines as tranquillizers in the traditional sense, one of their most paradoxical effects is that of potentiating amphetamine-induced locomotion (Rushton and Steinberg, 1966). On the other hand, this finding is entirely compatible with our hypothesis that benzodiazepines enhance prepotent behaviours. The argument is made more compelling in a paradigm which demonstrates amphetamine's sensitivity to environmental effects. Amphetamine-induced stereotypic behaviour typically has been quantified by behavioural intensity scales which obscure the incidence of specific behaviours (Ernst, 1967). This is so, even though it has been known for some time that the topography of the amphetamine-induced stereotypic behaviour varies considerably depending on the testing environment. This is true for both humans (Kokkinidis and Anisman, 1980) and rats (Ellinwood and Kilbey, 1975; Mumford et al., 1979; Pope et al., 1980). For example, an enclosed maze elicits more amphetamine-induced rearing than does an elevated maze (Mumford et al., 1979). A plausible hypothesis is that the ongoing behaviour of the normal animal elicited by the environment becomes incorporated into the stereotypic response. However, none of the cited studies convincingly demonstrated this assertion because no study compared the behaviour of saline- and amphetamine-treated rats in more than one environment.

Experiment 6: Amphetamine potentiates orientating responses appropriate to specific environments

We did this and recorded the ensuing behaviour using continuous coding in two situations: a wire mesh cage and an elevated table top (Beck et al., 1986b). Saline-treated rats in the wire cage thrust their noses into the mesh, whereas those placed on the table exhibited little snout contact but preferred to look over the edge of the table. Rats administered amphetamine acutely (7.0 mg/kg, i.p., immediate) evinced potentiation of the respective behaviours (Figure 2, from Beck et al., 1986b). Thus those in the cage incorporated snout contact into their stereotypy, whereas those on the table perseveratively peered over the edge. While the amphetamine-treated rats persisted in these behaviours over the 90 min session, the controls habituated to the novelty and assumed resting postures. Moreover, when the apparatus was modified at 30 min post injection, rats treated with amphetamine were unable to accommodate their behaviour to the new environment (Figure 2). In another group, a change of apparatus at 10 min post injection was only able to elicit a modest behavioural shift in stereotypy commensurate with the new configuration of the apparatus (Figure 2). By contrast, saline-treated rats evinced noticeable shifts in orientation (see non-snout contact in the cage/table group and snout contact in the table/cage group). Thus, amphetamine potentiated those orientating behaviours which had been made prepotent by the structure of the testing environment present early in the postinjection period. Presumably, this observation is related to the general proposition that amphetamine stereotypic responses are of behaviours prepotent in the animal's repertoire, whether they were originally learned or unlearned (Lyons and Robbins, 1975; Robbins et al., 1990).

Experiment 7: Diazepam pretreatment enhances the amphetamine-induced effect on environmentally specific orientating

The general parallel with the benzodiazepine prepotency hypothesis is obvious. The design of Experiment 6 may have some possibilities for testing the direct effect of benzodiazepines on explicitly elicited behavioural prepotencies. To our knowledge there is no evidence in the benzodiazepine literature for an equivalent period of heightened sensitivity to environmental influence early in the time-course of the drug, although there is support for a similar effect of ethanol (Reid et al., 1985). It is a curious characteristic of most drug studies, including those involving benzodiazepines, that the drug is administered at least 30 min before testing begins. This may have prevented an initial temporal effect from being detected.

The effects of benzodiazepine treatment on amphetamine stereotypy have been assessed in the same paradigm (Beck and Chow, unpublished). Diazepam (2.5 mg/kg, i.p.), administered alone 30 min before testing, increased the specific types of orientation seen when the apparatus was changed at 10 min

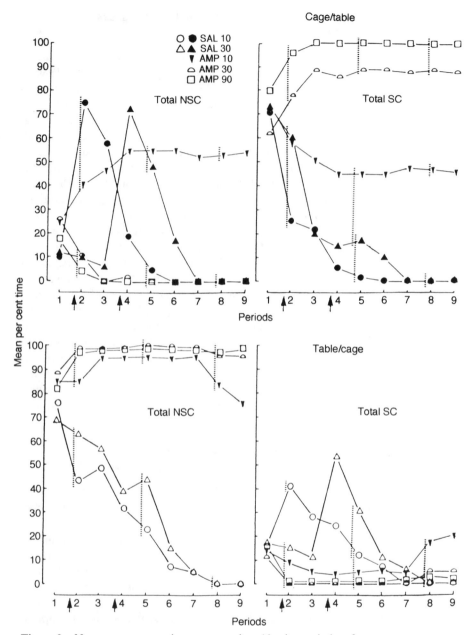

Figure 2 Mean percentage time across nine 10 min periods of non-snout contact behaviour (total NSC, e.g. hanging over the edge) and snout contact (total SC, e.g. sniffing the floor) for two types of apparatus change (cage/table, top graphs; and table/cage, bottom graphs) for five groups (*n* = 10) in each condition. The groups were: injection with isotonic saline and apparatus change at 10 min (SAL 10, open and filled circles) or at 30 min (SAL 30, open and filled triangles); or injection with amphetamine

into the session (Figure 3). The benzodiazepine-treated rats also habituated to the change more rapidly than did the rats administered saline. Diazepam potentiated the two forms of amphetamine (3.0 mg/kg, i.p., immediate) stereotypy relative to the effect of amphetamine treatment alone (Figure 3). The combined effect of the diazepam and a low dose of amphetamine was that of a higher dose of amphetamine alone. Thus the rats treated with both drugs showed no increase in non-snout contact but persisted in their snout contact in the cage environment, whereas those tested on the table top refused to engage in snout contact but persisted in hanging over the edge. This paradigm affords

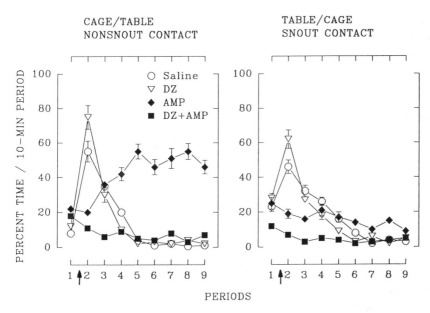

Figure 3 Mean percentage time and s.e.m.s of non-snout contact (left graph) and of snout contact (right graph) across nine 10 min periods for two types of apparatus change at 10 min post injection: cage/table (left graph) and table/cage (right graph) for four groups ($n = 8$) in each condition; injection with one of isotonic saline (open circles), diazepam (DZ, 2.5 mg/kg i.p., ×1, −30 min, open triangles), amphetamine (AMP, 3.0 mg/kg i.p., ×1, immediate, filled diamonds), or diazepam plus amphetamine (DZ + AMP, filled squares). Two-way ANOVA effects for group-by-period interactions were $F(15, 160) = 6.77$, $P < 0.001$ for the cage/table and $F(15, 160) = 2.07$, $P < 0.01$ for the table/cage condition. Arrows on the abscissae indicate the time of apparatus change.

(7 mg/kg, i.p., ×1, immediate) with apparatus change at 10 min (AMP 10, filled arrow), 30 min (AMP 30, open semicircle), or 90 min (AMP 90, open square). Means linked by dotted lines are not different (Tukey tests, $P < 0.05$). Dotted lines to the left of trials 2, 5 and 8 represent the comparison of groups over three-trial blocks. Arrows on the abscissae indicate the times of apparatus change. (After Beck *et al.*, 1986b.)

an opportunity to titrate the relative strengths of the opposing tendencies, and should be incorporated into a study of the temporal variable with benzodiazepines.

Both amphetamine stereotypy and polydipsia may be forms of sensitization

There are hints in the literature that the process whereby acute amphetamine treatment promotes environmentally elicited orientating behaviours may be related to the mechanism of sensitization produced by chronic amphetamine treatment. The latter phenomenon is characterized by an enhancement of stereotypy to a small challenge dose of amphetamine. It is thought to be mediated by dopaminergic receptor changes in the striatum, maximal effects being achieved with chronic intermittent dosing in female rats (Robinson and Becker, 1986; Robinson *et al.*, 1982). Ellinwood and Escalante (1972) suggested that the environmentally reflective orientating responses seen acutely become more enduring with repeated amphetamine treatment. If there are any changes in behaviour, they are in the direction of further focusing on specific environmental cues, simplification of the response into fewer elements, a shortening of the cycle time of the stereotypic response, and an increase in the degree to which the response occupies the postinjection period.

These behavioural changes are similar to those that occur in the acquisition of schedule-induced polydipsia (SIP). Food-deprived rats exposed to an intermittent schedule of food pellet delivery for ten 50 min sessions increase their water drinking up to four-fold relative to normal intake (Falk, 1967). The effect has been ascribed to sensitization (Beck *et al.*, 1989; Wetherington, 1982) because of its behavioural similarities with the sensitization process (Petrinovich, 1984). SIP, like sensitization, develops gradually (Falk, 1967), the development requiring repeated intermittent delivery of the eliciting stimulus, i.e. food pellet (Falk, 1967). The rate of water intake increases and drinking comes to occupy a larger portion of the interpellet interval. The SIP-sensitized animal exhibits heightened arousal (Beck *et al.*, 1989; Brett and Levine, 1981), an abrupt failure to manifest the response if the eliciting cue is omitted even though secondary cues are present (Beck *et al.*, 1989), a preference for performing a particular response, i.e. drinking, not just any oral response (Beck and Burger, 1992; Roper 1981); a selective sensitivity to the eliciting stimulus, e.g. drinking to a pellet but not to food powder or to small food granules (Beck *et al.*, 1989; Mumby and Beck, 1988), and an enduring sensitivity to the effects of the eliciting stimulus (Wetherington and Riley, 1986).

Beyond these common properties of sensitization, amphetamine-induced sensitization and SIP sensitization share other features. Both are characterized by large differences in expression between individual animals (Beck *et al.*, 1989; Mittleman and Valenstein, 1985; Tazi *et al.*, 1988); there is cross-sensitization between the two processes (Mittleman *et al.*, 1986; Mittleman and

Valenstein, 1984), and both are reduced by pretreatment with dopaminergic blockers (Todd et al., 1992; Janssen et al., 1963). It is noteworthy that both the effects of SIP and acute amphetamine are enhanced by benzodiazepine pretreatment (Rushton and Steinberg, 1966; Sanger and Blackman, 1975). At this time, it is not certain whether benzodiazepines themselves can sensitize directly or can accelerate sensitization induced by amphetamine or SIP.

In sum, it is clear that schedule-induced polydipsia and the sequelae of amphetamine treatment share many characteristics of the sensitization process. Since it is difficult to substitute non-oral activity such as wheel-running for schedule-induced drinking, it has been argued that drinking, as an ingestive activity, has a prepotency in the SIP regimen because of the drive state, i.e. food deprivation, and because the food pellet is the sensitizing stimulus (Roper, 1981). Seen in this light, the excessive drinking in the SIP paradigm is yet another example of reduced behavioural variation incurred by the potentiation of a prepotent tendency. However, differences from benzodiazepine effects are obvious. Whereas the behavioural biases enhanced by benzodiazepines were varied and complex, ranging from position habits to conditioned defensive reactions, those altered by amphetamine were orientating reactions and those sensitized by schedule induction were ingestive.

THE BEHAVIOUR OF APOMORPHINE-TREATED ADULTS AND SUCKLING RAT PUPS

Apomorphine-induced stereotypy is less responsive to the environment than is amphetamine-induced stereotypy

Like amphetamine, apomorphine induces stereotyped behaviour. The stereotypies are grossly similar, so that the same scale of stereotypic intensity has often been used to measure the effects of both drugs (Ernst, 1967). However, striking differences are also apparent. Whereas amphetamine-induced stereotypy is environmentally sensitive (Beck et al., 1986b), the same is not true of apomorphine stereotypy (Beck, 1992; Robbins et al., 1990; Szechtman, 1986). In the wire cage/table-top paradigm previously described for amphetamine (Beck et al., 1986b), rats treated acutely with apomorphine (5.0 mg/kg, i.p., immediate) maintained an indiscriminate nosing of the substrate irrespective of the apparatus structure (Beck, 1992). Indeed, the pervasiveness of the apomorphine-induced snout-contact response has been used to identify categorically the onset and termination of apomorphine stereotypy over a wide range of doses (Beck et al., 1986a; Szechtman et al., 1982). The environment present at the time of apomorphine injection was not preferred later in the session (Beck, 1992). However, the influence of the environment has been demonstrated in different substrains of rats (Szechtman et al., 1982). Following acute apomorphine treatment, rats from one substrain preferred engaging in oral activity on horizontal surfaces whereas rats from another substrain persisted in making non-oral snout contact with vertical surfaces. Again snout contact was a universal characteristic. Finally, yawning in response to low doses of apomorphine was increased in frequency by a novel setting (Dourish and Cooper, 1990). Taken together, the data suggest that apomorphine stereotypy permits only minor modification of a specific response, e.g. snout contact or yawning, and that the neural mechanism permitting this plasticity is genetically prewired.

Experiment 8: The behaviour of suckling rat pups resembles that of adults administered apomorphine

The relative inflexibility of expression of the behavioural characteristics of apomorphine administration are also reflected in the consistency of the morphogenesis of apomorphine-induced behaviour. Kinematic analysis of the topographic changes in behaviour over the time-course of the apomorphine postinjection period has led to the description of movement sequences with considerable explanatory power and some generality to other behaviours (Szechtman et al., 1988). The generic pattern has been referred to as a mobility gradient involving motoric shut-down in the case of apomorphine stereotypy or its reverse process, warm-up, in the case of the rat pup's locomotor development (Golani et al., 1981; Golani, 1992). For example, following an acute apomorphine injection, the rat's range of movement is restricted and it loses its ability to move first in the vertical plane, then in forward movement, and finally in movement in the horizontal plane (Szechtman et al., 1985). The reverse sequence occurs in the ontogeny of the rat pup's movements, first showing lateral movements on day 1 after birth, then forward movements on day 2, and finally vertical movements on day 8 (Eilam and Golani, 1988).

If apomorphine induces changes in locomotion and trunk movements in adult animals because the drug activates a mechanism controlling the same behaviours in rat pups, possibly other instructive parallels can be found in the rat pup model. We undertook some experiments to test the hypothesis that apomorphine in the adult potentiates behaviours prepotent in the repertoire of the suckling infant (Carter and Beck, unpublished). Whereas Eilam and Golani (1988) used the lone rat pup on a hard surface as their model, we used the rat pup searching for a teat in the company of litter-mates and the dam. This appeared worthwhile on ethological grounds and because others have observed day 1 and day 3 vertical movements in rat pups anticipating or receiving milk, suggesting an environmental sensitivity of these behaviours (Hall, 1979; Pedersen and Blass, 1981; Terry and Johanson, 1987).

We coded the behaviour of three litters of 10 pups each, from videotapes of the first 18 days of life (Carter and Beck, unpublished). Each coding session was long enough to ensure that 5 min of data were obtained per day from each pup during periods when the dam was nursing and was not nursing. Video recordings were obtained from top-down and bottom-up views of the nursing litters in clear plastic cages. This enabled the observer to view the behaviour of the pups beside or under the dam. The coded behaviours included: *dorsal nod*—dorsiflexion of trunk without lateral movements; this was upwards when the pup was prone and downwards when the pup was supine; *ventral nod*—ventroflexion of the trunk without lateral movements; *dorsal scan*—dorsiflexion of the trunk with side-to-side scanning movements; *ventral scan*—ventroflexion of the trunk with lateral scanning; *turn*—body turns 90°; *forward*—body moves forward by one pup-head length; *backward*—body moves backward one head length; *prone*—moves to a belly-down position; *supine*—moves to a belly-up position; *on teat*—attaches to teat; *off teat*—detaches from teat; *forepaw tread*—treading with forepaws; *push*—pushes another pup; *climb*—climbs over or under pup; *flank*—lies in passive contact with another pup.

Across days, the general pattern of development was in the order previously described (Eilam and Golani, 1988), i.e. with lateral and forward movements predominating before vertical movements (Figure 4). However, all movements were present on day 1, so the ordering was not in the order of appearance but rather in the daily incidence. Thus in non-nursing, i.e. pup–pup interactions, the dorsal (vertical) movements were rare at the outset but increased gradually over days following day 8, when Eilam and Golani (1988) noted their first appearance. Also consonant with Eilam and Golani's report, ventral nod (forward) increased after day 1, whereas ventral scan (lateral) was present from the beginning. Across days, ventral nod declined and ventral scan increased in incidence. In interaction with the nursing dam, all three types of movement were present on day 1, with the dorsal movements (vertical) again being the least frequent. In contrast to the pup–pup interactions, there was a surprising degree of stability across days in the incidence of the behaviours. In sum, changes in pup movements over days are complex, and differ in incidence depending on the setting, i.e. alone on bare surface (Eilam and Golani, 1988), with pups, and with pups and the dam (present study).

Observing the suckling pup–dam interaction, it became apparent that a sequence other than development over days might be useful as a model for apomorphine effects. Specifically, just as warm-up was studied in 11-day-old pups within a day (Golani *et al.*, 1981), we chose to observe pups of the same age searching for and finding the dam, and then searching for and finding the teat. There are some striking parallels between this sequence and that of the time-course of behaviour following apomorphine administration to the adult rat.

Both teat-searching in pups and the effects of apomorphine in adults involve motoric shut-down, both showing an ever-constricting range of movement. Thus, when the pup searches for its dam, the pup moves relatively rapidly about the cage, using more forward locomotion than turning, with the head position varying between head up and snout contact, following the surface whether it curves up or down (Figures 5 and 6, from Carter and Beck, unpublished; Hall, 1979). The same kinds of behavioural response occur in

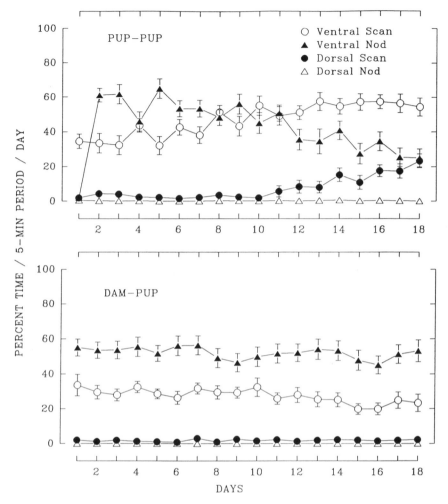

Figure 4 Mean percentage time and s.e.m.s per 5 min period per day, over days 1–18 of life under two conditions: pup–pup interactions (upper graph) and dam–pup interactions (lower graph). Means are of data collapsed across three litters of 10 pups each ($n = 30$) since the ANOVA litter effects were non-significant. In the pup–pup condition, one-way ANOVA effects for days were obtained for ventral scan, $F(17, 483) = 2.96$, $P < 0.01$, ventral nod, $F(17, 483) = 6.90$, $P < 0.001$, and dorsal scan, $F(17, 483) = 2.58$, $P < 0.05$. No other period effects were significant.

adults in the first few minutes of the time-course of action of apomorphine (Szechtman *et al.*, 1985).

Electrophysiological recordings have shown that the snout contact is accompanied by sniffing (Vanderwolf and Szechtman, 1987). This is significant because the rat pup is guided to the dam by odour (Schapiro and Salas, 1970;

Litter A1: Pup - Pup
$Sv^{27}{\rightarrow}$ $Nv^{4}{\rightarrow}$ $Sv^{35}{\rightarrow}$ $Nv^{28}{\rightarrow}$ $Sv^{78}{\rightarrow}$ $Nv^{78}{\rightarrow}$ Im^{100}
$Sv^{18}{\rightarrow}$ Sd^{14} /
$Sv^{18}{\rightarrow}$ $Sd^{9}{\rightarrow}$ $Sv^{29}{\rightarrow}$ Sd^{18} ./
$Sv^{17}{\rightarrow}$ Nv^{9} /
$Sd^{9}{\rightarrow}$ $Sv^{9}{\rightarrow}$ $Sd^{14}{\rightarrow}$ $Sv^{27}{\rightarrow}$ $Sd^{11}{\rightarrow}$ Sv^{22}/

Litter A2: Pup - Pup
$Nv^{10}{\rightarrow}$ $Sv^{15}{\rightarrow}$ $Nv^{9}{\rightarrow}$ $Sv^{38}{\rightarrow}$ $Nv^{26}{\rightarrow}$ $Sv^{75}{\rightarrow}$ $Nv^{71}{\rightarrow}$ Im^{100}
$Sd^{10}{\rightarrow}$ $Sv^{23}{\rightarrow}$ $Nv^{13}{\rightarrow}$ $Sv^{24}{\rightarrow}$ Sd^{14} /
$Sd^{10}{\rightarrow}$ $Sv^{15}{\rightarrow}$ Sd^{13} /
$Sd^{60}{\rightarrow}$ $Sv^{31}{\rightarrow}$ $Nv^{35}{\rightarrow}$ $Sd^{24}{\rightarrow}$ $Sv^{30}{\rightarrow}$ $Sd^{17}{\rightarrow}$ Sv^{29}/
$Sv^{9}{\rightarrow}$ $Sd^{8}{\rightarrow}$ $Sv^{13}{\rightarrow}$ $Sd^{5}{\rightarrow}$ $Sv^{21}{\rightarrow}$ Nv^{12} /

Litter A1: Dam - Pup
$Sv^{15}{\rightarrow}$ $Nv^{11}{\rightarrow}$ $Sv^{21}{\rightarrow}$ $Nv^{28}{\rightarrow}$ $Sv^{60}{\rightarrow}$ $Nv^{87}{\rightarrow}$ $Te^{100}{\rightarrow}$ $Nv^{89}{\rightarrow}$ St^{100}
$Nv^{4}{\rightarrow}$ Fl^{14} /
$Sv^{15}{\rightarrow}$ $Nv^{12}{\rightarrow}$ Fl^{11}./
$Nv^{4}{\rightarrow}$ $Sv^{11}{\rightarrow}$ $Nv^{16}{\rightarrow}$ Fl^{22}./
$Sv^{14}{\rightarrow}$ $Nv^{14}{\rightarrow}$ $Sv^{28}{\rightarrow}$ $Nv^{31}{\rightarrow}$ Fl^{26}./

Litter A2: Dam - Pup
$Sv^{12}{\rightarrow}$ $Nv^{12}{\rightarrow}$ $Sv^{8}{\rightarrow}$ $Nv^{27}{\rightarrow}$ $Sv^{50}{\rightarrow}$ $Nv^{88}{\rightarrow}$ $Te^{100}{\rightarrow}$ $Nv^{85}{\rightarrow}$ St^{100}
$Nv^{8}{\rightarrow}$ Fl^{7} /
$Sv^{45}{\rightarrow}$ $Nv^{32}{\rightarrow}$ Fl^{25}/
$Nv^{4}{\rightarrow}$ $Sv^{21}{\rightarrow}$ $Nv^{9}{\rightarrow}$ Fl^{27}/
$Sv^{7}{\rightarrow}$ $Nv^{7}{\rightarrow}$ $Sv^{44}{\rightarrow}$ $Nv^{33}{\rightarrow}$ Fl^{39} ./

Figure 5   Mean percentage of behaviours in a particular sequence observed in 11-day-old pups in litter A1 ($n = 10$) and litter A2 ($n = 10$) in pup–pup and dam–pup conditions. Behaviours included in this analysis were scan ventrally (Sv), nod ventrally (Nv), scan dorsally (Sd), nod dorsally (Nd), immobile (Im), flip from prone to supine (Fl), attach to teat (Te), and stretch response to milk let down (St). Sequences are event lagged to immobile in the pup–pup condition and to stretch in the dam–pup condition. As such, each represents the more probable trunk movement sequences to motoric shutdown. The superscript numbers are the percentage of sequences of that length or greater which were that particular sequence. So in pup–pup interactions for litter A1, on the third line, 'Sd¹⁸' means that 18% of the sequences of four or more behaviours were Sd, Sv, Nv and finally Im. Overall, note that ventral nodding is the most common antecedent to immobility, to teat attachment, and to stretch. Dorsiflexion occurs only in scanning and only in the pup–pup condition.

Terry and Johanson, 1987). Forward propulsion is reduced considerably when the pup locates the dam, head-up movements give way to snout contact, the pup burrows under the dam and after a variable interval of ventral searching, flips over to a supine position and continues ventral searching (Figures 5 and 6). Similarly, after a few minutes, the apomorphine-treated adult exhibits predominantly snout contact, with declining forward locomotion (Szechtman et al., 1985). While the apomorphine-treated adult will not go supine unaided, it will, if given antigravity support, follow a curved surface to ambulate

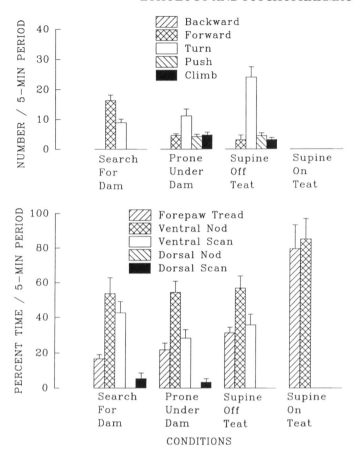

Figure 6 Upper graph: mean number and s.e.m.s per 5 min period of behaviours of 11-day-old pups ($n = 30$) under four conditions: search for the dam, prone under the dam, supine under the dam but not attached to the teat, and attached to the teat. The behaviours and their one-way ANOVA condition effects were backward, non-significant F, forward, $F(3, 87) = 7.89$, $P < 0.001$, turn, $F(3, 87) = 15.66$, $P < 0.001$, push, $F(3, 87) = 3.01$, $P < 0.05$, climb, $F(3, 87) = 2.91$, $P < 0.05$. Flank is not shown but it was 100% when the pup was supine on the teat and otherwise non-existent. Lower graph: mean percentage time and s.e.m.s per 5 min period of behaviours of six-day-old pups ($n = 30$) under the same four conditions. The behaviours and their one-way ANOVA condition effects were forepaw tread, $F(3, 87) = 11.01$, $P < 0.001$, ventral nod, $F(3, 87) = 4.00$, $P < 0.01$, ventral scan, $F(3, 87) = 5.92$, $P < 0.01$, dorsal nod, non-significant F, dorsal scan, $F(3, 87) = 2.84$, $P < 0.05$.

upside-down on a ventral surface while it continues making searching movements (Szechtman *et al.*, 1985). Critically, in both the supine pup and the supine apomorphine-treated adult, the righting reflex is suppressed. Both of these effects can be mimicked by laying the animal supine in the palm of the hand and gently massaging the mouth and forepaws (Figure 7).

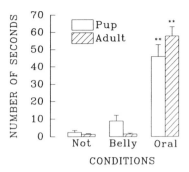

Figure 7 Mean number of seconds lying supine by 11-day-old pups ($n = 30$) and apomorphine-treated (7.0 mg/kg, i.p., ×1, −10 min) adult rats ($n = 10$) in three conditions: not stimulated tactilely, stimulated tactiley on the belly, and stimulated tactilely on the mouth and forepaws. Maximum time was 60 s. One-way ANOVA for conditions was, for pups, $F(2, 58) = 12.36$, $P < 0.001$, and for adults, $F(2, 58) = 10.41$, $P < 0.001$.

As the pup moves over the belly of the dam, pivoting increases along with an increase in small stepping movements of the forepaws and decreased forward movement, as is the case with the apomorphine-treated adult in the middle of the time-course of the drug's action (Figures 5 and 6; Szechtman et al., 1985). During this period the pup is asocial in the sense that it will not lie immobile in contact with another pup as it will when it has found a teat or when the dam is absent (Alberts, 1978). Rather, the pup pushes past the litter-mate as if it were an obstacle (Figure 6). Similarly, apomorphine in the adult eliminates social behaviour directed towards an uninjected conspecific (Chow and Beck, 1984a). The increased aggression which has been observed following apomorphine injection of both members of a pair is initially characterized by prolonged bouts of boxing (McKenzie, 1971). The enhancement of boxing is possibly a fortuitous consequence of the boxing posture, enabling mutual snout contact and forepaw-treading. This suggests that apomorphine initially potentiates a social manifestation of snout contact rather than aggression.

When a teat is located, attachment to it occurs, forepaw stepping continues but the animal remains in place, ventral nodding movements increase in frequency and mouthing movements occur (Figures 5 and 6) (Hall, 1979). Forepaw-treading and snout-probing (ventral nodding) by the pup have been implicated in the inhibition of the nursing dam's movements and in the facilitation of milk letdown (Stern and Johnson, 1990). In the apomorphine-treated adult this stage of the postinjection time-course is marked by small forepaw-stepping movements (Szechtman et al., 1988), and increased nodding and mouthing movements (Chow and Beck, 1984a; Gordon and Beck, 1984). The mouthing movements which occur in the apomorphine-treated animal have been electrophysiologically characterized as being relevant to liquid ingestion rather than to consumption of solids (Lambert *et al.*, 1986). If the dose of apomorphine is large, and if the substrate is hard and rough, the mouthing may become gnawing, an effect attributed to facilitative feedback from tactile stimulation through snout contact (Szechtman *et al.*, 1985; Szechtman *et al.*, 1988). An unusual feature of the young pup's milk ingestion is that it does not satiate and will virtually drown at the nipple (Hall, 1979). Congruently, the lack of a functional end-point for apomorphine-induced behaviour has led to its description as being insatiable, perseverative and aimless (Ernst, 1967). During the approximately 5 s of milk letdown the pup's body goes into rigid extension, called the stretch response (Drewett *et al.*, 1974; Hall, 1979). We have been unable to induce the stretch response experimentally in adults treated with apomorphine or to discover a published report of the same. Finally, when the snout contact is broken, indicating the end of the main effect of the drug, the rat yawns and goes to sleep (Dourish and Cooper, 1990; Szechtman *et al.*, 1982). The same sequence of cessation of snout contact, yawning and sleeping is also characteristic of the rat pup when the dam completes a bout of nursing (Drewett *et al.*, 1974; Hall, 1979; Hall and Rosenblatt, 1977). In sum, apomorphine administered to an adult rat elicits an elaborate sequence of behaviours with striking similarity to that evinced by the rat pup in search of a teat. Unfortunately for Freudian psychoanalysts, apomorphine is an emetic in humans.

Implications of the suckling pup model

There is ample evidence that the behavioural sequence precipitated by apomorphine is mediated primarily by dopaminergic pathways of the striatum and limbic system (cf. Golani, 1992). If the pup behaviour is also supported by dopaminergic systems then the teat-search sequence should be facilitated by dopamine agonists and impaired by dopamine antagonists. We were unable to find evidence in the literature for or against this conjecture. The inhibition of suckling which occurs at weaning may be mediated in part by serotonin since serotonin blockers induce typical suckling behaviour in postweanling pups (Williams *et al.*, 1979). Similarly, serotonin inhibitors enhance apomorphine-induced locomotor and oral activity in adults (Chow and Beck, 1984b; Weiner *et al.*, 1975). The implication is that these serotonin mechanisms may be immature and hence non-functional in the suckling rat pup. It is interesting that serotonin plays a critical role in controlling meal length in mature animals (Blundell, 1991). The immaturity of this mechanism in pups may account for the suckling pup's failure to satiate in its milk intake. Normally, milk ingestion is limited by the dam's supply.

Finally, the model may shed new light on some pathologies. Dopaminergic pathways are believed to be involved in oral dyskinesias which are exacerbated by treatment with L-dopa, the precursor of dopamine, and by withdrawal from neuroleptic (antidopaminergic) treatment (Baldessarini and Tarsy, 1976). The involvement of dopamine in the excessive drinking of schedule-induced poly-dipsia has been noted (Todd *et al.*, 1992). Dopamine pathways of the limbic system are known to play a critical role in stress effects (Costall *et al.*, 1982; Robinson and Becker, 1986). Accordingly, it is conceivable that stress might induce elements of suckling behaviour in adults. There is a curious stereotypy known as wind-sucking or crib-biting in mature horses stressed by confine-ment without exercise (Hosoda, 1950). It consists of standing with the forelegs spread apart in extension, extending the neck, and making thrusting tongue movements while grasping the stall with the teeth and gulping air. The behaviour resembles that of suckling by a foal. Wind-sucking is alleviated by treatment with opiate blockers and possibly also by treatment with dopaminer-gic antagonists (Dodman *et al.*, 1987).

CONCLUSION

This chapter began with a description of the role of variability in behaviour. A distinction was made between the processes of variation and redundancy but the difference was not operationally defined. Beyond identifying redundancy generation with reward, no clear description of the mechanism involved in the generation of variability was presented. We simply do not have one. This makes it difficult to determine whether a decrease in behavioural variability is the result of down-regulation in a neural substrate producing variation or up-regulation of a mechanism producing redundancy. The importance of the distinction is illustrated by recourse to the model of genetic evolution.

Genetic variation occurs as a change in the genes themselves through gene mutation and recombination. By contrast, redundancy develops in, or natural selection acts on, reproducing clusters of genes, the genome. By analogy, behavioural variation may be expressed through selective changes in any dimension or element of a response, whereas the redundancy process affects all dimensions of a response simultaneously, reinforcing a constellation of response elements. The evidence presented in this chapter illustrates how difficult it is to dissociate these processes. In every instance of reduced behavioural variability there were related intrusions of enhanced behavioural biases, clearly manifestations of a redundancy process. The same mix of reduced behavioural variability and enhancement of behavioural packages is described in the chapter in this volume by Eilam and Golani on amphetamine effects on spatial exploration. Taken together, the data suggest that systemic administration of drugs may not be a suitable tool for dissociating the processes of redundancy and variation. In addition, delineation of the proces-ses was made more difficult by the lack of independent and dependent behavioural variables which would permit selective manipulation and assess-ment of behavioural variation and redundancy. In summary, the attempt to separate these processes has not been successful.

On the other hand, the results do illuminate the differences between the behavioural biases potentiated by diazepam, amphetamine and apomorphine. Diazepam's effects were subtle, enhancing the behavioural bias of the moment, shifting with changing contingencies. The effects were equivocal enough to have been confused with anxiolytic and amnesic sequalae. Amphetamine administration biased behavioural output in favour of any normal behaviour which happened to occur early in the time-course of the drug's action. The topography and spatial distribution of the behaviours were influenced by the structure of the environment and by prior learning. Apomorphine potentiated one or more specific elements of an unlearned sequence of behaviours. The full sequence was approximated by the teat search and suckling routine of a pup. The behaviours selected for expression from the sequence were the result of an interaction of drug dose, interval in the time-course of the drug's action and the configuration of the environment. Future research employing intracranial administration of receptor-specific ligands will enable us to fractionate these effects so as to reveal their common and disparate substrates.

ACKNOWLEDGEMENT

Funding for the research described was provided by the Alberta Mental Health Research Council to C.H.M. Beck.

REFERENCE NOTES

Beck, C.H.M. and Chow, H.L. (unpublished). Diazepam enhances different amphetamine-induced behaviors depending on the initial environment.
Carter, L.J. and Beck, C.H.M. (unpublished). Variability of the perseverative teat-search sequence and righting reflex in the rat pup.

REFERENCES

Alberts, J.R. (1978) Huddling by rat pups: multisensory control of contact behavior. *J. Comp. Physiol. Psychol.*, **92**, 220–230.
Amsel, S. and Roussel, J. (1952) Motivational properties of frustration: effect on a running response of the addition of frustration to the motivational complex. *J. Exp. Psychol.*, **43**, 363–368.
Baldessarini, R.J. and Tarsy, D. (1976) Mechanisms underlying tardive dyskinesia. In: *The Basal Ganglia* (ed. M.D. Yahr), Raven Press, New York, pp. 433–446.
Beck, C.H.M. (1992) The environment modulates the mobility gradient, temporally if not sequentially. *Behav. Brain Sci.*, **15**, 268–269.
Beck, C.H.M. and Burger, L. (1992) Food granules elicit heavy drinking in polydipsic rats independently of meal duration. *Physiol. Behav.*, **51**, 419–423.
Beck, C.H.M., Chow, H.L. and Cooper, S.J. (1986a) Dose-related response of male rats to apomorphine: snout contact in the open field. *Physiol. Behav.*, **37**, 819–825.
Beck, C.H.M., Chow, H.L. and Cooper, S.J. (1986b) Initial environment influences amphetamine-induced stereotypy: subsequently environment change has little effect. *Behav. Neural Biol.*, **46**, 383–397.
Beck, C.H.M. and Cooper, S.J. (1986a) The effect of the β-carboline, FG 7142, on the

behavior of male rats in a living cage: an ethological analysis of social and nonsocial behavior. *Psychopharmacology*, **89**, 203–207.

Beck, C.H.M. and Cooper, S.J. (1986b) β-Carboline FG 7142-reduced aggression in male rats: reversed by the benzodiazepine receptor antagonist, RO 15-1788. *Pharmacol. Biochem. Behav.*, **24**, 1645–1649.

Beck, C.H.M. and Fibiger, H.C. (1992) Selective activation of the cerebral cortex of rats during conditioned and unconditioned stress: revealed by the immediate early gene, c-fos. *Soc. Neurosci. Abstr.*, **18**, 1565.

Beck, C.H.M. and Kalynchuk, L.E. (1992) Analysis of the ongoing behavior of rats in nonmatching-to-sample: improved acquisition and performance is related to facilitation of investigation. *Behav. Brain Res.*, **48**, 171–176.

Beck, C.H.M. and Loh, E.A. (1990) Reduced variability in extinction: effect of chronic treatment with the benzodiazepine, diazepam or with ethanol. *Psychopharmacology*, **100**, 323–327.

Beck, C.H.M., Huh, J.S., Mumby, D.G. and Fundytus, M.E. (1989) Schedule-induced behavior in rats: pellets versus powder. *Anim. Learning Behav.*, **17**, 49–62.

Berridge, K.C. and Treit, D. (1986) Chlordiazepoxide directly enhances positive ingestive reactions. *Pharmacol. Biochem. Behav.*, **24**, 217–221.

Blundell, J. (1991) Pharmacological approaches to appetite suppression. *Trends Pharmacol. Sci.*, **12**, 147–157.

Bolles, R.C. (1970) Species-specific defense reactions and avoidance learning. *Psychol. Rev.*, **77**, 32–48.

Brett, L.P. and Levine, S. (1981) The pituitary–adrenal response to 'minimized' schedule-induced drinking. *Physiol. Behav.*, **26**, 153–158.

Broekkamp, C.L., Le Pichon, M. and Lloyd, K. (1984) The comparative effects of the benzodiazepines, progabide and PK 9084 on acquisition of passive avoidance in mice. *Psychopharmacology*, **78**, 8–18.

Buckland, C., Mellanby, J. and Gray, J.A. (1986) The effects of compounds related to gamma-aminobutyrate and benzodiazepine receptors on behavioural responses to anxiogenic stimuli in the rat: extinction and successive discrimination. *Psychopharmacology*, **88**, 285–295.

Chow, H.L. and Beck, C.H.M. (1984a) The effect of apomorphine on the open-field behavior of rats: alone and in pairs. *Pharmacol. Biochem. Behav.*, **21**, 85–88.

Chow, H.L. and Beck, C.H.M. (1984b) p-Chlorophenylalanine and p-chloroamphetamine pretreatment of apomorphine-challenged rats: effects on solitary and social behavior. *Eur. J. Pharmacol.*, **102**, 297–304.

Conti, L.H., Maciver, C.R., Ferkany, J.W. and Abreu, M.E. (1990) Footshock-induced freezing behavior in rats as a model for assessing anxiolytics. *Psychopharmacology*, **102**, 492–497.

Cooper, S.J. (1980) Effects of chlordiazepoxide and diazepam on feeding performance in a food-preference test. *Psychopharmacology*, **69**, 73–78.

Corey, D.T. (1978) The determinants of exploration and neophobia. *Neurosci. Biobehav. Rev.*, **2**, 235–253.

Costall, B., Domeney, A.M. and Naylor, T. (1982) Behavioral and biochemical consequences of persistent overstimulation of mesolimbic dopamine systems in the rat. *Neuropharmacology*, **21**, 327–335.

Cotman, C.W. and McGaugh, J.L. (1980) *Behavioral Neuroscience*. Academic Press, New York.

Crow, L.T. (1970) Is variability a unifying concept? *Psychol. Rec.*, **27**, 783–790.

Davies, C. and Steinberg, H.A. (1984) A biphasic effect of chlordiazepoxide on animal locomotor activity. *Neurosci. Lett.*, **46**, 247–251.

Dember, W.N. and Fowler, H. (1958) Spontaneous alternation behavior. *Psychol. Bull.*, **55**, 412–428.

Devenport, L. (1983) Spontaneous behavior: inferences from neuroscience. In: *Animal Cognition and Behavior* (ed. R.L. Mellgren). North-Holland, Amsterdam, pp. 83–124.

Devenport, L. (1989) Sampling behavior and contextual change. *Learn. Motiv.*, **20**, 107–114.

Dodman, N.H., Shuster, L. and Court, M.H. (1987) Investigation into the use of narcotic antagonists in the treatment of a stereotypic behavior pattern (crib-biting) in the horse. *Am. J. Vet. Res.*, **48**, 311–319.

Dourish, C.T. and Cooper, S.J. (1990) Neural basis of drug-induced yawning. In: *Neurobiology of Stereotyped Behaviour* (eds S.J. Cooper and C.T. Dourish). Clarendon Press, Oxford, pp. 91–116.

Drewett, R.F., Statham, C. and Wakerley, J.B. (1974) A quantitative analysis of the feeding behavior of suckling rats. *Anim. Behav.*, **22**, 907–913.

Edelman, G.M. (1987) *Neural Darwinism*. Basic Books, New York.

Eilam, D. and Golani, I. (1988) The ontogeny of exploratory behavior in the house rat (*Rattus rattus*): the mobility gradient. *Dev. Psychobiol.*, **21**, 679–710.

Ellinwood, E.H., Jr and Escalante, O.D. (1972) Chronic methamphetamine intoxication in three species of experimental animals. In: *Current Concepts in Amphetamine Abuse* (eds E.H. Ellinwood Jr and S. Cohen). US Government Printing Office, Washington, pp. 59–68.

Ellinwood, E.H., Jr and Kilbey, M.M. (1975) Amphetamine stereotypy: the influence of environmental factors and prepotent behavioral patterns on its topography and development. *Biol. Psychiatry*, **10**, 3–16.

Ernst, A.M. (1967) Mode of action of apomorphine and dexamphetamine on gnawing compulsion in rats. *Psychopharmacologia*, **28**, 35–41.

Falk, J.L. (1967) Control of schedule-induced polydipsia: type, size and spacing of meals. *J. Exp. Anal. Behav.*, **10**, 199–206.

Fanselow, M.J. and Helmstetter, F.J. (1988) Conditional analgesia, defensive freezing, and benzodiazepines. *Behav. Neurosci.*, **102**, 233–243.

File, S.E. (1982) Colony aggression: effects of benzodiazepines on intruder behavior. *Physiol. Psychol.*, **10**, 413–416.

Frick, F.C. and Miller, G.A. (1951) A statistical description of operant conditioning. *Am. J. Psychol.*, **64**, 20–36.

Golani, I. (1992) A mobility gradient in the organization of vertebrate movement: the perception of movement through symbolic language. *Behav. Brain Sci.*, **15**, 249–308.

Golani, I., Bronchti, G., Moualem, D. and Teitelbaum, P. (1981) 'Warm-up' along dimensions of movements in the ontogeny of exploration in rats and other infant mammals. *Proc. Natl Acad. Sci. USA*, **78**, 7226–7229.

Gordon, D. and Beck, C.H.M. (1984) Subacute apomorphine injections in rats: effects on components of behavioral stereotypy. *Behav. Neural Biol.*, **41**, 200–208.

Hall, W.G. (1979) The ontogeny of feeding in rats: I. Ingestive and behavioral response to oral infusions. *J. Comp. Physiol. Psychol.*, **93**, 977–1000.

Hall, W.G. and Rosenblatt, J.S. (1977) Suckling behavior and intake control in the developing rat pup. *J. Comp. Physiol. Psychol.*, **91**, 1232–1247.

Hommer, D.W., Skolnick, P. and Paul, S.M. (1987) The benzodiazepine/GABA receptor complex and anxiety. In: *Psychopharmacology: The Third Generation of Progress* (ed H.Y. Meltzer). Raven Press, New York, pp. 977–984.

Hosoda, T. (1950) On the heritability and susceptibility to wind-sucking in horses. *Jpn. J. Zootech. Sci.*, **21**, 25–28.

Itoh, H. and Takaori, S. (1968) Effects of psychotropic agents on rats in a Y-shaped box. *Jpn. J. Pharmacol.*, **18**, 344–352.

Janssen, P.A., Niemegeers, C.J.E., Schellekens, K.H.L. and Lenaerts, F.M. (1963) Is it possible to predict the clinical effects of neuroleptic drugs (major tranquilizers) from animal data? Part IV: An improved experimental design for measuring the inhibitory effects of neuroleptic drugs in amphetamine-induced 'chewing' and 'agitation' in rats. *Arzneimittelforschung*, 17, 841–854.

Kalynchuk, L.E. and Beck, C.H.M. (1992) Behavioral analysis of diazepam-induced memory deficits: evidence for sedation-like effects. *Psychopharmacology*, **106**, 297–302.

Klemm, W.R. (1990) The behavioral readiness response. In: *Brainstem Mechanisms of Behavior* (eds W.R. Klemm and R.P. Vertes). Wiley, New York, pp. 105–145.

Kokkinidis, L. and Anisman, H. (1980) Amphetamine models of paranoid schizophrenia: an overview and elaboration of animal experimentation. *Psychol. Bull.*, **88**, 551–579.

Koob, G.F., Braestrup, C. and Thatcher-Britton, K. (1986) The effects of FG 7142 and RO 15-1788 on the release of punished responding by chlordiazepoxide and ethanol in the rat. *Psychopharmacology*, **90**, 176–178.

Lambert, R.W., Goldberg, L.J. and Chandler, S.H. (1986) Comparison of mandibular movement trajectories and associated patterns of oral muscle electromyographic activity during spontaneous and apomorphine-induced rhythmic jaw movements in the guinea pig. *J. Neurophysiol.*, **55**, 301–319.

Loh, E.A. and Beck, C.H.M. (1989) Rats treated chronically with the benzodiazepine, diazepam or with ethanol exhibit reduced variability of behavior. *Alcohol*, **6**, 311–316.

Lyons, M. and Robbins, T. (1975) The action of central nervous system stimulant drugs: a general theory concerning amphetamine effects, Vol. 2. In: *Current Developments in Psychopharmacology* (eds W. Essman and L. Valzelli). Spectrum, New York, pp. 79–163.

Mackintosh, N.J. (1969) Habit-reversal and probability learning: rats, birds, and fish. In: *Animal Discrimination Learning* (eds R.M. Gilbert and N.S. Sutherland). Academic Press, New York, pp. 175–185.

Mazmanian, D.S. and Roberts, W.A. (1983) Spatial memory in rats under restricted viewing conditions. *Learning Motivation*, **14**, 123–129.

McKenzie, G.M. (1971) Apomorphine-induced aggression in the rat. *Brain Res.*, **34**, 323–330.

Mellgren, R.L., Misasi, L. and Brown, S.W. (1984) Optimal foraging theory: prey density and travel requirements in *Rattus norvegicus*. *J. Comp. Psychol.*, **98**, 142–153.

Miczek, K.A. (1974) Intraspecies aggression in rats: effects of *d*-amphetamine and chlordiazepoxide. *Psychopharmacologia*, **39**, 275–301.

Mittleman, G. and Valenstein, E.S. (1984) Ingestive behavior evoked by hypothalamic stimulation and schedule-induced polydipsia are related. *Science*, **224**, 415–417.

Mittleman, G. and Valenstein, E.S. (1985) Individual differences in non-regulatory ingestive behavior and catecholamine systems. *Brain Res.*, **348**, 112–117.

Mittleman, G., Castaneda, E., Robinson, T.E. and Valenstein, E.S. (1986) The propensity for nonregulatory ingestive behavior is related to differences in dopamine systems: behavioral and biochemical evidence. *Behav. Neurosci.*, **100**, 213–200.

Mumby, D. and Beck, C.H.M. (1988) Schedule-induced polydipsia: attenuating effects of decreased size of food granulations. *Physiol. Behav.*, **43**, 375–381.

Mumford, L., Teixeira, A.R. and Kumar, A. (1979) Sources of variation in locomotor activity and stereotypy in rats treated with *d*-amphetamine. *Psychopharmacology*, **62**, 241–245.

Naruse, T. and Asami, T. (1987) Intravenous self-administration of diazepam in rats. *Eur. J. Pharmacol.*, **135**, 365–373.

Nicholson, A.N. and Wright, C.M. (1974) Inhibitory and disinhibitory effects of nitrazepam, diazepam and flurazepam hydrochloride on delayed matching behaviour in monkeys (*Macaca mulatta*). *Neuropharmacology*, **13**, 919–926.

Olds, M.E. (1966) Facilitatory action of diazepam and chlordiazepoxide on hypothalamic reward behavior. *J. Comp. Physiol. Psychol.*, **62**, 136–140.

Olivier, B. van Aken, H., Jaarsma, I. *et al.* (1984) Behavioural effects of psychoactive drugs on agonistic behaviour of male territorial rats (resident–intruder model). In: *Ethopharmacological Aggression Research* (eds K.A. Miczek, M.R. Kruk and B. Olivier). Liss, New York, pp. 137–156.

Page, S. and Neuringer, A. (1985) Variability as an operant. *J. Exp. Psychol. Anim. Behav. Proc.*, **11**, 429–452.

Pedersen, P.E. and Blass, E.M. (1981) Olfactory control over suckling in albino rats. In: *Development of Perception: Psychobiological Perspectives* (eds R.N. Aslin, J.R. Alberts and M.R. Peterson). Academic Press, New York, pp. 201–219.

Pellow, S. and File, S.E. (1986) Anxiolytic and anxiogenic drug effects in exploratory activity in an elevated plus maze: a novel test of anxiety in the rat. *Pharmacol. Biochem. Behav.*, **24**, 525–529.

Petrinovich, L. (1984) A two-factor dual-process theory of habituation and sensitization. In: *Habituation, Sensitization and Behavior* (eds H.V.S. Peeke and L. Petrinovich). Academic Press, Orlando, FL, pp. 15–55.

Pico, R.M. and Davis, J.L. (1984) The radial maze performance of mice: assessing the dimensional requirements for serial order memory in animals. *Behav. Neural. Biol.*, **49**, 2–26.

Poling, A., Picker, M., Vande Polder, D. and Clark, R. (1986) Chronic effects of ethosuximide, phenytoin, clonazepam, and valporic acid on delayed-matching-to-sample performance of pigeons. *Psychopharmacology*, **88**, 301–304.

Pope, S.G., Dean, P. and Redgrave, P. (1980) Dissociation of *d*-amphetamine-induced locomotor activity and stereotyped behavior by lesions of the superior colliculus. *Psychopharmacology*, **70**, 297–302.

Pringle, J.W.S. (1951) On the parallel between learning and evolution. *Behaviour*, **3**, 174–215.

Reid, L.D., Hunter, G.A., Beaman, C.M. and Hubbell, C.L. (1985) Toward understanding ethanol's capacity to be reinforcing: a conditioned place preference following injections of ethanol. *Pharmacol. Biochem. Behav.*, **22**, 483–487.

Robbins, T.W., Mittleman, G., Molloy, A.G. *et al.* (1990) In: *Neurobiology of Stereotyped Behaviour* (eds S.J. Cooper and C.T. Dourish). Clarendon Press, Oxford, pp. 25–63.

Robinson, T.E. and Becker, J.B. (1986) Enduring changes in brain and behavior produced by chronic amphetamine administration: a review of animal models of amphetamine psychosis. *Brain Res. Rev.*, **11**, 157–198.

Robinson, T.E., Becker, J.B. and Presty, S.K. (1982) Long-term facilitation of amphetamine-induced rotational behavior and striatal dopamine release produced by a single exposure to amphetamine: sex differences. *Brain Res.*, **253**, 231–241.

Robinson, T.E. and Berridge, K.C. (1993) The neural basis of drug craving: an incentive-sensitization theory of addiction. *Brain Res. Rev.*, **18**, 247–291.

Rodrigo, G. and Lusiardo, M. (1988) Effects on memory following a single dose of diazepam. *Psychopharmacology*, **95**, 263–267.

Roper, T.J. (1981) What is meant by the term 'schedule-induced,' and how general is schedule induction? *Anim. Learning Behav.*, **9**, 433–440.

Rushton, R. and Steinberg, H. (1966) Combined effects of chlordiazepoxide and dexamphetamine on activity of rats in an unfamiliar environment. *Nature*, **211**, 1312–1313.

Russell, W.M.S. (1962) Evolutionary concepts in behavioral science: IV. The analogy between organic and individual behavioral evolution, and the evolution of intelligence. *Gen. Systems*, **7**, 157–193.

Sanger, D.J. and Blackman, D.E. (1975) The effects on the development of adjunctive drinking in rats. *Q. J. Exp. Biol.*, **27**, 499–505.

Schapiro, S. and Salas, M. (1970) Behavioral response of infant rats to maternal odours. *Physiol. Behav.*, **5**, 815–817.

Seligman, M.E.P. (1970) On the generality of the laws of learning. *Psychol. Rev.*, 77, 406–418.

Spyraki, C. and Fibiger, H.C. (1988) A role for the mesolimbic dopamine system in the reinforcing properties of diazepam. *Psychopharmacology*, 94, 131–137.

Spyraki, C., Kazandjian, A. and Varonos, D. (1985) Diazepam-induced place preference conditioning: appetitive and antiaversive properties. *Psychopharmacology*, 87, 225–232.

Staddon, J.R. (1976) Learning as adaptation. In: *Handbook of Learning and Cognitive Processes*, Vol. 2 (ed. W.K. Estes). Erlbaum, New York, pp. 37–98.

Steele, C.M. and Southwick, L. (1985) Alcohol and social behavior. I: The psychology of drunken excess. *J. Pers. Soc. Psychol.*, 48, 18–34.

Stern, J.M. and Johnson, S.K. (1990) Ventral somatosensory determinants of nursing behavior in Norway rats. I. Effects of variations in the quality and quantity of pup stimuli. *Physiol. Behav.*, 47, 993–1011.

Szechtman, H. (1986) Behavior performed at onset of drug action and apomorphine stereotypy. *Eur. J. Pharmacol.*, 121, 49–56.

Szechtman, H., Ornstein, K., Teitelbaum, P. and Golani, I. (1982) Snout-contact fixation, climbing and gnawing during apomorphine stereotypy in rats from two substrains. *Eur. J. Pharmacol.*, 80, 385–392.

Szechtman, H., Ornstein, K., Teitelbaum, P. and Golani, I. (1985) The morphogenesis of stereotyped behavior induced by the dopamine receptor agonist apomorphine in the laboratory rat. *Neuroscience*, 14, 783–798.

Szechtman, H., Eilam, D., Teitelbaum, P. and Golani, I. (1988) A different look at measurement and interpretation of drug-induced stereotyped behavior. *Psychobiology*, 16, 164–173.

Tan, S., Kirk, R.C., Abraham, W.C. and McNaughton, N. (1990) Chlordiazepoxide reduces discriminability but not rate of forgetting in delayed conditional discrimination. *Psychopharmacology*, 101, 550–554.

Tazi, A., Dantzer, R. and Le Moal, M. (1988) Schedule-induced polydipsia experience decreases locomotor response to amphetamine. *Brain Res.*, 445, 211–215.

Terry, L.M. and Johanson, I.B. (1987) Olfactory influences on the ingestive behavior of infant rats. *Dev. Psychobiol.*, 20, 313–352.

Thiebot, M.H., Le Bihan, C., Soubrie, P. and Simon, P. (1985) Benzodiazepines reduce the tolerance to reward delays in rats. *Psychopharmacology*, 86, 147–152.

Todd, K.G., Beck, C.H.M. and Martin-Iverson, M.T. (1992) Effects of D1 and D2 antagonists on behavior of polydipsic rats. *Pharmacol. Biochem. Behav.*, 42, 381–388.

Treit, D., Pinel, J.P.J. and Fibiger, H.C. (1981) Conditioned defensive burying: a new paradigm for the study of anxiolytic agents. *Pharmacol. Biochem. Behav.*, 15, 619–626.

Vanderwolf, C.H. and Szechtman, H. (1987) Electrophysiological correlates of stereotyped sniffing in rats injected with apomorphine. *Pharmacol. Biochem. Behav.*, 26, 299–304.

Vogel, J.R. and Principi, K. (1971) Effects of chlordiazepoxide on depressed performance after reward reduction. *Psychopharmacologia*, 21, 8–12.

Weiner, W.J., Goetz, C. and Klawans, H.L. (1975) Serotonergic and antiserotonergic influences on apomorphine-induced stereotyped behavior. *Acta Pharmacol. Toxicol.*, 36, 155–159.

Wetherington, C.L. (1982) Is adjunctive behavior a third class of behavior? *Neurosci. Biobehav. Rev.*, 6, 329–350.

Wetherington, C.L. and Riley, A.L. (1986) Diminution of schedule-induced polydipsia after a long rest period. *Physiol. Behav.*, 37, 375–378.

White, N.M. (1989) Reward or reinforcement: what's the difference? *Neurosci. Biobehav. Rev.*, 13, 181–186.

Widgiz, S.L.M. and Beck, C.H.M. (1990) Diazepam effects on the exploratory behavior of rats in an elevated runway: evidence for biphasic effects of benzodiazepines. *Behav. Brain Res.*, **40**, 109–118.

Williams, C.L., Rosenblatt, J.R. and Hall, W.G. (1979) Inhibition of suckling in weaning-age rats: a possible serotonergic mechanism. *J. Comp. Physiol. Psychol.*, **93**, 414–429.

15 Neurochemical Mechanisms Underlying Maternal Behaviour in the Rat

S. HANSEN

Department of Psychology, University of Göteborg, Sweden

INTRODUCTION

This chapter summarizes two sets of experiments from our laboratory. Their common denominator is that they focus on the behaviour of female rats during lactation. The first set highlights the way in which dopaminergic mechanisms may contribute to 'traditional' components of maternal behaviour, such as pup retrieval, nest-building and nursing. It will be suggested that the mesolimbic dopamine (DA) system primarily mediates activational aspects of maternal motivation and that mesolimbic DA dysfunction is associated with a peculiar form of maternal neglect which can be interpreted as a perceived devaluation of the intrinsic incentive properties of the pups.

The second set of experiments to be described is concerned with a less well-studied behavioural phenomenon observed during lactation in the rat: the apparent change in the affective appraisal of threatening stimuli, such that the mother acts less fearfully or anxiously than otherwise. Studies will be presented which suggest that it is the infants that alter their mother's emotionality, and that they may do so in part by modulating γ-aminobutyric acid (GABA) mechanisms in the mother's brain.

THE MEDIAL PREOPTIC AREA AND MATERNAL BEHAVIOUR

Like several other steroid hormone-dependent behaviours, maternal responsiveness appears to depend upon the integrity of the hypothalamus. There are at least three pieces of evidence which point to a special role for the medial preoptic area (mPOA), comprising the anterior part of the hypothalamus, in this regard. First, it has been clear for some time that lesions placed in the mPOA of postpartum lactating rats disrupt most aspects of maternal behaviour, including retrieving, nest-building and nursing responses (reviewed by Numan, 1990). More recently, Numan *et al.* (1988) demonstrated that axon-sparing excitotoxic degeneration of the mPOA reproduces the effect of

Ethology and Psychopharmacology. Edited by S.J. Cooper and C.A. Hendrie
© 1994 John Wiley & Sons Ltd

non-specific lesions on maternal behaviour. Damage to other major hypothalamic nuclei, such as the paraventricular nucleus (Numan and Corodimas, 1985) or the ventromedial nucleus (Hansen, 1989), exert minor effects on maternal responsiveness. Thus, lesion studies strongly suggest that medial preoptic cell bodies, and their efferent connections, appear to be most important for parental responsiveness in the rat.

The second source of evidence relates to the importance of the ovarian secretion of oestradiol and progesterone during the end of pregnancy for the initiation of maternal behaviour, at least in the nulliparous female rat. About two days before parturition the circulating levels of progesterone drop precipitously to low levels, whereas the circulating levels of oestradiol increase gradually during the latter half of pregnancy to reach peak levels at the time of delivery (Bridges, 1984, 1990). A number of studies show that this hormonal profile, and particularly the strong oestradiol signal, provides a necessary hormonal stimulus for the initiation of maternal behaviour (reviewed by Bridges, 1990). Intracerebral implants of oestradiol, if placed in the mPOA, stimulate the onset of maternal behaviour (Numan et al., 1977; Fahrbach and Pfaff, 1986). The mPOA contains numerous neurones with oestrogen receptors (e.g. Simerly et al., 1990).

A third, and recent, line of evidence linking the mPOA to maternal behaviour is the demonstration of enhanced expression of the immediate-early gene c-fos in cells of this region in females interacting with pups (Numan and Numan, 1992; see also Da Costa et al., 1992). According to Fleming et al. (1992), the mPOA is the only hypothalamic region showing significant activation, although increased c-fos immunoreactivity was present in parts of the limbic system (amygdala) and paralimbic cortex (piriform cortex). Observations such as these suggest that infants can activate medial preoptic neurones in their caretakers.

Considering these lesion, hormone implant and immunohistochemical studies, there can be little doubt that the medial preoptic area is at the heart of the neuronal circuitry mediating maternal behaviour.

PREOPTIC–VENTRAL TEGMENTAL AREA CONNECTIONS

The anatomical connections of the mPOA have been carefully mapped out (Simerly and Swanson, 1986, 1988; Swanson and Mogenson, 1981). Interestingly, this work shows that among the widespread mPOA projections there are direct connections of the preoptic region to the ventral tegmental area (VTA), which contains the A10 DA cell group, which, in turn, innervates the ventral striatum (including the nucleus accumbens), limbic areas and paralimbic cortical regions (see Swanson and Mogenson, 1981). The VTA neurones, which receive preoptic input, are probably mostly DAergic and project principally to the ventral striatum (Swanson, 1982).

Thus, there are anatomical pathways that permit hormone-sensitive preoptic mechanisms to modulate the functioning of the mesolimbic DA system with its pervasive involvement in incentive motivational mechanisms (Blackburn et al., 1992; Everitt, 1990; Robbins et al., 1989; Salamone, 1992). What, then, is the evidence that DA in general, and mesolimbic DA in particular, participates in the control of maternal behaviour?

DOPAMINE INVOLVEMENT IN MATERNAL BEHAVIOUR

Effects of non-specific lesions and dopamine antagonists

The behavioural consequences of early-lesion studies suggested that the meso-limbic DA system matched the mPOA in its importance for maternal behaviour. Consider for instance the study by Gaffori and Le Moal (1979; see also Numan and Smith, 1984), who investigated parturient female rats bearing radiofrequency lesions in the VTA. About a third of the lesioned rats cannibalized their young at parturition; the remaining subjects showed no interest whatsoever in the pups, no nursing, nest-building or pup retrieval being observed during the postoperative period. Consider also the high incidence of cannibalism and the severely disorganized maternal behaviour observed in mothers following lesions of the ventral striatum (Smith and Holland, 1975), and the lack of effect on maternal behaviour of dorsal striatal lesions (Kirkby, 1967).

Needless to say, the non-specific lesioning methods employed in these early studies do more than destroy DA neurones in the damaged area and so it is impossible to tell the extent to which the syndromes are derived from DA deficiency. However, studies in which lactating rats are treated with fairly selective DA receptor antagonists do reveal disturbances in pup-caring activities, though not quite as dramatic as the lesion studies would seem to indicate. For example, Giordano et al. (1990) found that haloperidol, in doses as low as 0.05–0.1 mg/kg, disrupted pup retrieval and nest-building. At the doses employed, the drug did not affect locomotor activity or food pellet carrying; importantly, neither nursing behaviour nor pup-licking were affected by the DA antagonist (Giordano et al., 1990). Subsequent work (Hansen et al., 1991a; Stern, 1991; Stern and Taylor, 1991) confirmed the vulnerability to DA receptor blockade of active maternal responses such as pup retrieval, and the relative resistance of nursing behaviour to the same treatment.

Interaction with pups enhances ventral striatal dopamine release

Considering the disruptive effects of DA receptor blockade on aspects of maternal behaviour, we wished to know whether mesostriatal DA neurones are activated when mother rats interact with pups. Lactating females were im-planted with a microdialysis probe in the ventral striatum and allowed to recover overnight while being separated from their infants (Hansen et al.,

1993). Microdialysis samples were then collected when no pups were present in her cage (baseline condition in Figure 1). The litter was then reunited with their mother for 1 h while sampling continued. Nursing was the predominant behaviour of the mother during this period and Figure 1 shows a concomitant rise in the levels of DA and its metabolites (clean pups). In order to elicit more active maternal behaviours, the pups were removed from the cage, smeared with flowerpot soil mixed with water and returned to the mother. The presence of dirty pups activated the mother behaviourally and stimulated ventral striatal DA release even further (Figure 1).

These data indicate that the mesolimbic DA system of maternal rats is activated by cues from newborns. The results suggest that infants in acute demand of active parental care—by being dirty, outside the nest, perhaps also cold and vocalizing due to the smearing procedure—are particularly effective in this regard.

The specific way in which pups modulate DA activity in the mother is unknown. One hypothesis is that olfactory mechanisms are involved; indeed it has been shown in other contexts that conspecific odours or activation of the accessory olfactory system stimulate mesolimbic DA transmission (Damsma *et al.*, 1992; Louilot *et al.*, 1991; Mitchell and Gratton, 1992a, 1992b). Another possibility is that snout contact with the young, which is crucial for maternal behaviour in rats (Kenyon *et al.*, 1983), in connection with sniffing, licking and retrieval activities plays a role because it has been demonstrated that tactile

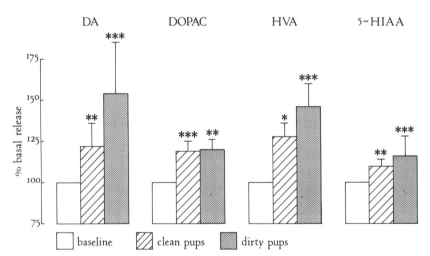

Figure 1 Changes in the extracellular concentrations of dopamine (DA), 3,4-dihydroxyphenylacetic acid (DOPAC), homovanillic acid (HVA) and 5-hydroxy-indoleacetic acid (5-HIAA) in the ventral striatum of maternal rats interacting with their pups after a period of separation. $*p < 0.05$, $**p < 0.02$, $***p < 0.01$ (Wilcoxon matched-pairs signed ranks test). (Reprinted from *Pharmacology, Biochemistry and Behaviour*, **45**, Hansen *et al.*, Interaction with pups enhances dopamine transmission in the ventral striatum of material rats: a microdialysis study, 673–676, 1993, with kind permission of Pergamon Press.)

information from the perioral region stimulates striatal DA release (Adams *et al.*, 1991). Endocrine mechanisms associated with suckling may also be involved: for example, there is evidence that prolactin, the levels of which are enhanced in the cerebrospinal fluid of nursing females (Rubin and Bridges, 1991), stimulates striatal DA release in the rat (Laping *et al.*, 1991).

Regardless of mechanism, the demonstration that infants can activate DA release in the ventral striatum of their mothers is yet another example of how social cues from significant others regulate forebrain DA activity in rodents. For example, guinea-pig mothers modulate DA turnover in the septum in their infants (Tamborski *et al.*, 1990), aggressive male rats enhance DA release in the nucleus accumbens of submissive individuals (Louilot *et al.*, 1986), and sexually attractive female rats increase ventral striatal DA release in males (Damsma *et al.*, 1992). Thus, a rather wide range of social circumstances cause elevated DA release in the ventral striatum, and it is unlikely, therefore, that this neuronal event is concerned with motivational specificity and the activation of the specific behaviours appropriate to the situation; it seems more plausible that DA serves a facilitatory role that serves to enhance the general readiness to respond (e.g. Blackburn *et al.*, 1992). Mechanisms related to response selection and the directedness of behaviour are more likely to involve non-DA limbic and cortical afferents to the ventral striatal target neurones (e.g. Cador *et al.*, 1991).

6-OHDA-induced mesolimbic dopamine lesions disrupt pup retrieval

Because pup exposure seems to be associated with enhanced DA release in maternal rats (Hansen *et al.*, 1993), it would be of interest to know the behavioural consequences of specific damage to the mesolimbic DA system. We addressed this question by investigating the effect of the selective catecholamine neurotoxin 6-OHDA, infused either into the VTA (the A10 DA cell body region) or into the ventral or dorsal striatum (DA terminal areas). The females were lesioned on day 2–3 post partum, allowed two days of recovery and given six daily observations for maternal behaviours. The tests included observations of nursing (crouching over the pups in the nest), nest-building (constructing and maintaining a nest out of shredded newspaper) and pup retrieval (carrying stray pups back into the nest).

Figure 2 shows that females receiving midbrain 6-OHDA were indistinguishable from sham-operated controls with regard to nursing and nest-building. By contrast, the latency to retrieve pups into the nest was greatly prolonged in the lesioned females. On many tests the experimental mothers failed to carry young altogether, and occasionally non-retrieving 6-OHDA mothers were observed to carry nest material in their mouths during the retrieval tests (Hansen *et al.*, 1991a).

6-OHDA infusions in the ventral striatum (an important target area for VTA DA fibres) resulted in a similar behavioural syndrome. Thus, nursing and nest-building appeared intact whereas the time taken to retrieve displaced

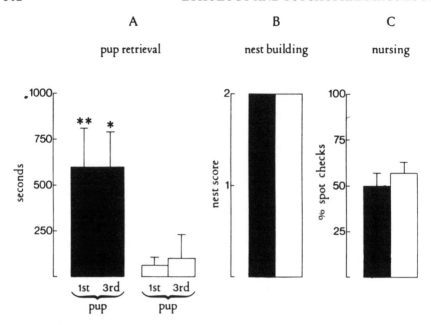

Figure 2 Maternal behaviours of rats that received 6-OHDA (shaded bars) or vehicle (open bars) into the ventral tegmental area three to four days post partum. The data are expressed as medians ± semi-interquartile ranges. (A) Latency to receive pups in 10 min tests. (B) Quality of nest, as rated on a three-point scale. (C) percentage of spot checks on which the females were crouching over the litter in the nest. $*p < 0.05$, $**p < 0.02$ versus vehicle (Mann–Whitney U-test). (Reproduced from Hansen *et al.*, 1991a, by permission of the American Psychological Association.)

pups was much longer than in control mothers; as was the case for mothers receiving VTA 6-OHDA infusions, the subjects with ventral striatal lesions often failed to retrieve any pup during the 10 min observations. 6-OHDA lesions in the dorsal striatum, which is mainly innervated by DA fibres originating in the substantia nigra, did not affect pup retrieval or any other parameter of maternal behaviour (Hansen *et al.*, 1991b).

Apart from the observation that non-retrieving 6-OHDA rats would approach and sniff the pups in the beginning of a test, we had little idea as to the preferred activity of DA-depleted mothers. Their behaviour was therefore monitored during an extended (30 min) pup retrieval test (Hansen, 1993b). It was found that feeding was the predominant behaviour, occupying over 70% of the testing time. In the absence of studies indicating hyperphagia in 6-OHDA-treated rats, it seems reasonable to assume, in accordance with McFarland's (1974) time-sharing theory, that the high levels of feeding were caused indirectly by the pup retrieval deficit. Hence, because 6-OHDA mothers are unlikely to retrieve their pups, they are more liable to engage in some other motivated activity relevant to motherhood. Since lactation is accompanied by considerable hyperphagia in the rat (e.g. Lindén *et al.*, 1990), feeding con-stitutes an easily elicited behaviour during lactation that might readily sub-stitute for pup retrieval in the 6-OHDA mother.

These findings suggest that the strong tendency of maternal rats to retrieve infants placed outside the nest depends upon the integrity of the mesolimbic DA system.

Restoration of pup retrieval of 6-OHDA mothers by increasing maternal motivation

Research on DA mechanisms in other motivational contexts suggests that activation of the mesolimbic DA system heightens the responsiveness to incentive properties of biologically significant stimuli, which in turn induces a general readiness to perform active behaviours (e.g. Blackburn *et al.*, 1992). The involvement of DA in this process is perhaps most clearly displayed in situations requiring some degree of perceptual, cognitive or motor effort and endurance (e.g. Salamone, 1987). Accordingly, it is possible to view the pup retrieval deficit of mothers with mesolimbic DA dysfunction as being caused by a perceived devaluation of the intrinsic incentive properties of distressed pups in an unsheltered area. We reasoned that if this interpretation was correct, then alterations of the test procedure that enhance, for instance, the pups' salience or the mother's motivation might remedy the pup retrieval deficit.

In our standard tests for pup retrieval, the entire litter is typically removed from the home cage, and three of the pups are then placed in the corner opposite to the nest within 1–3 min (Hansen *et al.*, 1991a, 1991b). The next experiment (Hansen, 1993b) assessed three modifications of the standard test procedure, all of which arguably enhance in various ways the incentive value of the displaced infants. In the *first* condition the stimulus pups were treated with clonidine—a drug that stimulates the emission of ultrasonic vocalizations (e.g. Hansen, 1993a)—before the retrieval test. Because infant distress calls stimulate maternal searching behaviour and facilitate pup retrieval, it was hoped that the retrieval performance of 6-OHDA females might improve under this condition. In the *second* condition the interval between litter removal and testing was lengthened from a few minutes to 3 h; an unnaturally long period of separation from the infants that might increase the motivation to carry pups and initiate nursing. *Third*, we considered the possibility that since the whole litter is removed from the nest before conducting the actual pup-retrieval test, the nest site might rapidly lose its status as a preferred place with special affective significance, and thereby impair pup retrieval; indeed, the mesolimbic DA system appears crucial for the formation of affective bonds to particular places (reviewed by Carr *et al.*, 1989). Thus part of the litter was allowed to remain in the nest during the pup-retrieval test.

Figure 3 shows that prolonged separation (3 h) improved pup retrieval in the

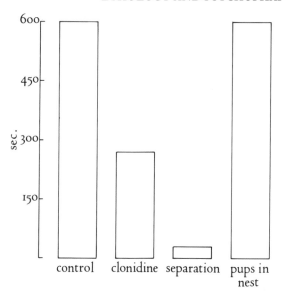

Figure 3   Median latency to retrieve pups of maternal rats with 6-OHDA lesions in the ventral striatum. The mothers were observed under standard test conditions (control); when the stimulus pups were exposed to clonidine to stimulate ultrasonic callings (clonidine); following 3 h of separation from the pups (separation); and allowing part of the litter to remain in the nest during testing (pups in nest). The latency to retrieve following separation was significantly shorter than under the other conditions ($p < 0.01$; Wilcoxon matched-pairs signed ranks test). (From Hansen, 1993b.)

6-OHDA mother rats. None of the other treatments were effective, though a non-significant trend towards shorter retrieval latencies was seen in tests with clonidine-treated stimulus pups (Figure 3).

The observation that prolonged pup separation restores pup retrieval in mothers with mesolimbic DA dysfunction is consistent with the idea that ventral striatal DA deficiency reduces the perceived incentive qualities of pups, that normally activate rapid pup retrieval. In the absence of a response-promoting DA system (cf. Blackburn *et al.*, 1992), the performance of mothers becomes dependent upon additional activating cues (arising from prolonged separation from the litter) that play little role in the normal mother. This line of reasoning is not unlike that which underlies studies demonstrating that supplementary environmental stimulation can override the motor symptoms of rats with nigrostriatal lesions (reviewed by Salamone, 1992).

However, the exact mechanism whereby prolonged pup separation reactivates pup retrieval remains to be specified. One possibility is that separation increases general drive, which might activate any well-established response. However, 6-OHDA mothers deprived of food rather than pups for several hours showed no improvement in pup retrieval, suggesting that the restoration of pup retrieval was due to an increase in maternal motivation specifically (Hansen, 1993b). Given that lengthy separation from infants is associated with milk engorgement of the mammary glands, another possibility is that this maternal form of visceral arousal helps the mother to attend to the sensory cues emitted by the infants and thereby promotes pup retrieval.

A theoretically important question for further research is to disentangle the neurobiological mechanism whereby separation from pups remedies the pup-retrieval deficit in mothers with ventral striatal DA lesions. One possibility is that the effect depends on residual DA mechanisms: for example, pup separation may be associated with enhanced release of DA, which, by acting on DA receptors on striatal neurones, temporarily normalizes neuronal function and thereby restores pup-carrying. An alternative is that pup separation affects neuronal activity in limbic and paralimbic brain areas which influence the ventral striatum by non-DA mechanisms (cf. McGeorge and Faull, 1989). Thus, abnormally long pup separations might heighten the activity in limbic areas concerned with maternal behaviour to such an extent that facilitatory DA mechanisms become unnecessary.

AFFECTIVE BEHAVIOUR IN THE MOTHER RAT

Behavioural and neuroendocrine responses to threat in lactating rats

In addition to the direct caring for of the infants, motherhood in the rat is also associated with alterations in several other realms of behaviour, such as emotional and affective behaviours. These behavioural adaptations probably complement direct pup-caring activities. For example, the unusual aggressiveness towards foreign adult conspecifics that is normally seen in lactating rats (e.g. Hansen and Ferreira, 1986a, 1986b) probably serves to protect the litter from non-parental, potentially hostile conspecifics that might harm the infants. The neural circuitry mediating offensive maternal aggression is at least partly separate from that controlling maternal pup-caring activities: it includes, for instance, the ventromedial hypothalamic nucleus, the peripeduncular region of the lateral midbrain and the supraoptic decussations connecting these areas (Hansen, 1989; Hansen and Ferreira, 1986a, 1986b; Hansen et al., 1985). Olfactory mechanisms and perhaps also suckling stimulation seem important for maternal aggression (Ferreira and Hansen, 1986; Ferreira et al., 1987; Hansen and Ferreira, 1986b).

Recent evidence also suggests that mother rats are less fearful of threats than cycling females. This was first reported by Fleming and Luebke (1981), who observed the behaviour of parturient and virgin females placed in a start box connected to an unfamiliar open-field arena. They found that mothers, in comparison with virgins, entered the novel arena with shorter latency and that they ambulated and reared more in the open field. More evidence for reduced fear during motherhood was presented in a study by Hård and Hansen (1985), in which the freezing responses of mothers and virgins subjected to a brief auditory signal were compared. Mothers were found to freeze for a shorter period of time than virgins; indeed, 50% of the lactating females failed to freeze at all. Freezing is one of several manifestations of the defensive motivational system, the activation of which is considered as fear (Bolles, 1970). Another expression of this motivational system—shock-induced defensive fighting (Blanchard and Blanchard, 1984)—is similarly suppressed in the lactating rat (Thoman et al., 1970).

There are neuroendocrine parallels to the apparent reduction in the behavioural response to threats during lactation; for example, stressful stimuli, such as exposure to ether vapours or immobilization, elicit release of adrenocortical steroids and of oxytocin in virgin rats, but these hormonal responses are considerably reduced in mothers (Carter and Lightman, 1986; Thoman et al., 1970).

Behaviour of lactating rats in conflict tests

Studies on the neurochemistry of fear and anxiety have predominantly employed conflict tests—in which the achievement of a desired goal is thwarted by aversive events—to induce an anxiety-like state in the rat (reviewed by Iversen, 1983). Conflict can, for example, be generated by allowing thirsty rats to drink from an electrified water spout (Vogel et al., 1971) or by allowing hungry rats to feed in unfamiliar, brightly lit surroundings (Britton and Britton, 1981). In these situations, normal rats typically show little drinking or eating. However, treatment with anxiolytics (e.g. a benzodiazepine) releases activities suppressed by punishment or novelty, such that drugged animals accept more shocks to obtain water (Vogel et al., 1971) and eat more in the open field (Britton and Britton, 1981). Although the interpretation of such anticonflict effects is not always straightforward (Treit, 1985), it is known that many drugs with this action relieve anxiety in people.

Given the evidence that lactating rats are less fearful than normal, we expected to see a naturally occurring anticonflict effect in mothers not unlike that observed in non-lactating subjects treated with a benzodiazepine. This hypothesis was assessed by comparing the behaviour of mothers and virgins in conflict situations, such as punished drinking and feeding in a novel arena (Britton and Britton, 1981; Vogel et al., 1971).

Figure 4 shows that thirsty (24 h of water deprivation) lactating females (tested one day after parturition) accepted more shocks than virgins to obtain water in the punished drinking test, the anticonflict effect being particularly pronounced when the pups were present in the test cage (Ferreira et al., 1989). Control experiments indicated that the anticonflict effect was not attributable to differences between virgins and mothers in pain sensitivity, thirst or housing conditions (Ferreira et al., 1989). Mothers and virgins also differed in the test for food intake in a novel arena: parturient females tested in the

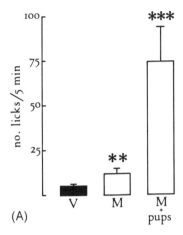

(A)

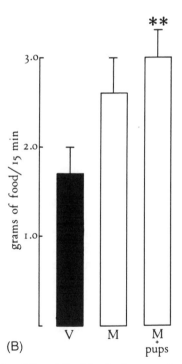

(B)

Figure 4 Punished drinking (A) and food intake in a novel arena (B) in virgin (V) and mother (M) rats (tested with or without pups) following 24 h of water or food deprivation. **$p < 0.02$, ***$p < 0.002$ versus virgins, Mann–Whitney U-test). (Reproduced from Ferreira *et al.*, 1989, by permission of the American Psychological Association.)

presence of pups ate significantly more food than did virgin controls following a 24 h fast (Figure 4; Ferreira et al., 1989). However, in a third conflict test—shock probe exploration (Meert and Colpaert, 1986)—the behaviour of mothers and virgins was similar (Ferreira et al., 1989).

These results suggest that mother rats differ from virgins in the way in which they assess and deal with anxiety-provoking conflict situations which elicit concurrent approach and avoidance tendencies. Bitran et al. (1991) recently reported the occurrence of reduced timidity in yet another animal test for anxiety, the elevated plus-maze. They found that parturient females were more prone to enter the open arms than were cycling or pregnant controls. Thus, an apparent anticonflict effect during motherhood can be demonstrated in several preclinical tests for anxiolytic activity.

Neurochemical studies of the maternal anticonflict effect

The anticonflict effect of benzodiazepines has been related to enhancement of GABA neurotransmission (reviewed by Haefely, 1985). Ferreira et al. (1989) therefore investigated whether lactation is associated with alterations in the binding of various ligands to the GABA receptor complex in brain tissue obtained from limbic and cortical areas. However, the binding characteristics of flunitrazepam, muscimol or TBPS did not differ between lactating and virgin females (Ferreira et al., 1989). In addition, the removal of the ovaries or adrenals—glands that secrete hormones with anticonflict actions (e.g. Crawley et al., 1986)—did not affect punished responding in mother rats (Hansen, 1990).

On the other hand, Qureshi et al. (1987) found that the cerebrospinal fluid concentration of GABA was considerably elevated in lactating rats, while pup removal decreased it within 6 h. Thus, increased availability of an endogenous ligand of the GABA receptor complex during lactation may underlie the tendency of maternal female rats to disregard aversive aspects in conflict situations. Needless to say, additional neurochemical mechanisms are also likely to be involved. For example, increased attention is being directed to serotonergic (e.g. Åsberg et al., 1987; Engel et al., 1984) and neuropeptide Y (Wahlestedt et al., 1993) mechanisms in anxiety. Adjustments during lactation in these and other systems may contribute to the altered emotionality of the puerperal rat. Further examination of the neurochemical processes underlying the effective changes of parturient rats may contribute to the understanding of the neurobiology of anxiety disorders, and may also help to explain the greatly enhanced risk for mental disorder observed in pre-disposed puerperal women (McNeil, 1987).

ACKNOWLEDGEMENTS

This work was supported by the Swedish MRC and The Bank of Sweden Tercentenary Foundation. I should like to thank my collaborators, including Annabel Ferreira,

Christina Harthon, Mogens Nielsen, Elisabeth Wallin-Wahlström and Kjell Svensson. Professor Steven J. Cooper gave valuable comments on a previous version of the manuscript.

REFERENCES

Adams, F., Schwarting, R.K.W., Boix, F. and Huston, J.P. (1991) Lateralized changes in behavior and striatal dopamine release following unilateral tactile stimulation of the perioral region: a microdialysis study. *Brain Res.*, **553**, 318–322.

Åsberg, M., Schalling, D., Träskman-Bendz, L. and Wägner, A. (1987) Psychobiology of suicide, impulsivity, and related phenomena. In: *Psychopharmacology: The Third Generation of Progress* (ed. H.Y. Meltzer). Raven Press, New York, pp. 655–668.

Bitran, D., Hilvers, R.J. and Kellogg, C.K. (1991) Ovarian endocrine status modulates the anxiolytic potency of diazepam and the efficacy of γ-aminobutyric acid–benzodiazepine receptor-mediated chloride ion transport. *Behav. Neurosci.*, **105**, 653–662.

Blackburn, J.R., Pfaus, J.G. and Phillips, A.G. (1992) Dopamine functions in appetitive and defensive behaviours. *Prog. Neurobiol.*, **39**, 247–279.

Blanchard, D.C. and Blanchard, R.J. (1984) Inadequacy of pain–aggression hypothesis revealed in naturalistic settings. *Aggressive Behav.*, **10**, 33–46.

Bolles, R.C. (1970) Species-specific defence reactions and avoidance learning. *Psychol. Rev.*, **77**, 32–48.

Bridges, R.S. (1984) A quantitative analysis of the roles of dosage, sequence, and duration of estradiol and progesterone exposure in the regulation of maternal behavior in the rat. *Endocrinology*, **114**, 930–940.

Bridges, R.S. (1990) Endocrine regulation of parental behavior in rodents. In: *Mammalian Parenting* (eds N.A. Krasnegor and R.S. Bridges). Oxford University Press, New York, pp. 93–117.

Britton, D.R. and Britton, K.T. (1981) A sensitive open field measure of anxiolytic drug activity. *Pharmacol. Biochem. Behav.*, **15**, 577–582.

Cador, M., Robbins, T.W., Everitt, B.J. *et al.* (1991) Limbic–striatal interactions in reward-related processes: modulation by the dopaminergic system. In: *The Mesolimbic Dopamine System: From Motivation to Action* (eds P. Willner and J. Scheel-Krüger). Wiley, New York, pp. 225–250.

Carr, G.D., Fibiger, H.C. and Phillips, A.G. (1989) Conditioned place preference as a measure of drug reward. In: *The Neuropharmacological Basis of Reward* (eds J.M. Liebman and S.J. Cooper). Clarendon Press, Oxford, pp. 264–319.

Carter, D.A. and Lightman, S.L. (1986) Oxytocin responses to stress in lactating and hyperprolactinaemic rats. *Abstr. 1st Int. Congr. Neuroendocr.*, **1**, 72.

Crawley, J.N., Glowa, J.R., Majewska, M.D. and Paul, S.M. (1986) Anxiolytic activity of an endogenous adrenal steroid. *Brain Res.*, **398**, 382–385.

Da Costa, A., Broad, K., Guevara, R. and Kendrick, K.M. (1992) Septal region and paraventricular nucleus: two neuroanatomical substrates controlling maternal behaviour in sheep. *Soc. Neurosci. Abstr.*, **22**, 369.7.

Damsma, G., Pfaus, J.G., Wenkstern, D. *et al.* (1992) Sexual behavior increases dopamine transmission in the nucleus accumbens and striatum of male rats: comparison with novelty and locomotion. *Behav. Neurosci.*, **106**, 181–191.

Engel, J.A., Hjorth, S., Svensson, K. *et al.* (1984) Anticonflict effect of the putative serotonin agonist 8-hydroxy-2-(di-*n*-propylamino)tetralin (8-OH-DPAT). *Eur. J. Pharmacol.*, **108**, 365–368.

Everitt, B.J. (1990) Sexual motivation: a neural and behavioural analysis of the mechanisms underlying appetitive and copulatory responses of male rats. *Neurosci. Biobehav. Rev.*, **14**, 217–232.

Fahrbach, S.E. and Pfaff, D.W. (1986) Effect of preoptic region implants of dilute estradiol on the maternal behavior of ovariectomized, nulliparous rats. *Horm. Behav.*, **20**, 354–363.

Ferreira, A. and Hansen, S. (1986) Studies on the sensory control of maternal aggression in *Rattus norvegicus*. *J. Comp. Psychol.*, **100**, 173–177.

Ferreira, A., Dahlöf, L.-G. and Hansen, S. (1987) Olfactory mechanisms in the control of maternal aggression, appetite, and fearfulness: effects of lesions to olfactory receptors, mediodorsal thalamic nucleus, and insular prefrontal cortex. *Behav. Neurosci.*, **101**, 709–717.

Ferreira, A., Hansen, S., Nielsen, S. *et al.* (1989) Behavior of mother rats in conflict tests sensitive to anxiolytic agents. *Behav. Neurosci.*, **103**, 193–201.

Fleming, A.S. and Luebke, C. (1981) Timidity prevents the virgin female rat from being a good mother: emotionality differences between nulliparous and parturient females. *Physiol. Behav.*, **27**, 863–870.

Fleming, A.S., Rusak, B. and Suh, E.J. (1992) *fos*-like immunoreactivity in brain of primiparous rats after mother–litter interactions. *Soc. Neurosci. Abstr.*, **22**, 364.20.

Gaffiori, O. and le Moal, M. (1979) Disruption of maternal behavior and appearance of cannabalism after ventral mesencephalic tegmentum lesions. *Physiol. Behav.*, **23**, 317–323.

Giordano, A.L., Johnson, A.E. and Rosenblatt, J.S. (1990) Haloperidol-induced disruption of retrieval behavior and reversal with apomorphine in lactating rats. *Physiol. Behav.*, **48**, 211–214.

Haefly, W. (1985) Tranquilizers. In: *Psychopharmacology 2, Part 1: Preclinical Psychopharmacology* (ed D.G. Grahame-Smith). Elsevier Science, Amsterdam, pp. 92–182.

Hansen, S. (1989) Medial hypothalamic involvement in maternal aggression of rats. *Behav. Neurosci.*, **103**, 1035–1046.

Hansen, S. (1990) Mechanisms involved in the control of punished drinking in the mother rat. *Horm. Behav.*, **24**, 186–197.

Hansen, S. (1993a) Effect of clonidine on the responsiveness of infant rats to maternal stimuli. *Psychopharmacology*, **111**, 78–84.

Hansen, S. (1993b) Maternal behavior of female rats with 6-OHDA lesions in the ventral striatum: characterization of the pup retrieval deficit. Submitted for publication.

Hansen, S. and Ferreira, A. (1986a) Food intake, aggression and fear behavior in the mother rat: control by neural systems concerned with milk ejection and maternal behavior. *Behav. Neurosci.*, **100**, 64–70.

Hansen, S. and Ferreira, A. (1986b) Effects of bicuculline infusions in the ventromedial hypothalamus and amygdaloid complex on food intake and affective behavior in mother rats. *Behav. Neurosci.*, **100**, 410–415.

Hansen, S., Ferreira, A. and Selart, M.E. (1985) Behavioural similarities between mother rats and benzodiazepine-treated non-lactating animals. *Psychopharmacology*, **86**, 344–347.

Hansen, S., Harthon, C., Wallin, E. *et al.* (1991a) Mesotelencephalic dopamine system and reproductive behavior in the female rat: effects of ventral tegmental 6-hydroxydopamine lesions on maternal and sexual responsiveness. *Behav. Neurosci.*, **105**, 588–598.

Hansen, S., Harthon, C., Wallin, E. *et al.* (1991b) The effects of 6-OHDA-induced dopamine depletions in the ventral or dorsal striatum on maternal and sexual behavior in the female rat. *Pharmacol. Biochem. Behav.*, **39**, 71–77.

Hansen, S., Bergvall, Å.H. and Nyiredi, S. (1993) Interaction with pups enhances dopamine transmission in the ventral striatum of maternal rats: a microdialysis study. *Pharmacol. Biochem. Behav.*, **45**, 673–676.

Hård, E. and Hansen, S. (1985) Reduced fearfulness in the lactating rat. *Physiol. Behav.*, **35**, 641–643.

Iversen, S.D. (1983) Animal models of anxiety. In *Benzodiazepines Divided* (ed. M.R. Trimble). Wiley, Chichester, pp. 87–99.

Kenyon, P., Cronin, P. and Keeble, S. (1983) Role of the infraorbital nerve in retrieving behavior in lactating rats. *Behav. Neurosci.*, **97**, 255–269.

Kirkby, R.J. (1967) Caudate nucleus lesions and maternal behavior in the rat. *Psychon. Sci.*, **9**, 601–602.

Laping, N.J., Dluzen, D.E. and Ramirez, V.D. (1991) Prolactin stimulates dopamine release from the rat corpus striatum in the absence of extra-cellular calcium. *Neurosci. Lett.*, **134**, 1–4.

Lindén, A., Uvnäs-Moberg, K., Forsberg, G. *et al.* (1990) Involvement of cholecystokinin in food intake: II. Lactational hyperphagia in the rat. *J. Neuroendocrinol.*, **2**, 791–796.

Louilot, A., Le Moal, M. and Simon, H. (1986) Differential reactivity of dopaminergic neurons in the nucleus accumbens in response to different behavioral situations: an in vivo voltammetric study in free moving rats. *Brain Res.*, **397**, 395–400.

Louilot, A., Gonzalez-Mora, J.L., Guadalupe, T. and Mas, M. (1991) Sex-related olfactory stimuli induce a selective increase in dopamine release in the nucleus accumbens of male rats. *Brain Res.*, **553**, 313–317.

McFarland, D.J. (1974) Time-sharing as a behavioral phenomenon. In: *Advances in the Study of Behavior*, Vol. 5 (eds D.S. Lehrman, J.S. Rosenblatt, R.A. Hinde and E. Shaw). Academic Press, New York, pp. 201–225.

McGeorge, A.J. and Faull, R.L.M. (1989) The organization of the projection from the cerebral cortex to the striatum in the rat. *Neuroscience*, **29**, 503–537.

McNeil, T.F. (1987) A prospective study of postpartum psychoses in a high-risk group. 2. Relationships to demographic and psychiatric history characteristics. *Acta Psychiatr. Scand.*, **75**, 35–43.

Meert, T.F. and Colpaert, F.C. (1986) The shock probe conflict procedure: a new assay responsive to benzodiazepines, barbiturates and related compounds. *Psychopharmacology*, **88**, 445–450.

Mitchell, J.B. and Gratton, A. (1992a) Mesolimbic dopamine release elicited by activation of the accessory olfactory system: a high speed chronoamperometric study. *Neurosci. Lett.*, **140**, 81–84.

Mitchell, J.B. and Gratton, A. (1992b) Partial dopamine depletion of the prefrontal cortex leads to enhanced mesolimbic dopamine release elicited by repeated exposure to naturally reinforcing stimuli. *J. Neurosci.*, **12**, 3609–3618.

Numan, M. (1990) Neural control of maternal behavior. In: *Mammalian Parenting* (eds N.A. Krasnegor and R.S. Bridges). Oxford University Press, New York, pp. 232–259.

Numan, M. and Corodimas, K.P. (1985) The effects of paraventricular hypothalamic lesions on maternal behavior in rats. *Physiol. Behav.*, **35**, 417–425.

Numan, M., Corodimas, K.P., Numan, M.J. *et al.* (1988) Axon-sparing lesions of the preoptic region and substantia innominata disrupt maternal behavior in rats. *Behav. Neurosci.*, **102**, 381–396.

Numan, M. and Numan, M.J. (1992) Maternal behavior in female rats is associated with increased numbers of *fos* containing neurons in the medial preoptic area. *Soc. Neurosci. Abstr.*, **22**, 370.12.

Numan, M., Rosenblatt, J.S. and Komisaruk, B.R. (1977) Medial preoptic area and onset of maternal behavior in the rat. *J. Comp. Physiol. Psychol.*, **91**, 146–164.

Numan, M. and Smith, H.G. (1994) Maternal behavior in rats: Evidence for the involvement of preoptic projections to the ventral tegmental area. *Behav. Neurosci.*, **98**, 712–727.

Qureshi, G.A., Hansen, S. and Södersten, P. (1987) Offspring control of cerebrospinal fluid GABA concentrations in lactating rats. *Neurosci. Lett.*, **75**, 85–88.

Robbins, T.W., Cador, M., Taylor, J.R. and Everitt, B.J. (1989) Limbic–striatal interactions in reward-related processes. *Neurosci. Biobehav. Rev.*, **13**, 155–162.

Rubin, B.S. and Bridges, R.S. (1991) Immunoreactive prolactin in the cerebrospinal fluid of estrogen-treated and lactating rats as determined by push–pull perfusion of the lateral ventricles. *J. Neuroendocrinol.*, **1**, 345–349.

Salamone, J.D. (1987) The actions of neuroleptic drugs on appetitive instrumental behaviors. In *Handbook of Psychopharmacology, Vol 19* (eds L.L. Iversen, S.D. Iversen and S.H. Snyder). Plenum, New York, pp. 575–608.

Salamone, J.D. (1992) Complex motor and sensorimotor functions of striatal and accumbens dopamine: involvement in instrumental behavior processes. *Psychopharmacology*, **107**, 160–174.

Simerly, R.B. and Swanson, L.W. (1986) The organization of neural inputs to the medial preoptic nucleus of the rat. *J. Comp. Neurol.*, **246**, 312–342.

Simerly, R.B. and Swanson, L.W. (1988) Projections of the medial preoptic nucleus: a *Phaseolus vulgaris* leucoagglutinin anterograde tract-tracing study in the rat. *J. Comp. Neurol.*, **270**, 209–242.

Simerly, R.B., Chang, C., Muramatsu, M. and Swanson, L.W. (1990) Distribution of androgen and estrogen receptor mRNA-containing cells in the rat brain: an in situ hydridization study. *J. Comp. Neurol.*, **294**, 76–95.

Smith, M.O. and Holland, R.C. (1975) Effects of lesions of the nucleus accumbens on lactation and postpartum behavior. *Physiol. Psychol.*, **3**, 331–336.

Stern, J.M. (1991) Nursing posture is elicited rapidly in maternally naive, haloperidol-treated female and male rats in response to ventral trunk stimulation from active pups. *Horm. Behav.*, **25**, 504–517.

Stern, J.M. and Taylor, L.A. (1991) Haloperidol inhibits maternal retrieval and licking, but enhances nursing behavior and litter weight-gains in lactating rats. *J. Neuroendocrinol.*, **3**, 591–596.

Swanson, L.W. (1982) The projections of the ventral tegmental area and adjacent regions: a combined fluorescent retrograde tracer and immunofluoresence study in the rat. *Brain Res. Bull.*, **9**, 321–353.

Swanson, L.W. and Mogenson, G.J. (1981) Neural mechanisms for the functional coupling of autonomic, endocrine and somatomotor responses in adaptive behavior. *Brain Res. Rev.*, **3**, 1–34.

Tamborski, A., Lucot, J.B. and Hennessy, M.B. (1990) Central dopamine turnover in guinea pig pups during separation from their mothers in a novel environment. *Behav. Neurosci.*, **104**, 607–611.

Thoman, E.B., Conner, R.L. and Levine, S. (1970) Lactation suppresses adrenal corticosteriod activity and aggressiveness in rats. *J. Comp. Physiol. Psychol.*, **70**, 364–369.

Treit, D. (1985) Animal models for the study of anti-anxiety agents: a review. *Neurosci. Biobehav. Rev.*, **9**, 203–222.

Vogel, J.R., Beer, B. and Clody, D.E. (1971) A simple and reliable conflict procedure for testing anti-anxiety agents. *Psychopharmacology*, **21**, 1–7.

Wahlestedt, C., Pich, E.M., Koob, G.F. *et al.* (1993) Modulation of anxiety and neuropeptide Y-Y1 receptors by antisense oligodeoxynucleotides. *Science*, **259**, 528–531.

16 The Neuropharmacology of Meal Patterning

PETER G. CLIFTON

Laboratory of Experimental Psychology, School of Biological Sciences, University of Sussex, Brighton, UK

INTRODUCTION

When considering any area of ethology it is always tempting to return to Niko Tinbergen's original conception of the four fundamental problems with which ethologists should be concerned (Tinbergen, 1951). One of these concerned the short-term causation of behaviour. Why for, example, are many behaviour patterns performed intensely, but for relatively short periods? What mechanisms allow an animal to produce organized sequences of behaviour? Why does an animal which is apparently motivated to either attack or flee break off from an agonistic encounter and produce a displacement activity such as grooming or feeding?

It is striking that ethologists' interest in causation has waned considerably over the last two decades, yet the interest in ethological techniques seen in the general area of behavioural neuroscience and psychopharmacology is on the increase. This shift has probably occurred, in part, because of theoretical advances in evolutionary biology that have driven empirical studies of the functional aspects of behaviour. At the same time it has seemed doubtful that purely observational techniques and experiments in which only behaviour is manipulated are likely to give a real understanding of causal mechanisms. However, the major advances in neuroanatomy and neurochemistry of recent years have begun to suggest increasingly detailed behavioural experiments in which ethological methods can have great value. Thus ethology's major contribution to the study of causation may be to provide appropriate techniques for the observation of behaviour which can then be combined with the manipulation of underlying neural or physiological substrates of behaviour. Tinbergen himself (e.g. Tinbergen, 1969) seems to have been sympathetic to such cross-fertilization, but other ethologists have felt much more reluctant to do other than to study and explain behaviour in its own terms, or in terms of a series of black boxes whose contents had better remain unseen (Baerends, 1970). The current lack of pure ethological studies of causation may denote a

Ethology and Psychopharmacology. Edited by S.J. and Cooper C.A. Hendrie
© 1994 John Wiley & Sons Ltd

dissatisfaction with this black box approach and the ascendancy of a more integrative approach to the study of behavioural causation.

OBSERVATIONAL STUDIES OF FEEDING

The initial phase of any ethological study is observational and this should apply to studies of ingestive behaviour. A descriptive study of feeding behaviour, even as seen in a rat housed in a relatively impoverished laboratory environment in which food and water are continuously available, shows a richness that is not apparent in a simple record of the number of grams of food eaten in a 30 min intake test after 23 h food deprivation.

Two components of such a description seem of especial relevance. First, even when food and water are continuously available, ingestive behaviour is concentrated into short periods of time when it occurs at high intensity. Explanations for this clustering may be sought at two levels. The short-term causal factors that elicit feeding are likely to persist over time, in part because there are delays between ingestion of food and its physiological consequences, and also because feeding may reinforce its own occurrence by, for example, bringing the animal into contact with reinforcing gustatory and olfactory cues. However, clustered feeding is also predicted by functional considerations. Gaining access to a food source may frequently entail risk, and it would therefore make sense to maximize the advantage obtained for a given risk. In addition, sources of food are likely, in all but laboratory environments, to be clustered in both temporal and spatial domains. Immediate presence of food will often indicate further food availability both nearby and in the next short period of time. Thus natural selection is likely to favour, in many species, causal mechanisms that cluster feeding behaviour.

As with any clustered behaviour, there is the difficulty of deciding just what constitutes a 'cluster' and whether there are several levels at which clusters can be recognized. In feeding, clusters at the levels of meals and bouts may be apparent. Log-survivorship analyses will suggest suitable time criteria to define such clusters (Slater and Lester, 1982; Clifton, 1987). The theoretical basis of the log-survivorship method rests on the fact that if feeding events were distributed at random in time then the intervals of time between feeding would have a Poisson distribution. If this distribution is replotted as a survivorship function, in which the numbers on the y-axis represent the numbers of intervals that survive to a given duration, then a Poisson distribution will give a straight line if the y-axis is logarithmic. Plots for feeding behaviour are rarely, if ever, fitted by a straight line and instead have a 'broken-stick' appearance that betrays the existence of at least two classes of interval: first, those intervals that occur within bouts of feeding and have a high probability of ending and, second, those intervals that occur between bouts of feeding and have a low probability of ending. For some data three underlying distributions may improve the fit to the data and suggest two levels of organization: *bouts* of feeding that occur within *meals*. Clifton (1987) and Sibly *et al.* (1990) discuss curve-fitting techniques which allow suitable criteria to be established for given data sets.

A second common component of descriptions of feeding is that it frequently occurs within a relatively limited behavioural context. Appetitive behaviour that provides access to food is followed by consummatory behaviour and behaviour indicative of satiety. Thus, in the laboratory rat, a period of bar-pressing may be succeeded by consumption of 45 mg food pellets, a period spent moving around the cage, an extended grooming sequence and rest. Lions may show similar sequences of hunting, food consumption, social grooming and rest in the wild (Schaller, 1972).

In the laboratory, satiety sequences were initially recorded by Antin *et al.* (1975) using a variant of one–zero recording. Presence or absence of each of a series of behavioural categories was recorded for each subject over successive 1 min periods. A disadvantage of this method is that the resulting scores do not provide good estimates of the proportion of time spent performing each behaviour. Instead scores for rare behaviour patterns are overestimates by comparison with those for common behaviour patterns. Montgomery and Wilner (1988) recorded which of several exclusively defined behaviour patterns were being performed by an individual at 15 s intervals. In practice the observer made a sequential scan through 12 individuals every 15 s making such judgements. Essentially the same method has been employed in a number of subsequent studies (Dourish *et al.*, 1989; Clifton *et al.*, 1989a; Willner *et al.*, 1990). The scores obtained from summing such scores over 5 or 10 min bins provide unbiased time budgets. The data are typically then analysed using standard parametric methods, although assumptions of normal distributions and continuously distributed data are usually not met and alternative techniques employing randomization methods may be more appropriate.

More detailed recordings of individual sequences of behaviour are required when detailed behavioural classification is appropriate. Such methods, often termed microstructural analysis, have been especially useful in the study of dopamine agonists where recognition of stereotypy and hyperactivity is crucial to theoretical interpretation of the data (e.g. Rusk and Cooper, 1989). However, the term microstructural analysis has also been used to describe detailed records of a single meal after prolonged food deprivation. In the latter studies feeding is monitored automatically and no observational data provided (e.g. Willner *et al.*, 1985).

There is one general problem, which seems not to have been seriously addressed before, when studying the short-lasting effects of acute drug treatment on sequences of behaviour that themselves last for many minutes or several hours. Effects of the drug may vary strongly during this period. Thus an increased latency to feed, reduced meal size and normal intermeal interval obtained after drug A compared with unchanged latency, reduced meal size and increased intermeal interval after drug B could be interpreted in two rather different ways. The changes might reflect drug A's action on 'hunger' (i.e. the initiation of food intake) and drug B's action on 'satiation' and 'satiety' (i.e. the termination of food intake), but might also simply reflect a short onset and offset of action by drug A contrasted with a longer onset and offset of action by drug B.

OBSERVATIONAL STUDIES AND CAUSATION

I have already referred to the general divergence of views within ethology regarding the level of explanation appropriate for causal questions. This is well illustrated by two aspects of feeding behaviour studied by ethologists and comparative psychologists.

Positive feedback and meal structure

Wiepkema (1971) reported that when mice fed they did so in a series of short bouts that formed part of a longer meal. Using direct observation after 23 h food deprivation, he noted that bout duration increased over the first part of a meal; intervals between bouts showed no change. He also showed that if the food was made unpalatable the increase in bout duration was abolished. From these observations he concluded that meals occur, in part, because feeding facilitates its own production. Curiously enough, although Wiepkema's work is frequently quoted, his observations have hardly ever been replicated. There are some limited human data suggesting that subjective changes in hunger follow a similar pattern (Hill *et al.*, 1984). There are no published data for the bout structure of meals, either after deprivation or during *ad libitum* feeding in the rat. This is unfortunate because, in combination with appropriate drug treatments, it would provide a direct way of testing the extent to which different neurochemical systems are involved in establishing a meal.

Prandial correlations

A second area in which behavioural observations were thought to reveal underlying causation was in the relationships, observed in free-feeding animals, between meal size and the intervals that preceded and followed feeding. The simplest expectation might be that the longer feeding is postponed, the larger the resulting meal size. Although this holds when animals are deprived of food, it is uncommon in free-feeding animals. Instead, meal size is positively correlated with the interval that follows a meal, though the correlations are fairly weak. Several views have been taken of such correlations, from the sceptical position that they are probably artifacts (Hirsch and Collier, 1974), to the idea that meal size is not strongly related to current deprivation state, although the postprandial duration of satiety is influenced by current meal size (LeMagnen, 1985).

In these examples two features are apparent. First, it is difficult to move from behavioural explanations to accounts in terms of underlying physiology and neurochemistry. Second, the mechanisms influencing food intake may be very different in deprivation-induced feeding and free feeding. In the remainder of this chapter I will consider the value and limitations of the behavioural methods described earlier in analysing the involvement of serotonin (5-HT), dopamine and certain neuropeptides in feeding behaviour.

5-HT AND FEEDING PATTERNS

Drugs that are likely to lead to non-specific stimulation of 5-HT systems include the amphetamine derivative fenfluramine and 5-HT reuptake inhibitors such as fluoxetine and sertraline. There are studies of each of these drugs examining meal patterning and satiety sequences. As Table 1 shows, meal patterning studies suggest several common features including reduced feeding rate and lowered meal size. Effects on intermeal interval are more variable, but it is likely that satiety ratio (the increment in intermeal interval seen for an increment in meal size) is reliably increased, although this parameter was not calculated in several of the quoted studies.

One important question of interpretation here is the extent to which we are dealing with separate effects. Although it is known that imposition of a reduced feeding rate in non-drugged animals will reduce meal size (Clifton et al., 1984), probably by interfering with positive feedback processes (Lucas and Timberlake, 1988), it requires a reduction of intake rate of 60% to produce a 50% reduction in meal size. In the studies shown in Table 1 a halving in meal size is typically associated with only a 20% reduction in intake rate. Thus reductions in meal size cannot be accounted for solely in terms of a reduction in feeding rate. An independent action of 5-HT that reduces meal size is the next simplest explanation.

Table 1   5-HT indirect agonists and meal patterns

	Meal size	Feeding rate	imi	Satiety ratio
dl-Fenfluramine	↓	↓	–	?
d-Fenfluramine	↓	↓	–	↑
Fluoxetine	↓	↓	–	↑
Sertraline	↓	↓	–	↑

Data summarized from Blundell and Latham (1978), Burton et al. (1981), Clifton et al. (1989a), Grignaschi and Samanin (1991). Meal size was generally measured directly, and feeding rate determined by dividing meal size by meal duration. Intermeal interval (imi) was the period between meals and satiety ratio was estimated by dividing mean intermeal interval by mean meal size. Since satiety ratios were estimated from tabulated values for other parameters, the indications of change in this table are speculative.

Pharmacological studies also suggest a separation of the feeding rate and meal size effects. Blundell and Latham (1978) suggested some time ago that the very different potencies of *dl*-fenfluramine and Organon 6582 in affecting meal size and feeding rate indicated that the two measures were under separate neurochemical control. Grignaschi and Samanin (1992) showed that while cyanopindolol (a 5-HT$_{1A}$ and 5-HT$_{1B}$ antagonist) returns meal size towards control values after *d*-fenfluramine treatment, it has little effect on feeding rate.* By contrast, ritanserin, a 5-HT$_2$ antagonist, was effective against changes in feeding rate, but not against meal size.

The decrease in meal size and increase in satiety ratio are both consistent with the general statement that these drugs enhance satiety or, to follow Blundell (1991), enhance both satiation (the process leading to a switch from feeding to non-feeding) and satiety (the process that inhibits a further switch from non-feeding to feeding). It's an open question as to whether the same neurochemical mechanisms are involved in both processes. Evidence for a distinction is provided by the finding that the cholecystokinin (CCK) antagonist devazepide blocks the reduction in meal size produced by *d*-fenfluramine, but fails to block the enhancement of intermeal interval for a meal of given size produced by this drug (Clifton and Cooper, 1992; Grignaschi *et al.*, 1993b).

Thus meal pattern studies tentatively suggest that fenfluramine independently reduces meal size (a 5-HT$_{1B}$, CCK-dependent mechanism), increases satiety ratio (probably a 5-HT$_{1B}$, CCK-independent mechanism) and decreases feeding rate (perhaps a 5-HT$_2$, CCK-independent mechanism). Satiety sequence studies are less advanced, since there has been some dispute as to whether fenfluramine simply shortens feeding and leads to earlier onset of resting (Blundell and Latham, 1980) or disturbs the sequence by enhancing activity and preventing the onset of rest (Montgomery and Willner, 1988; Willner *et al.*, 1990). A recent reanalysis of data collected from a study of satiety sequences obtained after repeated administration of *dl*-fenfluramine shows that behavioural disturbance is only evident on first administration of the drug and may represent a drug action unrelated to feeding (Clifton *et al.*, submitted 1993).

5-HT reuptake inhibitors, such as fluoxetine and sertraline, produce similar effects on meal patterning to those seen with *dl*-fenfluramine and *d*-fenfluramine (Table 1). 5-HT reuptake inhibitors have been less amenable to meal pattern studies in combination with antagonists. Indeed, simple intake studies have failed to reverse fluoxetine anorexia with any serotonin antagonist (Grignaschi and Samanin, 1992a) and have only been successful with sertraline on some occasions (Lucki *et al.*, 1988) and not others (Grignaschi and Samanin,

*Nomenclature of 5-HT receptors follows the latest recommendations of the Serotonin Club (Humphrey *et al.*, 1993). Thus the receptor previously known as 5-HT$_{1C}$ is referred to as 5-HT$_{2C}$, the 5-HT$_2$ receptor is referred to as 5-HT$_{2A}$ and general references to 5-HT$_2$ receptors include 5-HT$_{2A}$ and 5-HT$_{2C}$ receptors. Since agonists at 5-HT$_{1A}$ receptors *enhance* food intake (see below) it has been generally assumed that the action at 5-HT$_{2C}$ receptors must be leading to reduction of meal size.

1993), leading to the suggestion that non-serotonergic mechanisms must be involved in the effects of 5-HT reuptake inhibitors on food intake. Here behavioural data must be weighed against pharmacological data. There is a close parallel between actions of fenfluramine and fluoxetine on meal patterns (Burton et al., 1981; Clifton et al., 1989a) and on diet selection (Leibowitz et al., 1990; Weiss et al., 1991), and no other class of drug is known to produce this pattern of behavioural effects. The serotonergic basis of d-fenfluramine anorexia seems secure (Neill and Cooper, 1988). In addition there is one report that metergoline can partially antagonize fluoxetine anorexia (Lee and Clifton, 1992b). This was seen in two short-term intake tests and in a meal pattern study. The latter was of particular interest since metergoline partially antagonized the fluoxetine-induced reduction of meal size but actually enhanced the fluoxetine-induced reduction of feeding rate. In a subsequent study (Lee, unpublished) the effect on feeding rate became much greater as the dose of metergoline was increased. This would explain why previous studies (Grignaschi and Samanin, 1992a), which had employed high metergoline doses, failed to produce any behavioural antagonism on intake measures. The greatly slowed feeding rate, after combined treatment with fluoxetine and metergoline, would not allow any increase in meal duration to be reflected in an increase in food intake. The important theoretical conclusions from our studies, which mirror those for fenfluramine, is that the actions of fluoxetine on meal size and feeding rate are neurochemically separate and that the effect on meal size, at least, is mediated by serotonergic systems.

Although behavioural data strongly support the idea that 5-HT reuptake inhibitors such as fluoxetine and sertraline affect feeding through enhancement of central 5-HT activity, they do not speak to the contentious issue of whether an action on 5-HT reuptake or release is crucial. Caccia et al. (1992) have argued persuasively that the doses of fluoxetine that produce anorexia in food-deprived subjects are large enough to affect release of 5-HT as well as reuptake.

Studies with direct serotonin agonists present a patchy picture. Simansky and Vaidya (1990), using an observational technique similar to the standard one for satiety sequences, showed that mCPP or RU24969 produced relatively similar effects on feeding-associated behaviour to those produced by sertraline. These drugs are effective at 5-HT$_{1B}$ and 5-HT$_{2C}$ receptors. By contrast, a third agonist, DOI, which acts at 5-HT$_{2A}$ receptors, caused anorexia accompanied by a disruption of behaviour that was not characteristic of normal satiety. mCPP, in a meal pattern study, produced a similar pattern of reduced meal size and slowed feeding rate to the action of fluoxetine, though the effects were of much shorter duration (Clifton et al., 1993). Taken together, these studies focus attention on 5-HT$_{1B}$ and 5-HT$_{2C}$ receptors as having a crucial role in influencing feeding behaviour, but do not allow a clear neurochemical distinction to be made between the apparently independent effects that drugs such as fenfluramine have on satiation, satiety and feeding rate.

The 5-HT$_{1A}$ agonist 8-OH-DPAT paradoxically enhances food consumption and it has become clear that this reflects an action at autoreceptors in the raphe nuclei (Dourish et al., 1986). Although no meal pattern studies are available, satiety sequences support a specific action on feeding with delayed onset of grooming and rest (Muscat et al., 1988). Recent intake studies suggest a dopaminergic component in the action of 8-OH-DPAT after central adminstration (Fletcher, 1991), and more detailed behavioural analysis would be of great interest. Curiously it has turned out that some other putative 5-HT$_{1A}$ agonists are, in fact, also potent dopamine antagonists. Williams and Dourish (1992) describe how NAN-190, one such compound, enhances food intake, but also has the neuroleptic-like action of blocking apomorphine-induced stereotypy. In fact, the lengthening in duration of feeding bouts that was also produced by this drug is also a typical neuroleptic effect (see below; Blundell and Latham, 1978; Clifton et al., 1991).

Intake studies using serotonin antagonists have complemented those with agonists by demonstrating that, at least in satiated rats, food intake may increase (Fletcher, 1988). These studies have yet to be followed up with more detailed behavioural analysis.

There is a general consensus that one postsynaptic site action of serotonin on food intake is the paraventricular nucleus of the hypothalamus. Shor-Posner and Leibowitz (1986) demonstrated that both decreased meal size and slowed feeding rate resulted from infusion of 5-HT into the paraventricular and other nearby medial nuclei of the hypothalamus. They have also reported similar results for d-fenfluramine, fluoxetine and sertraline (Leibowitz et al., 1993). In addition they showed that the non-selective 5-HT antagonist metergoline injected into the paraventricular nucleus can enhance meal size and rate of feeding on the carbohydrate and fat components of a self-selected diet (Leibowitz et al., 1993). It is, perhaps, slightly unexpected that actions on feeding rate and meal size arise at the same site, given the extensive behavioural and pharmacological evidence that indicates separate neurochemical mechanisms. Effects at the same group of structures, though on simple intake measures, were reported by Hutson et al. (1986) for the serotonin agonists RU24969 and TFMPP. A recent failure to replicate some of these findings using smaller injection volumes (Fletcher et al., 1992) suggests that much more extensive exploration of non-hypothalamic sites using behavioural techniques of the kind described earlier would be very fruitful, especially in light of the widespread innervation of basal ganglia and cortex by serotonergic neurones (Palacios et al., 1990).

DOPAMINE AND FEEDING PATTERNS

As in the previous section I will start by considering studies using indirect agonists. d-Amphetamine enhances release and inhibits reuptake of catecholamines, primarily dopamine, noradrenaline and adrenaline. The drug, once clinically prescribed as an anorectic, but abondoned due to potential for abuse, has been used in a variety of systemic and central meal-patterning studies. Blundell and Latham (1978) demonstrated that 1 mg/kg d-amphetamine increased latency to the first meal and also increased subsequent intermeal intervals. This dose was associated with an unchanged feeding rate. Lower doses actually increased both feeding rate and total food intake, primarily by reducing intermeal intervals. Blundell and Latham (1978) argued that the results were probably best interpreted in terms of generalized effects, probably of dopamine, on activation. Low doses of d-amphetamine infused into the striatum elicit feeding under some conditions (Winn et al., 1982), but not others (Bakshi and Kelley, 1991b).

Studies with more selective direct dopamine agonists have produced similar results. Rusk and Cooper (1989) reported a microstructural analysis of single meals after administration of the selective dopamine D_2 agonist N-0437; they reported only a mild and low level of stereotypy which had no effect on the bout structure of a meal. In a meal pattern study low doses of N-0437 enhanced food intake and meal size, whereas higher doses lowered food intake and reduced meal size; meal frequency was unaffected (Clifton et al., 1989a). The anorexia that was observed resulted from a reduced rate of food intake. A similar pattern of change in meal patterning was produced by i.c.v. administration of low doses of either d-amphetamine or bromocriptine (Evans and Eikelboom, 1987). They interpreted their results in terms of a strengthening of the reinforcement provided by food. Clifton et al. (1989b) instead favoured an effect on satiety cues in which low doses of N-0437, by acting preferentially at autoreceptors, reduced the normal enhancement of satiety by the dopaminergic mechanism stimulated directly by higher doses of N-0437.

This difference of interpretation is not trivial. There is a very substantial literature pointing to the involvement of dopamine in reward processes, although the precise nature of this involvement is unclear (Taylor and Robbins, 1986). At low doses d-amphetamine might enhance interoceptive cues arising from food intake, which would perhaps be seen as an 'antisatiety' effect; it might also, given sensitive behavioural tests, be seen as enhanced positive feedback at the beginning of a meal. Alternatively dopamine might enhance the reinforcing impact of external stimuli associated with food intake; this suggestion is close to the idea of an effect of dopamine antagonists on preparatory aspects of food intake (Blackburn et al., 1987). At higher doses of amphetamine, activation of locomotion and stereotypy will interfere with feeding. Satiety sequence or microstructural recording would provide a useful screen for the intensity and duration of such effects but has not been widely used.

There is also evidence consistent with a specific anorexic effect of d-amphetamine. For example, Leibowitz et al. (1986) infused d-amphetamine into the lateral hypothalamus and recorded subsequent meal patterns. They noted delayed latencies to the first meal, together with reductions in the size and duration of the first two or three meals. Effects on intermeal interval depended upon whether the drug was administered during the dark (active) or light (inactive) phases of the diurnal cycle. During the dark intermeal intervals were shortened, but during the light they were unaffected. The delayed latency to feed is, as Leibowitz et al. suggest, compatible with an effect on the initiation of feeding or, loosely, 'hunger'. The shortened meals, by contrast, would be consistent with an effect on satiation (but not satiety, since intermeal intervals were shortened), and recent evidence does suggest the involvement of 5-HT in the anorexia that results from infusion of d-amphetamine into the lateral hypothalamus (Parada et al., 1992).

Selective and potent dopamine D_1 agonists have only recently become available. A microstructural study with the partial agonist SK&F 38393 (Cooper et al., 1990) revealed a small reduction in eating rate and a larger reduction in bout frequency. Similar results have been reported for the full agonist A68930 (Al-Naser and Cooper, 1994). A recent unpublished meal study with A68930 (Al-Naser et al., in preparation) confirms these findings. A68930, given at doses of 0, 0.10.3 and 1.0 mg/kg, did not reduce eating rate, but greatly reduced meal size.

Although there is considerable evidence that dopamine antagonists may decrease, or less usually increase, food intake (Blundell, 1991), more detailed behavioural studies have been rare. Blundell and Latham (1978) briefly reported that the relatively non-selective dopamine antagonist pimozide had no effect on total food intake, markedly slowed eating rate during meals and yet produced an enhancement of meal size. More recently Clifton et al. (1991) compared the effects of three selective D_2 antagonists and one selective D_1 antagonist on meal patterning. Although the durations of action of each drug differed, each of the D_2 antagonists produced an enhancement of meal size and slowed feeding rate (Table 2). They varied in their effects on food intake, suggesting that the magnitude of action on feeding rate and meal size might vary independently. Although the D_1 antagonsist SCH 23390 produced some slowing in feeding rate, there was no enhancement of meal size. Failure to enhance meal size cannot be attributed to blockade of $5\text{-}HT_2$ receptors, to which SCH 23390 also binds, since the same pattern of results has recently

Table 2 Dopamine antagonists and meal patterns

	Meal size	Feeding rate	imi	Satiety ratio
Pimozide	↑	↓	↑	−
YM-09151-2	↑	↓	↑	−
Raclopride	↑	↓	−	↓
Remoxipride	↑	↓	↑	−
SCH 23390	−	↓	−	−
SCH 39166	−	↓	−	−

Data are summarized from Blundell and Latham (1978), Clifton et al. (1991) and Clifton (unpublished, SCH 39166 only).

been obtained with a second D_1 antagonist, SCH 39166, that has no action at $5\text{-}HT_2$ receptors (Clifton, submitted).

The problems of interpretation that arise with these results parallel those for amphetamine and direct dopamine agonists. Should the increase in meal size be interpreted as an 'antisatiety effect'? Infusion of the dopamine antagonist sulpiride into the lateral hypothalamus enhances food intake and would support this view (Parada *et al.*, 1988). Alternatively might it represent a failure to attend to interoceptive cues that arise from food intake, or to make the behavioural switch from feeding to other activities? Bakshi and Kelley (1991a) demonstrated enhanced food intake and, more significantly, increased durations of feeding bouts after infusion of haloperidol into the nucleus accumbens and favoured this type of interpretation. One important issue for future consideration will be roles of dopamine D_3 and further receptor subtypes, which show differential distribution patterns over the brain areas discussed above (Sokoloff *et al.*, 1990). A second issue concerns the functional interaction of D_1 and D_2 receptors. In preliminary intake studies Cooper and Al-Naser (1993) have shown that D_1 agonists, at subthreshold doses for behavioural effects, may enhance the anorectic action of a D_2 agonist. However, there are no detailed behavioural studies to show whether the D_1 agonist acts to enhance an action of the D_2 agonist on feeding rate, or whether more complex changes in feeding behaviour are responsible for decreased food intake.

PEPTIDES AND FEEDING BEHAVIOUR

The nature of CCK-induced inhibition of feeding has been vigorously debated over the last two decades, and the interpretation of behavioural studies has been a central component of that debate (Smith and Gibbs, 1992). Antin *et al.* (1975) used the satiety sequence technique to distinguish relatively natural from stress- or sickness-induced reductions in food intake. The recent development of selective CCK antagonists allowed Dourish *et al.* (1991) to use the same technique in rats showing a hyperphagic response. The increase in food intake, which was most marked after CCK_B receptor antagonism with devazepide, strongly suggested a role for endogenous brain CCK in satiation. Hsiao and Wang (1982) continuously infused CCK and recorded meal patterns. The number of meals taken was reduced but the meal size was unaffected. This result was interpreted as an enhancement of satiety. However, it illustrates the difficulty of unambiguously interpreting meal size and intermeal interval changes. Had meal size remained the same, and intermeal interval increased, the same theoretical interpretation of increased satiety would probably have been suggested! The studies of Antin *et al.* (1975) and Dourish *et al.* (1991), as well as the more physiological work of McHugh and Moran (1985), would suggest a role for CCK in satiation, and hence predict a reduction in meal size. Continuous CCK infusion, by providing the peptide at times when endogenous release would be low, and perhaps also reducing the signal/noise ratio of meal-associated changes in plasma CCK levels, may have led to the unexpected behavioural response in Hsiao and Wang's experiment. Recent developments of selective CCK agonists should provide a valuable stimulus to this area.

Recent intake studies indicate important roles for other peptides, including neuropeptide Y, galanin and opioid peptides. Though more detailed behavioural studies have not appeared in any number, there can be little doubt that they will make a major contribution to our understanding of the roles of these substances and their complex interactions with other neurotransmitters.

CONCLUDING REMARKS

I have given a deliberately selective view of studies of feeding behaviour following various pharmacological manipulations. One general question that arises is whether there are distinct patterns of behavioural change that relate to pharmacological action. Simple intake studies are clearly very limited in this regard since they only specify the direction and magnitude of one variable (grams eaten/unit time). When more complete records of feeding behaviour are made several distinct patterns emerge.

It appears that drugs activating $5\text{-HT}_{1B/2C}$ receptors produce little change in the latency to feed, but reduce meal size and feeding rate; feeding is followed by a relatively rapid transition towards resting. This period of non-feeding behaviour lasts longer than would be expected for the reduced meal size. There is some evidence that these different behavioural effects are also heterogeneous in terms of their underlying neurochemistry. In particular, although definitive experiments are still required, meal size may be reduced by activation of 5-HT_{1B} receptors, whereas feeding rate may be more strongly reduced by 5-HT_{2C} receptor stimulation.

Moderate doses of dopamine agonists, especially those acting at D_2 receptors, may increase the latency to feed and reduce meal size and feeding rate; at low doses such drugs may paradoxically enhance feeding rate, meal size and total intake. A comparison of microstructural studies suggests that D_2 receptors may be more important in influencing feeding rate, whereas D_1 receptor stimulation has a greater effect on the number of bouts within a meal. High doses of dopamine agonists may have substantial effects on feeding, but these arise from stimulation of locomotor and stereotypic behaviour. Amphetamine, which has widespread effects on amine neurotransmitter systems, has similarly mixed effects on feeding behaviour. A delayed latency to feed is characteristic of dopaminergic activity, but smaller than expected meals with longer than expected intervals is a characteristic also shared by drugs with serotonergic activity. Dopamine D_2 antagonists produce a quite different group of behavioural changes, in particular enhanced meal size and slowed feeding rate, that is not found with any other group of drugs. The effects of D_1 antagonists on meal patterning, by contrast, are relatively limited, being restricted to small reductions in both feeding rate and meal size.

To what extent do these patterns of behavioural change reflect particular underlying mechanisms? My own intuition is that we have to take great care in this area. Do we understand the actions of serotonergic drugs well enough to assert that a particular pattern in a 'satiety' sequence represents changes in physiological and neural systems specific to feeding rather than to more general aspects of activity/rest cycles? Can the enhanced meal size seen after treatment with a dopamine antagonist be attributed to blockade of satiety rather than to more general interference in behavioural switching? In these and similar cases good behavioural analysis is just one piece of a more complex jigsaw that we are attempting to solve. As early ethologists also discovered, over-ambitious interpretation and labelling of behavioural data is likely to be an impediment rather than an aid to progress.

REFERENCES

Al-Naser, H.A. and Cooper, S.J. (1994) A-68930, a novel, potent dopamine D_1 receptor agonist: a microstructural analysis of its satiety effect in the rat. *Behav. Pharmacol.*, 5, 210–218.

Antin, J., Gibbs, J., Holt, J. *et al.* (1975) Cholecystokinin elicits the complete behavioral sequence of satiety in rats. *J. Comp. Physiol. Psychol.*, 89, 784–790.

Baerends, G.P. (1970) A model of the functional organisation of incubation behaviour in the herring gull. *Behav. Suppl.*, 17, 261–312.

Bakshi, V.P. and Kelley, A.E. (1991a) Dopaminergic regulation of feeding behaviour: I. Differential effects of haloperidol microinfusion into three striatal subregions. *Psychobiology*, 19, 223–232.

Bakshi, V.P. and Kelley, A.E. (1991b) Dopaminergic regulation of feeding behavior: II. Differential effects of amphetamine microinfusion into three striatal subregions. *Psychobiology*, 19, 233–242.

Blackburn, J.R., Phillips, A.G. and Fibiger, H.C. (1987) Dopamine and preparatory behavior: I. Effects of pimozide. *Behav. Neurosci.*, 101, 352–360.

Blundell, J.E. (1991) Pharmacological approaches to appetite suppression. *Trends Pharmacol. Sci.*, 12, 147–157.

Blundell, J.E. and Latham, C.J. (1978) Pharmacological manipulation of feeding behaviour: possible influences of serotonin and dopamine on food intake. In: *Central Mechanisms of Anorectic Drugs* (eds S. Garrattini and R. Samanin). Raven Press, New York, pp. 83–109.

Blundell, J.E. and Latham, C.J. (1980) Characterization of adjustments to the structure of feeding behaviour following pharmacological treatment: effects of amphetamine and fenfluramine and the antagonism produced by pimozide and methergoline. *Pharmacol. Biochem. Behav.*, 12, 717–722.

Burton, M.J., Cooper, S.J. and Popplewell, D.A. (1981) The effect of fenfluramine on the microstructure of feeding and drinking in the rat. *Br. J. Pharmacol.*, 72, 621–633.

Caccia, S., Bizzi, A., Coltro, G., Fracasso, C., Frittoli, E., Mennini, T. and Garattini, S. (1992) Anorectic activity of fluoxetine and norfluoxetine in rats: relationship between brain concentrations and in-vivo potencies on monoaminergic mechanisms. *J. Pharm. Pharmacol.*, 44, 250–254.

Clifton, P.G. (1987) Analysis of feeding and drinking patterns. In: *Feeding and Drinking* (eds F.A. Toates and N. Rowland) Elsevier, New York, pp. 19–35.

Clifton, P.G. and Cooper, S.J. (1992) CCK–5-HT interactions influence meal size in the free feeding rat. In: *Multiple Cholecystokinin Receptors in the CNS* (eds C.T. Dourish and S.J. Cooper). Oxford University Press, Oxford, pp. 286–289.

Clifton, P.G., Popplewell, D.A. and Burton, M.J. (1984) Feeding rate and meal patterns in the laboratory rat. *Physiol. Behav.*, 32, 369–374.

Clifton, P.G., Barnfield, A.M.C. and Philcox, L. (1989a) A behavioural profile of fluoxetine-induced anorexia. *Psychopharmacology*, 97, 89–95.

Clifton, P.G., Rusk, I.N. and Cooper, S.J. (1989b) Stimulation and inhibition of food intake by the selective dopamine D_2 agonist, N-0437: a meal pattern analysis. *Pharmacol. Biochem. Behav.*, 33, 21–26.

Clifton, P.G., Rusk, I.N. and Cooper, S.J. (1991) Effects of dopamine D_1 and dopamine D_2 antagonists on the free feeding and free drinking patterns of rats. *Behav. Neurosci.*, 105, 272–281.

Clifton, P.G., Barnfield, A.M.C., Curzon, G. (1993) Effects of food deprivation and mCPP treatment on the microstructure of ingestive behaviour of male and female rats. *J. Psychopharmacol.* 7, 257–264.

Cooper, S.J. and Al-Naser, H. (1993) D_1:D_2 dopamine receptor interactions in relation to feeding responses and food intake. In: *D_1:D_2 Dopamine Receptor Interactions* (ed. J.L. Waddington). Academic Press, New York, pp. 203–204.

Cooper, S.J., Francis, J. and Rusk, I.N. (1990) The anorectic effect of SK&F-38393, a selective dopamine-D1 receptor agonist: a microstructural analysis of feeding and related behavior. *Psychopharmacology*, 100, 182–187.

Dourish, C.T., Hutson, P.H. and Curzon, G. (1986) 8-OH-DPAT-induced hyperphagia: its possible neural basis and clinical relevance. *Appetite*, 7 (Suppl), 127–140.

Dourish, C.T., Rycroft, W. and Iverson, S.D. (1989) Postponement of satiety by blockade of brain cholecystokinin (CCK-B) receptors. *Science*, 245, 1509–1511.

Evans, K.R. and Eikelboom, R. (1987) Feeding induced by ventricular bromocriptine and amphetamine: a possible excitatory role for dopamine in eating behaviour. *Behav. Neurosci.*, 101, 591–593.

Fletcher, P.J. (1988) Increased food intake in satiated rats induced by the 5-HT antagonists methysergide, metergoline and ritanserin. *Psychopharmacology*, 96, 237–242.

Fletcher, P.J. (1991) Dopamine receptor blockade in nucleus accumbens or caudate nucleus differentially affects feeding induced by 8-OH-DPAT injected into the dorsal or median raphe. *Brain Res.*, 552, 181–189.

Fletcher, P.J., Ming, Z.H., Zack, M.H. and Coscina, D.V. (1992) A comparison of the effects of the 5-HT_1 agonists TFMPP and RU 24969 on feeding following peripheral or medial hypothalamic injection. *Brain Res.*, 580, 265–272.

Grignaschi, G. and Samanin, R. (1992a) Role of serotonin and catecholamines in brain in the feeding suppressant effect of fluoxetine. *Neuropharmacology*, 31, 445–449.

Grignaschi, G. and Samanin, R. (1992b) Role of serotonin receptors in the effect of d-fenfluramine on feeding patterns in the rat. *Eur. J. Pharmacol.*, 212, 287–289.

Grignaschi, G. and Samanin, R. (1993a) Role of serotonin receptors in the effect of sertraline on feeding behaviour. *Psychopharmacology*, 110, 203–208.

Grignaschi, G., Mantelli, B., Fracasso, C., Anelli, M., Caccia, S., Samanin, R. (1993b) Reciprocal interaction of 5-hydroxytryptamine and cholecystokinin in the control of feeding patterns in rats. *Br. J. Pharmacol.*, 109, 491–494.

Hill, A.J., Magson, L.D. and Blundell, J.E. (1984) Hunger and palatability: tracking ratings of subjective experience before, during and after the consumption of preferred and less preferred food. *Appetite*, 5, 361–371.

Hirsch, E. and Collier, G. (1974) The ecological determinants of reinforcement in the guinea pig. *Physiol. Behav.*, 12, 239–249.

Hsiao, S. and Wang, C.H. (1983) Continuous infusion of cholecystokinin and meal pattern in the rat. *Peptides*, **4**, 15–17.

Humphrey, P.P.A., Hartig, P. and Hoyer, D. (1993) A re-appraisal of 5-HT receptor classification. In: *Proceedings of the 2nd International Symposium on Serotonin: From Cell Biology to Pharmacology and Therapeutics.* Kluwer, Dordrecht.

Hutson, P.H., Donohoe, T.P. and Curzon, G. (1988) Infusion of the 5-hydroxytryptamine agonists RU24969 and TFMPP into the paraventricular nucleus of the hypothalamus causes hypophagia. *Psychopharmacology*, **95**, 550–552.

Lee, M.D. and Clifton, P.G. (1992a) Free-feeding and free-drinking patterns of male rats following treatment with opiate kappa agonists. *Physiol. Behav.*, **52**, 1179–1185.

Lee, M.D. and Clifton, P.G. (1992b) Partial reversal of fluoxetine anorexia by the 5-HT antagonist metergoline. *Psychopharmacology*, **107**, 359–364.

Leibowitz, S.F., Shor-Posner, G., Maclow, C. and Grinker, J.A. (1986) Amphetamine-effects on meal patterns and macronutrient selection. *Brain Res. Bull.*, **17**, 681–689.

Leibowitz, S.F., Weiss, G.F. and Suh, J.S. (1990) Medial hypothalamic nuclei mediate serotonin's inhibitory effect on feeding behaviour. *Pharmacol. Biochem. Behav.*, **37**, 735–742.

Leibowitz, S.F., Alexander, J.T., Cheung, W.K. and Weiss, G.F. (1993) Effects of serotonin and the serotonin blocker metergoline on meal patterns and macronutrient selection. *Pharmacol. Biochem. Behav.*, **45**, 185–194.

LeMagnen, J. (1985) *Hunger.* Cambridge University Press, Cambridge.

Lucas, G.A. and Timberlake, W. (1988) Interpellet delay and meal patterns in the rat. *Physiol. Behav.*, **43**, 259–264.

Lucki, I., Kreider, M.S. and Simansky, K.J. (1988) Reduction of feeding behaviour by the serotonin uptake inhibitor sertraline. *Psychopharmacology*, **96**, 289–295.

McGuirk, J., Muscat, R. and Willner, P. (1992) Effects of the 5-HT uptake inhibitors femoxitine and paroxetine, and the 5-HT1A agonist, eltoprazine, on the behavioural satiety sequence. *Pharmacol. Biochem. Behav.*, **41**, 801–805.

McHugh, P.R. and Moran, T.H. (1985) The stomach: a conception of its dynamic role in satiety. *Prog. Psychobiol. Phys. Psychol.*, **11**, 197–230.

Montgomery, A.M.J. and Willner, P. (1988) Fenfluramine disrupts the behavioural satiety sequence in rats. *Psychopharmacology*, **94**, 397–401.

Montgomery, A.M.J., Willner, P. and Muscat, R. (1988) Behavioral specificity of 8-OH-DPAT-induced feeding. *Psychopharmacology*, **94**, 110–114.

Neill, J.C. and Cooper, S.J. (1989) Evidence that *d*-fenfluramine anorexia is mediated by 5-HT$_1$ receptors. *Psychopharmacology*, **97**, 213–218.

Palacios, J.M., Waeber, C., Hoyer, D. and Mengod, G. (1990) Distribution of serotonin receptors. *Ann. NY Acad. Sci.*, **600**, 36–57.

Parada, M.A., Hernandez, L. and Degoma, E. (1986) Serotonin may play a role in the anorexia induced by amphetamine injections into the lateral hypothalamus. *Brain Res.*, **577**, 218–225.

Parada, M.A., Hernandez, L. and Hoebel, B.G. (1988) Sulpiride injections in the lateral hypothalamus induce feeding and drinking in the rat. *Pharmacol. Biochem. Behav.*, **30**, 917–923.

Rusk, I.N. and Cooper, S.J. (1989) Microstructural analysis of the anorectic effect of N-0437, a highly selective dopamine D$_2$ agonist. *Brain Res.*, **494**, 350–358.

Schaller, G. (1972) *The Serengeti Lion.* University of Chicago Press, Chicago.

Shor-Posner, G., Grinker, J.A., Marinescu, C., Brown, O. and Leibowitz, S.F. (1986) Hypothalamic serotonin in the control of meal patterns and macronutrient intake selection. *Brain Research Bull.*, **17**, 663–671.

Sibly, R.M., Nott, H.M.R. and Fletcher, D.J. (1990) Splitting behavior into bouts. *Anim. Behav.*, **39**, 63–69.

Simansky, K.J. and Vaidya, A.H. (1990) Behavioral mechanisms for the anorectic action of the serotonin (5-HT) uptake inhibitor sertraline in rats: comparison with directly acting agonists. *Brain Res. Bull.*, 25, 953–960.

Slater, P.J.B. and Lester, N.P. (1982) Minimising errors in splitting behaviour into bouts. *Behviour*, 79, 153–161.

Smith, G.P. and Gibbs, J. (1992) The development and proof of the CCK hypothesis of satiety. In: *Multiple Cholecystokinin Receptors in the CNS* (eds C.T. Dourish and S.J. Cooper). Oxford University Press, Oxford, pp. 166–182.

Sokoloff, P., Giros, B., Martres, M-P. *et al.* (1990) Molecular cloning and characterization of a novel dopamine receptor (D_3) as a target for neuroleptics. *Nature*, 347, 146–151.

Taylor, J.R. and Robbins, T.W. (1986) 6-Hydroxydopamine lesions of the nucleus accumbens, but not of the caudate nucleus, attenuate enhanced responding with reward-related stimuli produced by intra-accumbens *d*-amphetamine. *Psychopharmacology*, 90, 390–397.

Tinbergen, N. (1951) *The Study of Instinct.* Clarendon Press, Oxford.

Tinbergen, N. (1969) Ethology. In: *Scientific Thought* (ed. R. Harré). Clarendon Press, Oxford.

Weiss, G.F., Rogacki, N. and Fueg, A. (1991) Effect of hypothalamic and peripheral fluoxetine injection on natural patterns of macronutrient intake in the rat. *Psychopharmacology*, 105, 467–476.

Wiepkema, P.R. (1971) Positive feedback at work during feeding. *Behaviour*, 39, 266–273.

Williams, A.R. and Dourish, C.T. (1992) Effects of the putative 5-HT_{1A} receptor antagonist NAN-190 on free feeding and on feeding induced by the 5-HT_{1A} agonist 8-OH-DPAT in the rat. *Brain Res.*, 219, 105–112.

Willner, P., Towell, A. and Muscat, R. (1985) Apomorphine anorexia: a behavioural and neuropharmacological analysis. *Psychopharmacology*, 87, 351–356.

Willner, P., McGuirk, J., Phillips, G. and Muscat, R. (1990) Behavioural analysis of the anorectic effects of fluoxetine and fenfluramine. *Psychopharmacology*, 102, 273–277.

Winn, P., Williams, S.F. and Herberg, L.J. (1982) Feeding stimulated by very low doses of *d*-amphetamine administered systemically or by microinjection into the striatum. *Psychopharmacology*, 78, 336–341.

17 The Relevance of Ethology for Animal Models of Psychiatric Disorders: A Clinical Perspective

ALFONSO TROISI

Cattedra di Psichiatria, Università di Roma Tor Vergata, Rome, Italy

INTRODUCTION

Clinical psychiatrists adopt a double standard for judging the scientific status of animal models of psychiatric disorders. On one hand, clinicians use psychotropic drugs that have been screened in animal tests extensively. In doing so, they implicitly acknowledge the utility of animal models. On the other hand, when asked about the theoretical relevance of animal research, clinicians express scepticism and point to the poor validity and limited explanatory power of animal models when assessed against the complexities of human psychopathology.

Such an apparent contradiction becomes understandable if one realizes that animal models are conceptually heterogeneous because they are used for different purposes. Willner (1991) has recently proposed a taxonomy of behavioural models in psychopharmacology that distinguishes three classes: screening tests; behavioural bioassays; simulations. Screening tests are designed primarily to expedite the discovery of new drugs. In behavioural bioassays, the whole animal is used to measure a physiological action (e.g. changes in brain function resulting from chronic drug administration). Simulations attempt to simulate the clinical phenomenology of human psychiatric disorders.

Screening tests and behavioural bioassays are an inevitable step in the process of developing new drugs. In addition, any new drug is tested in human patients before it can be used in clinical practice. For these reasons, clinicians do not raise many objections to these types of models. It is the behavioural models referred to as simulations that are the real target of clinicians' criticism. What clinicians really question is the possibility of modelling the aetiology, pathogenesis and clinical phenomenology of human psychiatric disorders in animals. The clinicians' criticisms appear to be well founded, in view of the

Ethology and Psychopharmacology. Edited by S.J. Cooper and C.A. Hendrie
© 1994 John Wiley & Sons Ltd

limited contributions to a better understanding of mental illnesses made, so far, by simulation models.

The thesis of this chapter is that the clinicians' scepticism is excessive and that some of the limits of animal models can be overcome by incorporating concepts and methods from ethology into clinical and animal research. To argue in favour of the ethological approach, I will address three problems that have hampered the development of valid animal models. The first is he inadequate description and measurement of behaviour. The second is the selection of the level of clinical phenomenology to be studied. The third is the limited consideration given to the role of social factors in influencing responses to pharmacological interventions.

These problems complicate both clinical and animal research, and their solution requires parallel changes in all the disciplines involved in the development of animal models of psychiatric disorders, i.e. clinical psychiatry, experimental psychopathology and behavioural pharmacology. By reporting the results of some ethological studies in each of these fields of investigation, I will attempt to demonstrate that ethology is equally relevant to both types of research: human and animal, clinical and experimental.

THE NECESSITY FOR BEHAVIOURAL ANALYSIS

The lack of balance in clinical psychiatry between psychological assessment and behavioural analysis is a major obstacle for the development of valid animal models. The clinical phenomenology of psychiatric disorders includes both subjective psychological experiences and objective behavioural changes. Nevertheless, the diagnostic process in psychiatry is based almost exclusively on the evaluation of the psychological symptoms as voiced by the patient. Very little attention is paid to the description and measurement of behavioural changes. Conversely, not knowing how an animal feels or what its mental experiences might be restricts the animal researcher to inferences based on observable behaviour. Because of this difference between the methods employed in human and animal studies (i.e. psychometric assessment versus direct observation of behaviour), the integration of clinical and animal data is generally difficult and sometimes impossible.

Why is psychiatry so deficient in behavioural assessment? The long-standing prevalence of the psychodynamic and psychosocial orientations in the psychiatric thinking of this century only in part explains the neglect of the behavioural aspects of mental illnesses. In fact, even though the biomedical approach is now dominant in the psychiatric arena, the rapidly increasing precision and sophistication in neurobiological techniques have not been accompanied by comparable advances in the definition and measurement of behavioural variables, as clearly demonstrated by the following quotations:

> It is striking that, in an age of computerized axial tomographic scans, positron-emission tomography, and other technological advances in psychobiological

measurement, the assessment of basic phenomenological hallmarks in psychiatry, such as aggressive behavior, has remained elusive. (Kay *et al.*, 1988, p. 545)

Behavioral assessments are still the Achilles heel of biological psychiatric research. (van Praag *et al.*, 1987, p. 6)

In spite of the increasing awareness of the current inadequacy of behaviour assessment, psychiatric research has not yet offered a valid solution to the problem. The very reason for this is that psychiatry lacks a theoretical and methodological framework for studying behaviour. Ethology can provide such a framework. The ethological approach combines methodological advantages, such as direct observation of behaviour, operational definition of categories and quantitative recording, with a theoretical emphasis on those behaviours that are closely related to social functioning, and therefore are relevant to clinical psychiatry (Hutt, 1970).

In the past three decades, many studies have been published arguing for the application of ethological methods in psychiatry (e.g. White, 1974; McGuire and Fairbanks, 1977) or describing the behavioural profiles of various subgroups of patients (e.g. Jones and Pansa, 1979; McGuire and Polsky, 1980). However, ethological studies addressing the most debated clinical problems, such as prediction of drug response (Bouhuys *et al.*, 1987) and definition of diagnostic boundaries (Pitman *et al.*, 1987; Troisi *et al.*, 1991a), have appeared in the psychiatric literature only in the past few years. Two examples of this type of study are given here.

About one-third of depressed patients do not respond to pharmacotherapy, and clinical variables are not consistently related to the drug response (Fawcett and Kravitz, 1985). Troisi *et al.* (1989) studied the non-verbal behaviour of 22 depressed patients to determine whether their response to antidepressant treatment (50–100 mg per day of amitriptyline for five consecutive weeks) could be predicted on the basis of the ethological profile at baseline. Patients' behaviour during interview was video-recorded from behind a one-way mirror using a colour video system located in a small sound-proof room adjacent to the interviewer's office. The audio portion of the interview was not recorded. Subsequently, two trained observers (blind to the patient's clinical features and verbal reports) viewed the videotape, and transcribed the record into quantitative measurements relating to specific behavioural categories. The non-verbal behaviour of each patient was scored according to an ethological scoring system (derived from Grant, 1968) that included 37 different behaviours, mostly facial expressions and hand movements. In the data analysis, these behaviours were combined to form eight functional categories that reflected various aspects of the patient's emotional and social functioning. At the end of the study, the patients were divided into two treatment-outcome groups on the basis of their final scores on a rating scale for depression. Under baseline conditions responders and non-responders did not differ with respect to sex, age, education, clinical diagnosis or severity of depression. In contrast, the ethological profiles of the two treatment outcome groups were different, with non-responders showing significantly more assertive and affiliative behaviours.

In a second study, using the same procedure described above, Troisi *et al.* (1990) studied the non-verbal behaviour of 44 patients with different diagnostic subtypes of depression. Psychiatrists disagree as to whether depression is a single syndrome with varying degrees of severity or is a group of two or more discrete illnesses with differing aetiologies and clinical pictures (Kendell, 1976). The DSM-III Diagnostic Manual (American Psychiatric Association, 1980) recognizes different subtypes of depression, although the validity of these remains to be determined. Ethological assessment failed to find any evidence for the validity of the DSM-III subtyping of depression. Of the eight behavioural categories analysed in the study, none showed statistically significant differences among the different diagnostic groups.

Taken together, these findings indicate that the ethological approach is not limited simply to a mere translation into quantitative and objective data of what clinicians already know on the basis of their judgement or the use of rating scales. Rather, it produces new insights in controversial areas of psychiatric disorders. If the clinical phenomenology of mental illnesses could be reformulated in ethological terms, the same, or similar, definitions could then be applied to the development of animal models, and analogues for specific behaviours might then become more feasible. Of course, to bridge the gap between clinical and animal data, the ethological analysis of behaviour should be adopted more extensively in animal research as well. Most of the animal models currently used in behavioural pharmacology are more notable for their relative speed and low cost than their resemblance to human behavioural changes associated with psychiatric disorders.

SYMPTOMS, SYNDROMES AND BEHAVIOUR SYSTEMS

Medicine distinguishes three nosological entities that are ranked according to an increasing order of specificity and complexity: symptoms, syndromes, and diseases. Symptoms are the basic components of the clinical picture of a disease. Syndromes are discrete clusters of symptoms and signs (i.e. those symptoms that can be identified by direct examination of the patient) that occur together and have a predictable time-course. Finally, a disease is a pathological entity characterized by a specific aetiology and/or pathogenesis.

Unfortunately, the language of psychiatry, more than that of other medical disciplines, frequently adopts the same terms for indicating different nosological entities. For example, the term 'depression' is commonly used to indicate both the abnormal mood condition consisting of sadness, helplessness and despair (i.e. a symptom) and the cluster of psychological, behavioural and vegetative symptoms, the essential feature of which is depressed mood (i.e. a syndrome).

Such terminological confusions have implications for animal research.

Studies aimed at developing animal models of psychiatric disorders rarely clarify whether the object of investigation is a symptom or a syndrome. Probably, the reasons for such a lack of specification are two-fold. First, many animal researchers are not aware of the semantic problems that plague current psychiatric nosology. Second, modelling human psychiatric syndromes in animals is a difficult task compared to that of modelling individual symptoms. However, whatever the reason for the lack of specification about the object of investigation, most animal studies in practice focus on symptoms. By contrast, the design of almost all current psychiatric research involves the assignment of subjects to a syndromic category (Costello, 1992). This difference in the level of analysis does not favour the incorporation of animal data into psychiatric theory. Adhering to the diagnostic language of clinical psychiatry, students of animal models often interpret their data in terms of syndromes even if the evidence is ambiguous. For example, Healy (1987) held that learned helplessness is a model of endogenous depression whereas Overmier and Hellhammer (1988) viewed it as a model of reactive depression. Willner (1985), on the basis of his extensive review of the literature, concluded that it was not clear which depressive syndrome is modelled by learned helplessness.

The prevalence in contemporary psychiatry of the syndromal approach is understandable considering the atypical status of psychiatric classification when compared with that of the rest of medicine. In medicine, classification of pathological conditions has consistently moved over time from symptoms through syndromes to diseases. In contrast, because of the scarce knowledge of the causes and mechanisms of mental illnesses, psychiatric nosography is still based on differential diagnosis between syndromes (Kendell, 1975). Obviously, a classification based on the aetiology and pathogenesis of disorders is far more valid and useful than that relying upon the description of symptomatology. However, syndromes are better than symptoms for classifying patients into meaningful clinical groups; i.e. for predicting the course of the disorder and selecting a therapy. Therefore, the majority of clinical psychiatrists value research on syndromes and view with scepticism any investigation that focuses on symptoms, probably because these studies remind them of the sterile taxonomic exercises of the descriptive psychopathology of the last century. Such a theoretical position has influenced the view of what animal studies should model, as clearly indicated by the following statement:

> In the case of animal models of human psychopathology one seeks to develop *syndromes* in animals which resemble those in humans in certain ways in order to study selected aspects of human psychopathology. (McKinney, 1984, italics added)

The problem with the syndromal approach is that psychiatric syndromes are not only difficult to model in animals but also questionable in terms of construct and predictive validity, as indicated by the frequent modifications in diagnostic systems (e.g. Zimmermann, 1988). However, the alternative approach, i.e. modelling symptoms, has its shortcomings as well. First, almost all psychiatric symptoms are non-specific: the same symptom may be associated with a variety of different syndromes and diseases. For example, anxiety and depression are frequently found in patients suffering from affective disorders as well as in those affected by psychotic and personality disorders. This clinical reality makes relatively impractical the suggestion that, when the clinical syndrome is impossible to reproduce in animal models, animal researchers should at least attempt to simulate specific symptoms (Abramson and Seligman, 1977; Willner, 1991). Second, the validity of several symptoms, as currently classified in psychiatric literature, is dubious. Are social anxiety, separation anxiety and obsessive anxiety variants of the same psychopathological dimension or very different emotions improperly lumped by the same term? Third, the behavioural translation of some psychiatric symptoms, as currently defined by clinicians, is as difficult as that of syndromes. For example, what behaviours should animal researchers use to model *constricted affect*, defined as a reduction in intensity of feeling tone, or *euphoria*, defined as intense elation with feelings of grandeur (Kaplan and Sadock, 1989)?

The ethological approach is useful in dealing with the problem of the level of analysis in animal models. Ethology is mostly concerned with natural classes of behaviour or 'behaviour systems'. A behaviour system is a complex of behavioural elements and physiological mechanisms that work in an integrated manner in order to serve one or more biological functions. Focusing on behaviour systems rather than on symptoms or syndromes may offer important advantages to students of animal models of psychiatric disorders, as suggested by the following examples.

Dixon and co-workers have conducted a series of ethopharmacological studies (reviewed in Dixon *et al.*, 1990) of flight behaviour in rodents. They demonstrated that flight takes different forms that are coupled to different physiological events and that these forms appear to be differentially susceptible to drug action. In addition, they demonstrated that the inhibition of approach-orientated activities causes deficits in social behaviour that mimic those induced by an excessive activation of flight responses. Even though these studies were not designed to model a specific psychiatric symptom or syndrome, they have important implications for clinical psychiatry. The finding that deficits in social behaviour can be the result of two different processes suggests interesting analogies with the clinical hypothesis that social withdrawal in schizophrenia can originate from either defensive avoidance of social stimuli or primary lack of motivation for social interactions (Carpenter *et al.*, 1991). Another important implication is that new actions of potential therapeutic importance may go unnoticed if drugs are tested only for properties indicated by their conventional labels. In Dixon's studies, both anxiolytics and neuroleptics reduced flight responses in mice but such a behavioural change had little or nothing to do with the antianxiety or antipsychotic effects of the drugs (Dixon *et al.*, 1990).

A second example of the advantages of focusing on behaviour systems comes from a comparative analysis of the effects of endogenous opioid blockade in human and primate subjects. Naltrexone, an opioid receptor antagonist, is currently marketed as a narcotic antagonist for management of opioid dependency and abuse. The rationale for treating opiate abusers with naltrexone is that repeated exposure to the abused drug, while blocking the positively reinforcing properties (i.e. euphoria and pleasure), would extinguish drug use behaviour. Clinical trials with naltrexone have shown that it is not well-accepted by heroin addicts, as indicated by very high dropout rates (up to 80% by six months) (Kosten and Kosten, 1991). In addition, some studies have reported that a subset of normal subjects show dramatic emotional changes after the acute administration of the drug. However, the nature of the aversive psychological effects of naltrexone remains unclear. A variety of terms have been used to label these effects: dysphoria, depressed mood, anxiety, tension, irritability, hostility, mental confusion. The use of these terms reflects the attempt to relate the unpleasant feelings produced by opioid receptor blockade to conventionally defined psychiatric syndromes (Frecska and Davis, 1991).

Findings from primate studies suggest a different view. Schino and Troisi (1992) showed that the acute administration of naloxone, an analogue of naltrexone, induces behavioural manifestations of separation distress in group-living juvenile macaques. In the naloxone condition, the subjects increased their relative role in maintaining spatial proximity with their mothers, made more grooming solicitations, and spent less time in social play. Similarly, previous studies with other primate species had shown that endogenous opioid blockade increases distress vocalizations emitted by infants after maternal separation (Kalin and Shelton, 1989) and promotes a need for social comfort in adult animals (Fabre-Nys et al., 1982). To say that, in non-human primates, opioid blockade induces an anxiety or depressive syndrome does not explain adequately the complex and specific behavioural changes observed in the aforementioned studies. A more meaningful explanation is that, in a variety of species including primates, endogenous opioids act as a neurochemical substrate for social affect, and that opioid blockade causes a transient dysfunction of the attachment behaviour system (Panksepp et al., 1985). After naltrexone administration, comparable effects may occur in normal human subjects or, at least, in specific subpopulations of individuals who are more vulnerable to separation distress (Troisi and Schino, 1992). Such a vulnerability is unlikely to be related to a single psychiatric syndrome. In fact, separation anxiety is a psychopathological dimension implicated in different disorders including agoraphobia (Liotti, 1993), panic disorder (Free et al., 1993), depression (Harris and Bifulco, 1993) and child abuse (Troisi, in preparation).

A suggestion deriving from the above discussion is that animal researchers should be aware of the transient status of psychiatric diagnostic systems. Rather than attempting to create one model for a syndrome, researchers should attempt to analyse basic behavioural dysfunctions that cut across different types of conventionally defined syndromes. This research strategy would allow animal researchers to avoid the risk of modelling nosological entities the validity of which may be disproved by future research. It is worth noting that the same approach has also been advocated by clinical researchers who recognize the weakness of current psychiatric nosography (van Praag et al., 1987). This does not mean that symptoms and syndromes should be entirely disregarded by animal reseachers. Rather, the validity of these nosological entities should be critically re-examined in the light of the results of studies of biologically meaningful categories of behaviour.

SOCIAL FACTORS AND DRUG RESPONSE

Individual variability in drug responsiveness is a well-known phenomenon in clinical psychopharmacology. However, differences among patients are generally explained as the result of diagnostic errors or individual differences in drug absorption and rate of metabolism. The possibility that social variables may affect biological systems and thereby alter behavioural responses to pharmacological agents is virtually ignored. In fact, many observations indicate that social events may cause critical changes in physiological systems (McGuire and Troisi, 1987). Doubtless, in clinical settings, it is extremely difficult to identify the kinds of social factors that can have an impact on physiological function and then on drug response. Therefore, this area of research is an ideal candidate for the use of animal models. The interplay between social factors, environmental setting and subjects' behavioural responses to pharmacological interventions should be a prominent area of research in behavioural pharmacology. This is not the case, however:

> Most investigators, being well trained in experimental design, have tended to view individual differences in subject reaction to manipulations or treatments essentially as error variance. That variance is real, however, and the individual differences that contribute to it may turn out to be exceedingly meaningful. (Suomi, 1985, p. 236)

Unlike traditional approaches for screening psychotherapeutic drugs, ethopharmacological studies have repeatedly investigated the relationship between social variables and drug response in animal models. For example, there is abundant evidence that animals of different rank respond differently to the same dose of pharmacological agent. Miczek and Gold (1983) demonstrated that, in adult squirrel monkeys, the effects of d-amphetamine depended on the social status of the individual monkeys within their group: low doses of the drug reduced agonistic behaviour in dominant monkeys but induced complete social isolation in subordinate monkeys. Raleigh et al. (1985) showed that, in vervet monkeys, dominant and subordinate males differ in their sensitivity to drugs that enhance central serotonergic function: fluoxetine, quipazine and tryptophan increased approaching and grooming and decreased avoiding and vigilance much more in dominant than in subordinate males. Schino *et al.* (1991) showed that, in group-living macaques, acute administration of lorazepam reduced the frequency of scratching, an anxiety-related behavioural response (Troisi *et al.*), significantly more in low-ranking than in high-ranking females.

Social status is of course only one of many variables that affect social behaviour. Other social variables, including the group's age/sex composition and the subjects' early experiences, have been found to influence behavioural responses of non-human primates to pharmacological agents (see Miczek, 1983). These findings are of great interest to clinicians and can encourage their consideration of animal models. Driven by animal research, clinical psychopharmacology may find it increasingly important to examine the impact of social systems and social status on identifiable biochemical substrates and to take social factors into account both in selecting the appropriate recipient of pharmacological treatment and in assessing the efficacy of pharmacological intervention (McGuire *et al.*, 1982).

CONCLUSIONS

Put in its simplest form, the thesis of this chapter is that the development of valid animal simulations of psychiatric disorders requires the integration of clinical psychiatry and behavioural pharmacology with ethology. This is not a new idea, however (see, for example, Suomi, 1985; McGuire *et al.*, 1982). Despite these writings and others, ethological methods and research findings have had little impact on animal models of psychiatric disorders. Any attempt at integrating ethology with psychiatry and psychopharmacology cannot ignore the reasons for such a failure.

There are two main reasons that can explain the reluctance to adopt the ethological approach. The first reason is theoretical. Ethology is not merely a matter of techniques for measuring behaviour; more importantly, it emphasizes the evolutionary context in the study of behaviour. Because evolutionary theory is still not commonly taught or utilized in training programmes in psychiatry, experimental psychology or pharmacology, students educated in these disciplines have difficulty in adopting the ethological approach. The second reason is practical. Clinical psychiatry and industrial psychopharmacology share a pragmatic orientation that emphasizes the achievement of short-term goals at the expense of the generation of new ideas, as shown by the following quotations:

> Most statements of the characteristics of a good animal model emphasize homology with the human disorder; that is, animal symptoms should resemble human symptoms and the etiologies should be similar. In the pharmaceutical industry, on the other hand, elegance and homology are irrelevant if the model does not identify which members of a large set of compounds will be clinically useful. (Howard and Pollard, 1983, p. 308)

Clinicians, by and large are much more concerned to have effective treatments for their patients than to be given elegant explicatory hypotheses for their patients' ill. Consequently, they prefer animal models of, say, anxiety to be more useful in developing new drugs rather than provide fundamental insights into the mechanisms of that condition. (Lader, 1991, p. 76)

The ethological study of behaviour, both in human patients and animal models, is complex and time consuming compared with the techniques currently used in clinical psychiatry and behavioural pharmacology. The time needed for measuring patients' non-verbal communication or analysing monkeys' social interactions is at least 10 times that for filling in a rating scale or testing a rat in the elevated plus-maze. Until the ethological approach proves its practical utility on a vast scale, it is unlikely that clinicians and industrial psychopharmacologists will abandon current methods of behavioural assessment. In the meanwhile, the task of exploring the potential of ethology for clinical psychiatry and behavioural pharmacology is mainly entrusted to academic researchers. In doing so, they belie the caustic aphorism of Arthur Block about academic pharmacology: 'a drug is any substance that injected in a rat produces an article'.

ACKNOWLEDGEMENT

I thank Michael T. McGuire MD for his useful comments on an earlier version of this chapter.

REFERENCES

Abramson, L.Y. and Seligman, M.E.P. (1977) Modeling psychopathology in the laboratory: history and rationale. In: *Psychopathology: Animal Models* (eds J.D. Maser and M.E.P. Seligman). Freeman, San Francisco, pp. 1–26.
American Psychiatric Association (1980) *Diagnostic and Statistical Manual of Mental Disorders*, 3rd edn. American Psychiatric Association, Washington.
Bouhuys, A.L., Beersma, D.G.M., van de Hoofdakker, R. and Roossien, A. (1987) The prediction of short- and long-term improvement in depressive patients: ethological methods of observing behavior versus clinical ratings. *Ethol. Sociobiol.*, **8**, 117S–130S.
Carpenter, W.T., Buchanan, R.W. and Kirkpatrick, B. (1991) The concept of the negative symptoms of schizophrenia. In: *Negative Schizophrenic Symptoms: Pathophysiology and Clinical Implications* (eds J.F. Greden and R. Tandon). American Psychiatric Association, Washington, pp. 3–20.
Costello, C.G. (1992) Research on symptoms versus research on syndromes: arguments in favour of allocating more research time to the study of symptoms. *Br. J. Psychiatry*, **160**, 304–308.
Dixon, A. K., Fisch, H.U. and McAllister, K.H. (1990) Ethopharmacology: a biological approach to the study of drug-induced changes in behavior. *Adv. Stud. Behav.*, **19**, 171–204.
Fabre-Nys, C., Meller, R.E. and Keverne, E.B. (1982) Opiate antagonists stimulate affiliative behavior in monkeys. *Pharmacol. Biochem. Behav.*, **16**, 653–659.

Fawcett, J. and Kravitz, H.M. (1985) Treatment of refractory depression. In: *Common Treatment Problems in Depression* (ed A.F. Schatzberg) American Psychiatric Association, Washington DC, pp. 2–27.

Frecska, E. and Davis, K.L. (1991) The opioid model in psychiatric research. In: *Neuropeptides and Psychiatric Disorders* (ed. C.B. Nemeroff). American Psychiatric Association, Washington, pp. 169–192.

Free, N.K., Winget, C.N. and Whitman, M.R. (1993) Separation anxiety in panic disorder. *Am. J. Psychiatry*, 150, 595–599.

Grant, E.C. (1968) An ethological description of non-verbal behaviour during interviews. *Br. J. Med. Psychol.*, 41, 177–184.

Harris, T. and Bifulco, A. (1993) Loss of a parent in childhood, attachment style, and depression in adulthood. In: *Attachment Across the Life Cycle* (eds C.M. Parkes, J. Stevenson-Hinde and P. Marris). Routledge, London, pp. 234–267.

Healy, D. (1987) The comparative psychopathology of affective disorders in animals and humans. *J. Psychopharmacol.*, 1, 193–210.

Howard, J.L. and Pollard, G.T. (1983) Are primate models of neuropsychiatric disorders useful to the pharmaceutical industry? In: *Ethopharmacology: Primate Models of Neuropsychiatric Disorders* (ed. K.A. Miczek). Liss, New York, pp. 307–312.

Hutt, S.J. (1970) The role of behavior studies in psychiatry: an ethological viewpoint. In: *Behavior Studies in Psychiatry* (eds S.J. Hutt and C. Hutt). Pergamon Press, Oxford, pp. 1–23.

Jones, I.H. and Pansa, M. (1979) Some nonverbal aspects of depression and schizophrenia occurring during the interview. *J. Nerv. Ment. Dis.*, 167, 402–409.

Kalin, N.H. and Shelton, S.E. (1989) Defensive behaviors in infant rhesus monkeys: environmental cues and neurochemical regulation. *Science*, 243, 1718–1721.

Kaplan, H.J. and Sadock, B.J. (1989) Typical signs and symptoms of psychiatric illness. In: *Comprehensive Textbook of Psychiatry/V* (eds H.I. Kaplan and B.J. Sadock). Williams & Wilkins, Baltimore, pp. 469–475.

Kay S.R., Wolkenfeld, F. and Murrill, L. (1988) Profiles of aggression among psychiatric patients. I. Nature and prevalence. *J. Nerv. Ment. Dis.*, 176, 539–546.

Kendell, R.E. (1975) The concept of disease and its implications for psychiatry. *Br. J. Psychiatry*, 127, 305–315.

Kendell, R.E. (1976) The classification of depressions: a review of contemporary confusion. *Br. J. Psychiatry*, 129, 15–28.

Kosten, T.A. and Kosten, T.R. (1991) Pharmacological blocking agents for treating substance abuse. *J. Nerv. Ment. Dis.*, 179, 583–592.

Lader, M. (1991) Animal models of anxiety: a clinical perspective. In: *Behavioral Models in Psychopharmacology: Theoretical, Industrial and Clinical Perspectives* (ed. P. Willner). Cambridge University Press, Cambridge, pp. 76–88.

Liotti, G. (1993) Insecure attachment and agoraphobia. In: *Attachment Across the Life Cycle* (eds C.M. Parkes, J. Stevenson-Hinde and P. Marris). Routledge, London, pp. 216–233.

McGuire, M.T. and Fairbanks, L.A. (1977) Ethology: psychiatry's bridge to behavior. In: *Ethological Psychiatry: Psychopathology in the Context of Evolutionary Biology* (eds M.T. McGuire and L.A. Fairbanks). Grune & Stratton, New York, pp. 1–40.

McGuire, M.T. and Polsky, R.H. (1980) Ethological assessment of stable and labile social behaviors during acute psychiatric disorders: clinical applications. *Psychiatry Res.*, 3, 291–306.

McGuire, M.T. and Troisi, A. (1987) Physiological regulation–deregulation and psychiatric disorders. *Ethol. Sociobiol.*, 8, 9S–25S.

McGuire, M.T., Raleigh, M.J. and Brammer, G.L. (1982) Sociopharmacology. *Annu. Rev. Pharmacol. Toxicol.*, 22, 643–661.

McKinney, W.T. (1984) Animal models of depression: an overview. *Psychiatr. Dev.*, **2**, 77–96.

Miczek, K.A. (1983) *Ethopharmacology: Primate Models of Neuropsychiatric Disorders.* Liss, New York.

Miczek, K.A. and Gold, L.H. (1983) Ethological analysis of amphetamine action on social behavior in squirrel monkeys (*Saimiri sciureus*). In: *Ethopharmacology: Primate Models of Neuropsychiatric Disorders* (ed. K.A. Miczek). Liss, New York, pp. 137–155.

Overmier, J.B. and Hellhammer, D.H. (1988) The learned helplessness model of human depression. *Anim. Models Psychiatr. Disord.*, **2**, 177–202.

Panksepp, J., Siviy, S.M. and Normansell, L.A. (1985) Brain opioids and social emotions. In: *The Psychobiology of Attachment and Separation* (eds M. Reite and T. Field). Academic Press, New York, pp. 1–49.

Pitman, R.K., Kolb, B., Orr, S.P. and Singh, M.M. (1987) Ethological study of facial behavior in nonparanoid and paranoid schizophrenic patients. *Am. J. Psychiatry*, **144**, 99–102.

Raleigh, M.J., Brammer, G.L., McGuire, M.T. and Yuwiler, A. (1985) Dominant social status facilitates the behavioral effects of serotonergic agonists. *Brain Res.*, **348**, 274–282.

Schino, G., Troisi, A., Perretta, G. and Monaco, V. (1991) Measuring anxiety in nonhuman primates: effect of lorazepam on macaque scratching. *Pharmacol. Biochem. Behav.*, **38**, 889–891.

Schino, G. and Troisi, A. (1992) Opiate receptor blockade in juvenile macaques: effect on affiliative interactions with their mothers and group companions. *Brain Res.*, **576**, 125–130.

Suomi, S.J. (1985) Ethology: animal models. In: *Comprehensive Textbook of Psychiatry/IV* (eds H.I. Kaplan and B.J. Sadock). Williams & Wilkins, Baltimore, pp. 226–237.

Troisi, A. (in preparation) Maternal separation anxiety and child abuse: a comparative analysis in primates and humans.

Troisi, A. and Schino, G. (1992) Aversive effects of opioid antagonists: evidence from primate studies. *Neurosci. Lett.*, **43**, S112.

Troisi, A., Pasini, A., Bersani, G. *et al.* (1989) Ethological predictors of amitriptyline response in depressed outpatients. *J. Affect. Disord.*, **17**, 129–136.

Troisi, A., Pasini, A., Bersani, G. *et al.* (1990) Ethological assessment of the DSM-III subtyping of unipolar depression. *Acta Psychiatr. Scand.*, **81**, 560–564.

Troisi, A., Pasini, A., Bersani, G. *et al.* (1991a) Negative symptoms and visual behavior in DSM-III-R prognostic subtypes of schizophreniform disorder. *Acta Psychiatr. Scand.*, **83**, 391–394.

Troisi, A., Schino, G., D'Antoni, M. *et al.* (1991b) Scratching as a behavioral index of anxiety in macaque mothers. *Behav. Neural Biol.*, **56**, 307–313.

van Praag, H.M., Kahn, R.S., Asnis, G.M. *et al.* (1987) Denosologization of biological psychiatry or the specificity of 5-HT disturbances in psychiatric disorders. *J. Affect. Disord.*, **13**, 1–8.

White, N.F. (1974) Ethology and psychiatry. In: *Ethology and Psychiatry* (ed. N.F. White). University of Toronto Press, Toronto, pp. 3–25.

Willner, P. (1985) *Depression: A Psychobiological Synthesis*. Wiley, New York.

Willner, P. (1991) Behavioral models in psychopharmacology. In: *Behavioral Models in Psychopharmacology: Theoretical, Industrial and Clinical Perspectives* (ed. P. Willner). Cambridge University Press, Cambridge, pp. 3–18.

Zimmermann, M. (1988) Why are we rushing to publish DSM-IV? *Arch. Gen. Psychiatry*, **45** 1135–1138.

18 Ethology, Human Lifestyle and Health

M. KRŠIAK

Department of Pharmacology, 3rd Medical Faculty, Charles University, Prague, Czech Republic

INTRODUCTION

It is really a great pleasure to be at this conference held on the occasion of the 30th anniversary of publication of the classical paper by Ewan Grant and John Mackintosh (Grant and Mackintosh, 1963) and, after 25 years, to meet again most members of the Birmingham group which laid the foundations for a new scientific discipline now called ethopharmacology. That they can take major credit for the rise of ethopharmacology has been rightly appreciated both at this conference and elsewhere (Kršiak, 1991).

In my opinion, the Birmingham group can claim yet another credit. It is their demonstration of how a new scientific discipline begins: by the application of principally new *concepts* plus finding an adequate *method* plus demonstrating their *utility*. Michael Chance recognized the great potential of ethological concepts in the study of drug effects on behaviour. For example, he drew attention to the discovery of ethology that 'Behaviour is composed of species-specific acts and postures which represent natural units of behaviour' (Chance, 1968), which could be very useful in the study of behavioural effects of drugs. Ewan Grant and John Mackintosh observed and listed the principal motor acts and postures of small laboratory rodents (Grant and Mackintosh, 1963), and thus developed a method which enabled the application of this concept (this is the publication which has become a 'classic', since almost all lists of elements used in subsequent ethopharmacology experiments on common laboratory rodents have been based on this paper). Finally, Paul Silverman demonstrated the utility of the concept and the method: in a series of carefully done experiments he showed that the study of drug effects on a great number of acts and postures occurring in rats during social encounters is not only feasible but also instructive (Silverman, 1965, 1966, 1988).

The work of the Birmingham group provided the evidence to demonstrate what remarkable success could be achieved in applying the ethological approach in an area as unexpected as pharmacology. The purpose of this chapter is to show that the ethological attitude can also provide new perspectives,

Ethology and Psychopharmacology. Edited by S.J. and Cooper C.A. Hendrie
© 1994 John Wiley & Sons Ltd

concepts and framework of thought in other 'atypical' areas, such as in the study of human lifestyle, health and disease.

HUMAN ETHOLOGICAL NEEDS

Ethology has been traditionally interested in the species-specific features of behaviour, as well as in the species-specific way of life and stimuli in various animals. Knowledge acquired by the ethological approach has been useful not only in theory, but also in practice. For example, successful breeding of wild animals in captivity depends on meeting their ethological needs, such as composition of a group, size of territory, opportunities to exercise some activities, etc. The health and welfare of any given species seems to depend on satisfying its specific ethological needs. Thus, the European convention for the protection of vertebrate animals used for experimental and other scientific purposes (Council of Europe, 1986) requires that adequate attention is paid to satisfying ethological needs of laboratory animals. This evokes a question: 'What are human ethological needs?' Have human beings, like other species, ethological needs in terms of inborn capabilities and tendencies for a species-specific way of life? Of course, there are great individual and cultural variations in various aspects of human lifestyle, so that the human lifestyle may appear to be composed of arbitrary customs (Russell, 1966). Nevertheless, one cannot resist the feeling that in spite of these variations there exist some general tendencies ('ethological needs') common to the entire species of *Homo sapiens* which fundamentally form its lifestyle (Table 1).

It can be argued that many people can lead a contented life without (for example) any need for a close personal relationship or for authority. However, these ethological needs (which at first sight appear to require another person) can (perhaps) be satisfied by 'self-service': by keeping a positive personal relationship with oneself and having oneself as an authority.

The need for authority (to respect somebody) does not mean that man needs, for example, a dictator (such a conclusion would be as erroneous as the deduction that man needs poisoned food because he is hungry). Ethological needs, like physiological (and any other 'natural') needs are 'blind' (in terms of discrimination between 'good' and 'bad') and, hence, they cannot endorse stimuli. Whether the stimuli to which they respond are right or false can be

Table 1 Some putative human ethological needs

Examples of 'natural', inborn needs, which might form the human lifestyle

---

The need for positive personal relationship
The need for authority
The need for freedom
The need for enjoyment
The need for communication

---

seen from consequences. The need for freedom might balance the need for authority (and vice versa), rather like when agonist and antagonist muscles participate in aimed movements. The ethological need for enjoyment can be satisfied, for example, by play, hobby, entertainment, possession, attainment, etc.

'VITAMIN L'

Because discussion of each of the suggested human ethological needs would be beyond the scope of this chapter, I will focus only on one of them: the need for positive personal relationship.

It seems that the putative need for positive personal relationship cannot be satisfied by any positive personal relationship, but only by that which is (for example) stable, affectionate, intimate, independent of given personal attributes (e.g. external appearance, physical or mental capabilities, age, etc.) and mutual. Interestingly enough, such relations are always individually specific (e.g. relations between parents and children or between husband and wife).

It can be argued that what I am trying to describe here in a rather clumsy way could be simply called love. But I will deliberately avoid using that term here, because its meaning can be too ambiguous or special. Instead, I would prefer to use the expression 'Vitamin L' here in order (1) to specify the attributes of the positive personal relationship in question (Table 2) and because (2) it implies that this kind of relationship might be important for health.

As for the latter, I must admit that at present I have no hard facts to support my assumption that a mature adult man or woman needs the 'vitamin L' for his or her health. On the other hand, it is now well established that a lack of relationships corresponding to the 'vitamin L' in childhood is detrimental (Bowlby, 1959).

While during adulthood the presumed self-production of 'vitamin L' might often be sufficient under favourable conditions (e.g. in a stabilized, personally rewarding situation), there are circumstances when the need seems to be suddenly enhanced (e.g. after divorce, bereavement, imprisonment, accident or serious illness).

Table 2 Some attributes of 'vitamin L'

The putative need for positive personal relationship is satisfied only by relations which are (for example)	
Stable	
Affectionate	
Intimate	'Vitamin L'
Independent of external appearance, etc.	
Mutual	

Intuitively, we may feel that the deficiency of 'vitamin L' could harm health or increase propensity to contract various illnesses. Does it increase vulnerability to drug abuse? Heart attacks? Ulcers? Violence? However, unless we are able to measure 'vitamin L', such questions remain unanswerable. When Michael Chance advocated application of ethological concepts to the study of behavioural effects of drugs, he aptly stressed that 'The selection of adequate concepts ... must go hand in hand with the acquisition of facts' (Chance, 1968). The same holds for the application of ethological concepts in the study of human lifestyle. But how to measure 'vitamin L'? Besides psychological techniques, e.g. questionnaires (Rubin, 1970), ethological measures such as the number of joint actions, verbal and non-verbal contacts might be as useful.

It could be argued that the suggested measures would be superfluous because they would merely substitute for criteria such as 'divorced', 'married', etc., already well established in health and population statistics. However, while these familiar criteria are simple, objective and easily available (Figure 1), in this context, they represent composite indices which might not distinguish between different degrees of saturation with the putative 'vitamin L' (deficiency, norm, 'hypervitaminosis'). Consequently, the work with epidemiological data classified by conventional population criteria is not as creative in concept or theory as it might have been.

There is one obvious limitation concerning treatment with 'Vitamin L': because of its individual specificity (personal character) it cannot be fully provided by medical personnel (they cannot fully substitute for individual parents, spouses, etc.). That does not mean that study of this concept would be useless. Transplantation immunity is also individually specific but nobody doubts the usefulness of its investigation. If anything, study of the role of positive personal relationships in health and disease could increase our appreciation and understanding of this phenomenon. For example, it could lead to a

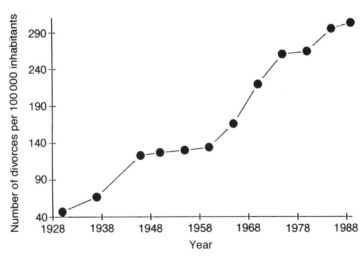

Figure 1 Divorce rate in the Czech Republic.

more general awareness that an appropriate level of positive relationship to oneself ('vitamin L_1'?) is necessary for rehabilitation in some patients. This might be the case, for example, in patients with marked face and body disfiguration after extensive burns (Königová, 1992). Or, that a lack of external positive personal relationship ('vitamin L_2'?) can be substituted to some extent by a convenient pet which is meeting at least some attributes of the 'vitamin L' (e.g. a dog or a cat).

HUMAN, MEDICAL AND CLINICAL ETHOLOGY

Therefore it may be quite useful to turn our attention to human ethological needs. The study of man from an ethological vantage point, with its typical focus on the species-specific way of life (e.g. directed to needs and stimuli-forming human lifestyle) could give an impulse to new patterns of research (Table 3). First, a 'new' human ethology might appear which could be in a better position to unravel specific ethological features of man than the traditional human ethology (which appears to be largely descriptive, preoccupied with recording human gestures, etc.). Second, the study of the role of ethological aspects of human lifestyle in health could originate a new area of research which might be called 'medical ethology'. Third, a similar study with respect to disease could constitute 'clinical ethology'.

However, what would be a clue and criterion in these studies? Obviously, we shall not be able to put proper questions, set viable hypotheses, get a meaningful message from the data, etc., in such studies without reference to ethical principles. But who is best qualified to decide ethical issues? Although we would be approaching the limits of science and skating on thin ice with the risk of breaking into unpleasant situations (e.g. ugly passionate disputes, solving nothing because of lack of a criterion), we could manage to remain on the 'safe' side of rational science because the clue (human logical and moral intuition) and the criterion (human health) is open to independent examination by others. If clinical ethics can exist and flourish as a separate discipline, why not a clinical ethology?

COULD ETHOLOGY BECOME AS IMPORTANT AS ECOLOGY?

Until the 1960s many laymen had not been aware of the dangers of environmental pollution. Then a relatively unknown academic discipline, ecology,

Table 3 Scope of medical and clinical ethology stemming from the 'new' human ethology

Discipline	Focused on ethological aspects of
'New' human ethology	Human lifestyle, needs, stimuli
Medical ethology	Health
Clinical ethology	Disease

brought enough evidence to convince the public (and politicians) that the capacity of the planet to recover is not limitless. Ecology has been a cliché in the mass media since the 1970s.

Many are afraid that human lifestyle has been steadily deteriorating during the last few decades. The widespread occurrence, and constant increase, of phenomena such as drug abuse, violence, family disintegration, etc., is given as evidence. Although these problems are studied by many experts from a great number of disciplines, their deeper understanding and effective treatment is still lacking. These disorders of human lifestyle appear to be one of the major research opportunities for ethology, and, vice versa, ethology seems to be one of the major scientific disciplines which could develop an adequate and fruitful paradigm for the study and understanding of these disorders. Should ethology be successful in convincing people that modern life threatens their innate needs and capabilities for the human way of life, and that it is necessary to protect and cultivate them for their health, then ethology could become a term as common in the mass media and rhetoric as ecology.

CONCLUDING REMARKS

Thus, ethology can evoke many intriguing questions and offer fundamentally new concepts in the study of human lifestyle, health and disease. Unusual questions may appear inappropriate, irrelevant or even ridiculous to many. Ethological concepts applied to unusual fields may appear odd, chimerical or even foolish. If I remember correctly, the exhortation to apply an ethological approach in the study of drug effects on behaviour in the 1960s and early 1970s (Chance and Silverman, 1964; Lát, 1964, 1965; Kršiak and Borgesová, 1972) also appeared eccentric. The Birmingham group had been offering not only ethological concepts, but also a convenient method and evidence of utility of this novel approach in pharmacology. Still it took about 10 years before this approach began to be utilized more widely (Kršiak, 1991).

Ethology offers principally new concepts which could guide the search for novel data as well as new methods and a climate of thought for the study of the human lifestyle. Whether they could represent a beginning of a new paradigm in this area in terms of Kuhn's conception (Kuhn, 1962) is open to question. New ethological concepts seem to be essential for this beginning, but now we mainly need to develop methods to apply them and to demonstrate their utility. Should somebody be successful in this, he or she might beget another classic.

ACKNOWLEDGEMENTS

I wish to thank Professor S.J. Cooper and Dr A.P. Silverman for kind comments and help with this manuscript. The present study was supported by a grant from the Czech Ministry of Health, IGA 0865-3.

REFERENCES

Bowlby, J. (1969) *Attachment and Loss Vol. 1. Attachment*. International Psycho-analytical Library No. 79, Hogarth Press, London.

Chance, M.R.A. (1968) Ethology and psychopharmacology. In: *Psychopharmacology: Dimensions and Perspectives* (ed. C.R.B. Joyce). Tavistock Publications, London, pp. 283–318.

Chance, M.R.A. and Silverman, A.P. (1964) The structure of social behaviour and drug action. In: *Animal Behavior and Drug Action* (eds. H. Steinberg, A.V.S. Reuck and J. Knight). J.A. Churchill, London, pp. 65–82.

Grant, E.C. and Mackintosh, J.H. (1963) A comparison of the social postures of some common laboratory rodents. *Behaviour*, **21**, 246–259.

Königová, R. (1992) The psychological problems of burned patients. The Rudy Hermans Lecture 1991. *Burns*, **18**, 189–199.

Kršiak, M. (1991) Ethopharmacology: a historical perspective. *Neurosci. Biobehav. Rev.*, **15**, 439–445.

Kršiak, M. and Borgesová, M. (1972) Drugs and spontaneous behaviour: why are detailed studies still so rare? *Activ. Nerv. Super. (Praha)*, **14**, 285–293.

Kuhn, T.S. (1962) *The Structure of Scientific Revolutions*. University of Chicago Press, Chicago.

Lát, J. (1964) Motivation from the point of view of the reflex theory, behaviorism and ethology (in Czech). *Čs. Fysiol.*, **13**, 316–331.

Lát, J. (1965) The spontaneous exploratory reactions as a tool for psychopharmaco-logical studies. In: *Pharmacology of Conditioning, Learning and Retention* (eds. M. Ya. Mikhel'son, V.G. Longo and Z. Votava). Pergamon Press, Oxford, pp. 47–66.

Rubin, Z. (1970) Measurement of romantic love. *J. Pers. Soc. Psychol.*, **16**, 265–273.

Russell, B. (1966) *Sceptical Essays*. Unwin Books, London.

Silverman, A.P. (1965) Ethological and statistical analysis of drug effects on the social behaviour of laboratory rats. *Br. J. Pharmacol.*, **24**, 579–590.

Silverman, A.P. (1966) The social behaviour of laboratory rats and the action of chlorpromazine and other drugs. *Behaviour*, **27**, 1–38.

Silverman, A.P. (1988) An ethologist's approach to behavioural toxicology. *Neurotoxicol. Teratol.*, **10**, 85–92.

Index

adrenal hyperplasia, congenital, 230
adrenaline, 320
adrenoceptor ligands, effects on anxiety,
    17–19
affective behaviour, 305–8
age variables, 26, 26
aggressive behaviour, 179–87
  analysis, implications for
      pharmacological research, 147–50
  animal models, 161–2
  anosmia affecting, 215–18
  antidepressant drugs in, 102–6
  benzodiazepines and, 274
  brain systems in, 143–6
  categories of, 179
  conflict and, 160–1
  definitions of, 160
  drug-induced enhancement, 49–50, 55
  DSM-III-R, 159
  environmental targets, 133–53
  ethopharmacological studies, 162–7
  female mice, 183–6
  human, and perinatal exposure to
      hormones, 229–30
  in mice, see mice, aggressive behaviour
  non-unitary nature of, 179
  odour-inhibited, 191–201
  Overt Aggression Scale, 161
  patterning, 148–9
  pheromones in, 205–20
  psychopharmacology in analysis of,
      150–2
  sensorimotor systems, 133–53
  serenics, see serenics
  testosterone-mediated, 228
    see also agonistic behaviour; offensive
      behaviour
  agonistic behaviour, 92–3, 161–2
  anosmia affecting, 215-18
  effect of olfactory signal inhibition,
      211–15
  male mice, 210–11
  pheromones in, 205–20
    see also aggressive behaviour;

defensive behaviour; submissive
  behaviour; threat behaviour
allopregnanolone, 17
alphaxalone, 17
alprazolam, 122, 123, 124, 151
  reduced SAP with, 71
amitriptyline, 23
amnesic effects, benzodiazepines, 275–6
amperozide, 20, 22
amphetamine, 85, 320, 336
  anorexic effect, 321–2
  enhancing prepotent behaviour, 277–80
  orienting responses and, 277
  stereotypy, 241–63, 276
    definitions, 246
    diazepam pretreatment, 277–80
    effects of dose, 261
    excursion rate, 253–5
    as form of sensitization, 280–1
    home bases and, 251–3
    number of routes, 256
    quantification measures, 242
    route sterotypy, 246–51
    stops, 253–5
    time course, 253–7
amylobarbitone, 17
analgesia
  call-induced, 117–20
  exercise-induced, 127
androgens
  aromatizable, 228
  early exposure to, 229, 230
animal models
  of anxiety, see anxiety, animal models
  of psychiatric disorders, 329–37
  validity of, 9–10, 13
anorexia, d-amphetamine in, 321–2
anosmia, affecting mouse agonistic
  behaviour, 215–18
antidepressants
  aggressive behaviour and, 102–6
  prediction from ethological analysis,
      85–106
  see also depressive illness